☆☆☆☆☆

Great Yoga Books

Mahanirvana
TANTRA

Cover & Graphic Design

Mattias Långström

Contact: oneofakindbooks@bhagwan.se

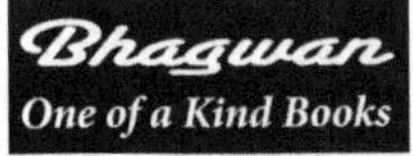

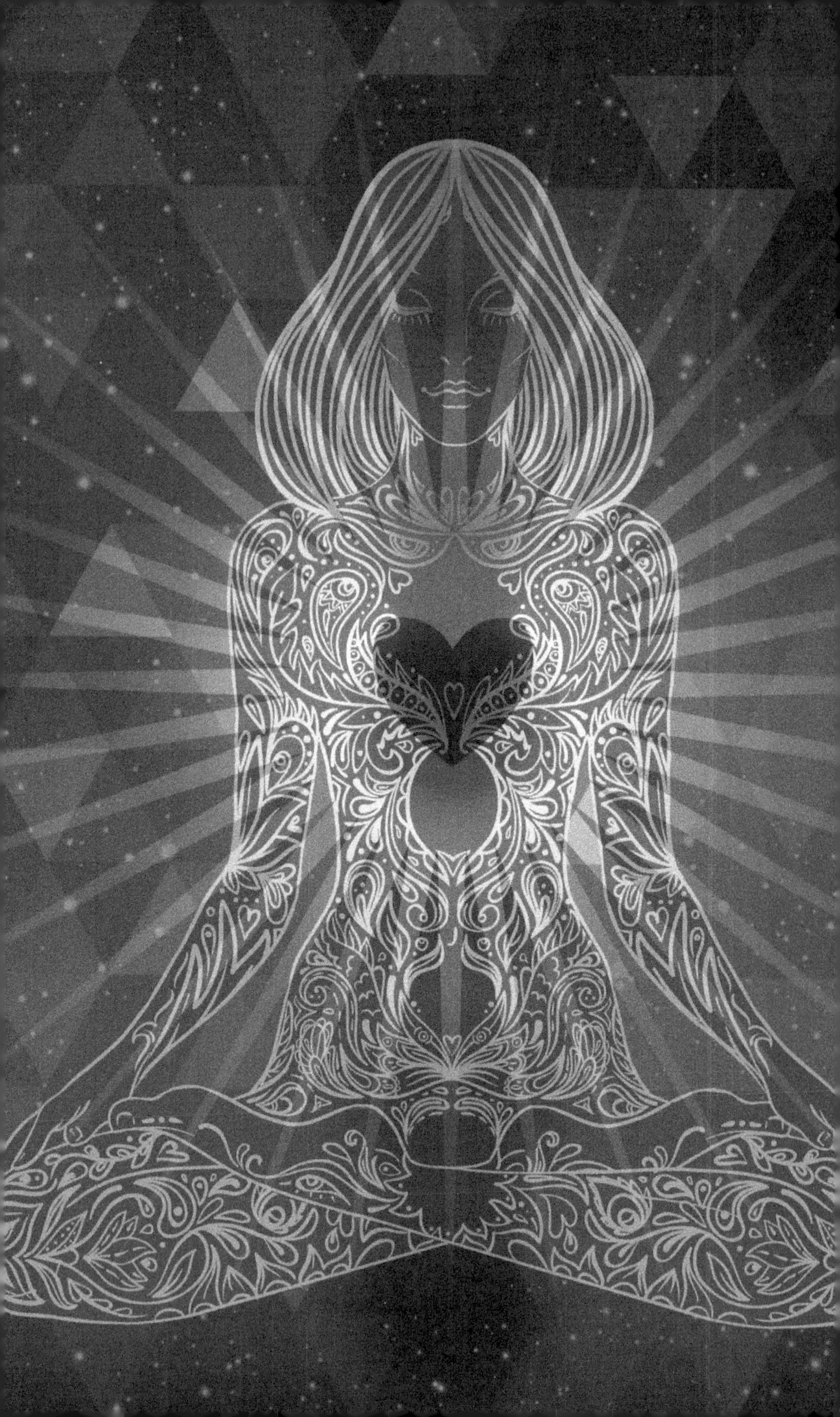

☆☆☆☆☆
Great Yoga Books

Mahanirvana

TANTRA

Copyright New Edition © Mattias Långström

ISBN: 9789198735765

Based on the Book

Mahanirvana Tantra

by Arthur Avalon

✳✳✳

PREFACE

*THE Indian Tantras, which are numerous, constitute
the Scripture (Shastra) of the Kaliyuga, and as such are
the voluminous source of present and practical orthodox
"Hinduism." The Tantra Shastra is, in fact, and whatever be its historical origin, a development of the Vaidika
Karmakanda, promulgated to meet the needs of that
age. Shiva says: "For the benefit of men of the Kali age,
men bereft of energy and dependent for existence on
the food they eat, the Kaula doctrine, O auspicious one!
is given" (Chap. IX., verse 12). To the Tantra we must
therefore look if we would understand aright both ritual, yoga, and sadhana of all kinds, as also the general
principles of which these practices are but the objective
expression.*

*Yet of all the forms of Hindu Shastra, the Tantra is that
which is least known and understood, a circumstance
in part due to the difficulties of its subject-matter and
to the fact that the key to much of its terminology and
method rest with the initiate. The present translation is,
in fact, the first published in Europe of any Indian Tantra. An inaccurate version rendered in imperfect English
was published in Calcutta by a Bengali editor some*

twelve years ago, preceded by an Introduction which displayed insufficient knowledge in respect of what it somewhat quaintly described as "the mystical and superficially technical passages" of this Tantra. A desire to attempt to do it greater justice has in part prompted its selection as the first for publication. This Tantra is, further, one which is well known and esteemed, though perhaps more highly so amongst that portion of the Indian public which favours "reformed" Hinduism than amongst some Tantrikas, to whom, as I have been told, certain of its provisions appear to display unnecessary timidity. The former admire it on account of its noble exposition of the worship of the Supreme Brahman, and in the belief that certain of its passages absolutely discountenance the orthodox ritual. Nothing can be more mistaken than such belief, even though it be the fact that "for him who has faith in the root, of what use are the branches and leaves." This anyone will discover who reads the text. It is true that, as Chap. VII., verse 94, says: "In the purified heart knowledge of Brahman grows," and Brahmajnane samutpanne krityakrityang na vidyate. But the statement assumes the attainment of Brahmajñana, and this, the Shastra says, can be attained, not by Vedantic discussions nor mere prayer, after the manner of Protestant systems of Christian worship; but by the Sadhana which is its main subject-matter. I have referred to Protestant systems, for the Catholic

Church possesses an elaborate ritual and a sadhana of its own which is in many points strikingly analogous to the Hindu system. The section of Tantrikas to whom I have referred are, I believe, also in error. For the design of this Tantra appears to be, whilst conserving commonly-recognized Tantrik principles, to secure that, as has sometimes proved to be the case, they are not abused. Parvvati says (Chap. I., verse 67): "I fear, 0 Lord! that even that which Thou hast ordained for the good of men will, through them, turn out for evil." Hitaya yane, karmani kathitani tvaya prabho Manyetani mahadeva viparitani manave. It is significant, in connection with these observations, to note that this particular Tantra was chosen as the subject of commentary by Shrimad Hariharananda Bharati, the Guru of the celebrated Hindu "reformer," Raja Ram Mohun Roy.

The Tantra has been assigned to the group of sixty-four known as those of the Rathakranta. It was first published by the Adi-Brahma-Samaja in 1798 Shakabda (A.D. 1876), and was printed in Bengali characters, with the notes of the Kulavadhuta Shrimad Hariharananda Bharati under the editorship of Anandachandra Vidyavagisha. The preface to this edition stated that three MSS. were consulted; one belonging to the library of the Samaja; the second supplied by Durgadasa Chandhuri, and the third taken from the library of Raja Ram

Mohun Roy. This text appears to be the basis of subsequent publications. It was again printed in 1888 by Shri Krishna Gopala Bhakta, since when there have been several editions with Bengali translations, including that of Shri Prasanna Kumara Shastri. The late Pandit Jivananda Vidyasagara published an edition in Devanagari character, with the notes of Hariharananda; and the Venkateshvara Press at Bombay have issued another in similar character with a Hindi translation.

The translation published is that of the first part only. It is commonly thought (and was so stated by the author of the Calcutta edition in English to which I have referred) that the second portion is lost. This is, however, not so, though copies of the complete Tantra are rare enough. The full text exists in manuscript, and I hope at a later date to have an opportunity of publishing a translation of it. I came across a complete manuscript some two years ago in the possession of a Nepalese Pandit. He would, however, only permit me to make a copy of his manuscript on the condition that the Shatkarmma Mantras were not published. For, as he said, virtue not being a condition precedent for the acquisition of siddhi in such Mantras, their publication might enable the evilly disposed to work harm against others, a crime which, he added, was, in his own country, where the Tantra was current, punishable by the civil power. I was unable to persuade him even with the observation that *the mere publication of the Mantra without knowledge of what is called the prayoga (which cannot be learned of books) would in any case be ineffectual. I could not give an undertaking which would have involved the publication of a mutilated text, and the reader must therefore for the present be content with a translation of the first part of the Tantra, which is generally known, and has, as stated, been several times printed. The incident has further value than the direct purpose for which I have told it. There are some to whom the Tantra, though they may not have read a line of it, is "nothing but black magic," and all its followers are "black magicians." This is of course absurd. In this connection I cannot avoid interposing the observation that certain practices are described in Tantra which, though they are alleged to have the results described therein, yet exist "for delusion." The true attitude of the higher Tantrika is illustrated by the action of the Pandit who, if he disappointed my expectations, at any rate by his refusal afforded an answer to these too general allegations.*

The second portion of the manuscript in his possession contained over double the number of Shlokas to be found in the first part here published.

The edition which has been used for the translation is that (now out of print) edited and published at Cal-

*cutta by Shri Krishna Gopala Bhakta in Chaitra 1295
Bengali era (April, 1888), with Commentary of Shrimad
Hariharananda Bharati, and with additional notes by
the learned and lately deceased Pandit Jaganmohana
Tarkalangkara, called Vriddha in order to distinguish
him from another celebrated Pandit of the same name.
A new edition of the same work is now, in course of
publication, with further notes by the latter's son, Pandit
Jnanendranatha Tantraratna.*

*This valuable Commentary is not, however, altogether
suitable for the general reader, for it assumes a certain
amount of knowledge on his part which he does not
possess. I have accordingly, whilst availing myself of its
aid, written my own commentary, and added an Introduction explaining certain matters and terms referred
to or presupposed by the text which, as they require a
somewhat more extended treatment, could not be conve-
niently dealt with in the footnotes. Some of the matters
there explained are, though common and fundamental,
seldom accurately defined. Nothing, therefore, is lost by
a re-statement of them with an intention to serve such
accuracy. Other matters are of a special character, and
are either not generally known or are misunderstood.
The Introduction, however, does not profess to be an
exhaustive treatment of that with which it deals. On the
contrary, it is but an extended note written to help some*

way towards a better understanding of the text by the ordinary reader. For a fuller exposition of general principles and practice the interested are referred to three works which I have in preparation, "Principles of Tantra" (Tantratattva), "Exposition of the Secret Worship" (Rahasyapujapaddhati), and "Description of the Six Centres" (Shatchakranirupana). There are, however, some matters in the Shastra or its accompanying oral tradition which he must, and if disposed thereto will, find out for himself. This, too, is implied by the saying in this Tantra that it is by merit acquired in previous births that the mind inclines to Kaula doctrine (Chapter VII., verse 99). However this may be, no one will understand the Shastra who starts his inquiry with a mind burdened with the current prejudices against it, whatever be the colour of truth some of them may possess by reason of actual abuse of Shastric principles.

In conclusion, I wish to thank my Indian friends for the aid they have given me in the preparation of this and other kindred works, and to whom I am indebted for much information gathered during many pleasant hours which we have spent together in the study of a subject of common interest to them and myself. The Tantras generally are written in comparatively simple Sanskrit. For their rendering, however, a working knowledge of their terminology and ritual is required, which can be only fully found in those to whom it is familiar through race, upbringing, and environment, and in whom there is still some regard for their ancient inheritance. As for others, they must learn to see through the Indian eye of knowledge until their own have been trained to its lines of vision. In this way we shall be in the future spared some of the ridiculous presentments of Indian beliefs common in the past and even now too current.

INTRODUCTION

Mount Kailasa.

The scene of the revelation of this Tantra is laid in Himalaya, the "Abode of Snow," a holy land weighted with the traditions of the Aryan race. Here in these lofty uplands, encircled with everlasting snows, rose the great mountain of the north, the Sapta Kula Parvata. Hence the race itself came, and there its early legends have their setting. There are still shown at Bhimudiyar the caves where the sons of Pandu and Draupadi rested, as did Rama and his faithful wife at the point where the Kosi joins the Sita in the grove of Asoka trees. In these mountains Munis and Rishis lived. Here also is the Kshetra of Shiva Mahadeva, where His Spouse Parvvati, the daughter of the Mountain King, was born, and where Mother Ganges also has her source. From time immemorial pilgrims have toiled through these mountains to visit the three great shrines of Gangotri, Kedarnath, and Badrinath. At Kangri, further north, the pilgrims make the parikrama of Mount Kailasa (Kang Rinpoche), where Shiva is said to dwell. This nobly towering peak rises to the north-west of the sacred Mansarowar

Lake (Mapham Yum-tso) from amidst the purple ranges of the lower Kangri Mountains. The paradise of Shiva is a summerland of both lasting sunshine and cool shade, musical with the song of birds and bright with undying flowers. The air, scented with the sweet fragrance of Mandara chaplets, resounds with the music and song of celestial singers and players. The Mount is Gana Parvata, thronged with trains of Spirits (devayoni), of which the opening Chapter speaks.

And in the regions beyond rises Mount Meru, centre of the world-lotus. Its heights, peopled with spirits, are hung with clusters of stars as with wreaths of Malati flowers. In short, it is written: "He who thinks of Himachala, though he should not behold him, is greater than he who performs all worship in Kashi (Benares). In a hundred ages of the Devas I could not tell thee of the glories of Himachala. As the dew is dried up by the morning sun, so are the sins of mankind by the sight of Himachala."

It is not, however, necessary to go to the Himalayan Kailasa to find Shiva. He dwells wheresoever his worshippers, versed in Kulatattva, abide, and His mystic mount is to be sought in the thousand-petalled lotus (sahasrara-padma) in the body of every human jiva, hence called Shivasthana, to which all, wheresoever situate, may repair when they have learned how to achieve the way thither.

Shiva promulgates His teaching in the world below in the works known as Yamala, Damara, Shiva Sutra, and in the Tantras which exist in the form of Dialogues between the Devata and his Shakti, the Devi in Her form as Parvvati. According to the Gayatri Tantra, the Deva Ganesha first preached the Tantra to the Devayoni on Mount Kailasa, after he had himself received them from the mouth of Shiva.

After a description of the mountain, the Dialogue opens with a question from Parvvati in answer to which and those which succeed it, Shiva unfolds His doctrine on the subjects with which this particular Tantra deals.

Shiva and Shakti.

That eternal immutable existence which transcends the turiya and all other states is the unconditioned Absolute, the supreme Brahman or Para-brahman, without Prakriti (nishkala) or Her attributes (nir-guna), which, as being the inner self and knowing subject, can never be the object of cognition, and is to be apprehended only through yoga by the realization of the Self (atmajñana), which It is. For as it is said, "Spirit can alone know Spi-

*rit." Being beyond mind, speech, and without name, the
Brahman was called "Tat," "That," and then "Tat Sat,"
"That which is." For the sun, moon, and stars, and all
visible things, what are they but a glimpse of light caught
from "That" (Tat)?*

*Brahman is both nishkala and sakala. Kala is Prakriti.
The nishkala Brahman or Para-brahman is the Tat,
when thought of as without Prakriti (prakriteranya).
It is called sakala when with Prakriti. As the substance
of Prakriti is the three gunas It is then su-guna, as in
the previous state It was nir-guna. Though in the latter
state It is thought of as without Shakti, yet (making
accommodation to human speech) in It potentially exists
Shakti, Its power and the whole universe produced by It.
To say, however, that the Shakti exists in the Brahman is
but a form of speech, since It and Shakti are, in fact, one,
and Shakti is eternal (Anadi-rupa). She is Brahma-rupa
and both vi-guna (nir-guna) and sa-guna; the Chai-
tanya-rupini-Devi, who manifests all bhuta. She is the
Ananda-rupini-Devi, by whom the Brahman manifests
Itself, and who, to use the words of the Sarada, pervades
the universe as does oil the sesamum seed.*

*In the beginning the Nishkala Brahman alone exi-
sted. In the beginning there was the One. It willed and
became many. Ahab bahu syam – "may I be many." In
such manifestation of Shakti the Brahman is known as*

the lower (apara) or manifested Brahman, who, as the subject of worship, is meditated upon with attributes. And, in fact, to the mind and sense of the embodied spirit (jiva) the Brahman has body and form. It is embodied in the forms of all Devas and Devils, and in the worshipper himself. Its form is that of the universe, and of all things and beings therein.

As Shruti says: "He saw" (Sa aikshata, aham bahu syam prajayeya). "He thought to Himself may I be many." "Sa aikshaya" was itself a manifestation of Shakti, the Para-mapurva-nirvana shakti, or Brahman as Shakti. From the Brahman, with Shakti (Para-shakti-maya) issued Nada (Shiva-Shakti as the "Word" or "Sound"), and from Nada, Vindu appeared. Kalicharana in his commentary on the Shatchakra-nirupana says that Shiva and Nirvana Shakti bound by a mayik bond and covering, should be thought of as existing in the form of Parang Vindu.

The Sarada says: Sachchidananda vibhavat sakalat parameshvarat asichchhaktistato nado, nadad vindu-samudbhavah ("From Parameshvara vested with the wealth of sachchidananda and with Prakriti (sakala) issued Shakti; from Shakti came Nada and from Nada was born Vindu"). The state of subtle body which is known as Kama-kala is the mula of mantra. The term mula-mantratmika, when applied to the Devi, refers to this subtle body of Hers known as the Kama-kala. The Tantra also speaks of three Vindus, namely Shiva-maya, Shakti-maya, and Shiva-shakti-maya.

The Parang-vindu is represented as a circle, the centre of which is the brahma-pada, or place of Brahman, wherein are Prakriti-Purusha, the circumference of which is encircling maya. It is on the crescent of nirvana-kala, the seventeenth, which is again in that of ama-kala, the sixteenth digit (referred to in the text) of the moon-circle (Chandramandala), which circle is situate above the Sun-Circle (Suryyamandala), the Guru and the hangsah, which are in the pericarp of the thousand-petalled lotus (sahasrarapadma). Next to the Vindu is the fiery Bodhini, or Nibodhika (v. post). The Vindu, with the Nirvana-kala, Nibodhika, and Ama-kala, are situated in the lightning-like inverted triangle known as "A, Ka, Tha," and which is so called because at its apex is A; at its right base is Za; and at its left base Tha. It is made up of forty-eight letters (matrika): the sixteen vowels running from A to Ka; sixteen consonants of the ka-varga and other groups running from A to Ka; and the remaining sixteen from Ka to Tha. Inside are the remaining letters (matrika), ha, la(second), and ksha. As the substance of Devi is matrika (matrika-mayi) the triangle represents the "Word" of all that exists. The triangle is itself encircled by the Chandramandala. The Vindu is symbolically described as being like a grain of gram (chanaka), which under its encircling sheath contains a divided seed. This Parang-vindu is Prakriti-Purusha, Shiva-Shakti. It is known as the Shabda-Brahman (the Sound Brahman), or Aparabrahman. A polarization of the two Shiva and Shakti Tattvas then takes place in Parashaktimaya. The Devi becomes Unmukhi. Her face turns towards Shiva. There is an unfolding which bursts the encircling shell of Maya, and creation then takes place by division of Shiva and Shakti or of "Hang" and "Sah." The Sarada says: "The Devataparashaktimaya is again Itself divided, such divisions being known as Vindu, Vaja, and Nada. Vindu is of the nature of Nada or Shiva, and Vaja of Shakti, and Nada has been said to be the relation of these two by those who are versed in all the Agamas." The Sarada says that before the bursting of the shell enclosing the brahma-pada, which, together with its defining circumference, constitute the Shabda-brahman, an indistinct sound arose (avyaktat-maravobhavat). This avyaktanada is both the first and the last state of Nada, according as it is viewed from the standpoint of evolution or involution. For Nada, as Raghava-bhatta says, exists in three states. In Nada are the guna (sattva, rajas, and tamas), which form the substance of Prakriti, which with Shiva It is. When tamo-guna predominates Nada is merely an indistin-ct or unmanifested (dhvanyat – mako'vykta-nadah) sound in the nature of dhvani. In this state, in which

*it is a phase of Avyaktanada, it is called Nibodhika, or
Bodhini. It is Nada when rajoguna is in the ascendant,
when there is a sound in which there is something like a
connected or combined disposition of the letters. When
the sattva-guna preponderates Nada assumes the form
of Vindu. The action of rajas on tamas is to veil. Its own
independent action effects an arrangement which is only
perfected by the emergence of the essentially manifesting sattvika guna set into play by it. Nada, Vindu, and
Nibodhika, and the Shakti, of which they are the specific
manifestation, are said to be in the form of Sun, Moon,
and Fire respectively. Jñana (spiritual wisdom) is spoken
of as fire as it burns up all actions, and the tamoguna is
associated with it. For when the effect of cause and effect
of action are really known, then action ceases. Ichchha
is the Moon. The Moon contains the sixteenth digit, the
Ama-kala with its nectar, which neither increases nor
decays, and Ichchha, or will, is the eternal precursor of
creation. Kriya is like the Sun, for as the Sun by its light
makes all things visible, so unless there is action and
striving there cannot be realization or manifestation. As
the Gita sways: "As one Sun makes manifest all the loka."*

*The Shabda-Brahman manifests Itself in a triad of
energies – knowledge (jñanashakti), will (ichchha-shak-
ti), and action (kriya-shakti), associated with the three
gunas of Prakriti, tamas, sattva, and rajas. From the*

*Parang-Vindu, who is both vindvat-maka and kalatma
– i.e., Shakti – issued Raudri, Rudra, and his Shakti,
whose forms are fire (vahni), and whose activity is
knowledge (jñana); Vama, and Vishnu and his Shakti, whose form is the sun, and whose activity is kriya
(action): and Jyeshtha and Brahma and his Shakti,
whose form is the Moon and whose activity is desire.
The Vamakeshvara Tantra says that Tri-pura is threefold, as Brahma, Vishnu, and Isha; and as the energies
desire, wisdom, and action, the energy of will when
Brahman would create; the energy of wisdom when She
reminds Him, saying "Let this be thus" ; and when, thus
knowing, He acts, She becomes the energy of action. The
Devi is thus Ichchha-shakti-jñana-shakti-kriya-shak-
ti-svaru-pini.*

*Para-shiva exists as a septenary under the form, firstly,
of Shambhu, who is the associate of time (kala-bandhu).
From Him issues Sada-shiva, Who pervades and manifests all things, and then come Ishana and the triad,
Rudra, Vishnu, and Brahma, each with their respective
Shakti (without whom they avail nothing) separately
and particularly associated with the gunas, tamas,
sattva and rajas. Of these Devas, the last triad, together
with Ishana, and Sada-shiva, are the five Shivas who
are collectively known as the Maha-preta, whose vija
is "Hsauh." Of the Maha-preta, it is said that the last
four form the support, and the fifth the seat, of the bed*

on which the Devi is united with Parama-shiva, in the room of chintamani stone, on the jewelled island clad with clumps of kadamba and heavenly trees set in the ocean of Ambrosia.

Shiva is variously addressed in this work as Shambhu, Sada-shiva, Shankara, Maheshvara, etc., names which indicate particular states, qualities, and manifestations of the One in its descent towards the many; for there are many Rudras. Thus Sada-shiva indicates the predominance of the sattva-guna. His names are many, 1,008 being given in the sixty-ninth chapter of the Shiva Purana, and in the seventeenth chapter of the Anushasana Parvan of the Mahabharata.

Shakti is both maya, that by which the Brahman creating the universe is able to make Itself appear to be different from what It really is, and mula-prakriti, or the unmanifested (avyakta) state of that which, when manifest, is the universe of name and form. It is the primary so called "material cause," consisting of the equipoise of the triad of guna or "qualities" which are sattva (that which manifests) rajas (that which acts), tamas (that which veils and produces inertia). The three gunas represent Nature as the revelation of spirit, Nature as the passage of descent from spirit to matter, or of ascent from matter to spirit, and Nature as the dense veil of spirit. The Devi is thus guna-nidhi ("treasure-house of guna"). Mu-

la-prakriti is the womb into which Brahman casts the seed from which all things are born. The womb thrills to the movement of the essentially active rajo-guna. The equilibrium of the triad is destroyed, and the guna, now in varied combinations, evolve under the illumination of Shiva (chit), the universe which is ruled by Maheshvara and Maheshvari. The dual principles of Shiva and Shakti, which are in such dual form the product of the polarity manifested in Parashakti-maya, pervade the whole universe, and are present in man in the Svayambhu-Linga of the muladhara and the Devi Kundalini, who, in serpent form, encircles it. The Shabda-Brahman assumes in the body of man the form of the Devi Kundalini, and as such is in all prani (breathing creatures), and in the shape of letters appears in prose and verse. Kundala means coiled. Hence Kundalini, whose form is that of a coiled serpent, means that which is coiled. She is the luminous vital energy (jiva-shakti) which manifests as prana, She sleeps in the muladhara, and has three and a half coils corresponding in number with the three and a half vindus of which the Kubjika Tantra speaks. When after closing the ears the sound of Her hissing is not heard death approaches.

From the first avyakta creation issued the second mahat, with its three guna distinctly manifested. Thence sprung the third creation ahangkara (selfhood), which is of threefold form – vaikarika, or pure sattvika ahangkara;

*the taijasa, or rajasika ahangkara; and the tamasika,
or bhutadika ahangkara. The latter is the origin of the
subtle essences (tan-matra) of the Tattvas, ether, air, fire,
water, earth, associated with sound, touch, sight, taste
and smell, and with the colours – pure transparency,
shyama, red, white, and yellow. There is some difference
in the schools as to that which each of the three forms
produces, but from such threefold form of Ahang-kara
issue the indriya ("senses"), and the Devas Dik, Vata,
Arka, Prachetas, Vahni, Indra, Upendra, Mitra, and
the Ashvins. The vaikarika, taijasa, and bhutadika are
the fourth, fifth, and sixth creations, which are known
as prakrita, or appertaining to Prakriti. The rest, which
are products of these, such as the vegetable world with
its upward life current, animals with horizontal life
current, and bhuta, preta and the like, whose life current
tends downward, constitute the vaikrita creation, the
two being known as the kaumara creation.*

*The Goddess (Devi) is the great Shakti. She is Maya, for
of Her the maya which produces the sangsara is. As Lord
of Maya She is Mahamaya. Devi is a-vidya (nescience)
because She binds and vidya (knowledge) because She
liberates and destroys the sangsara. She is Prakriti, and
as existing before creation is the Adya (primordial)
Shakti. Devi is the vachaka-shakti, the manifestation
of chit in Prakriti, and the vachya-shakti, or Chit itself.
The Atma should be contemplated as Devi. Shakti or*

Devi is thus the Brahman revealed in Its mother aspect (shri-mata) as Creatrix and Nourisher of the worlds. Kali says of Herself in Yogini Tantra "Sachchidanan-da-rupaham brahmaivaham sphurat-prab-ham." So the Devi is described with attributes both of the qualified Brahman; and (since that Brahman is but the mani-festation of the Absolute) She is also addressed with epithets, which denote the unconditioned Brahman. She is the great Mother (Ambika) sprung from the sacrificial hearth of the fire of the Grand Consciousness (chit); decked with the Sun and Moon; Lalita, "She who plays"; whose play is world-play; whose eyes playing like fish in the beauteous waters of her Divine face, open and shut with the appearance and disappearance of countless worlds now illuminated by her light now wrapped in her terrible darkness.

The Devi, as Para-brahman, is beyond all form and guna. The forms of the Mother of the Universe are thre-efold. There is first the Supreme (para) form, of which, as the Vishnu-yamala says, "none know." There is next her subtle (sukshma) form, which consists of mantra. But as the mind cannot easily settle itself upon that which is formless, She appears as the subject of contemp-lation in Her third, or gross (sthula), or physical form, with hands and feet and the like as celebrated in the De-vi-stotra of the Puranas and Tantras. Devi, who as Pra-kriti is the source of Brahma, Vishnu, and Mahesh-vara, has both male and female forms. But it is in Her female forms that She is chiefly contemplated. For though existing in all things, in a peculiar sense female beings are parts of Her. The Great Mother, who exists in the form of all Tantras and all Yantras, is, as the Lalita says, the "unsullied treasure-house of beauty"; the Sapphire Devi, whose slender waist, bending beneath the burden of the ripe fruit of her breasts, swells into jewelled hips heavy with the promise of infinite maternities.

As the Mahadevi She exists in all forms as Sarasvati, Lakshmi, Gayatri, Durga, Tripura-sundari, Anna-purna, and all the Devi who are avatara of the Brahman.

Devi, as Sati, Uma, Parvvati, and Gauri, is spouse of Shiva. It was as Sati prior to Daksha's sacrifice (daksha-yajna) that the Devi manifested Herself to Shiva in the ten celebrated forms known as the dasha-mahavidya referred to in the text – Kali, Bagala, Chhinnamasta, Bhuvaneshvari, Matangini, Shodashi, Dhumavati, Tripura-sundari, Tara, and Bhairavi. When, at the Daksha-yajna She yielded up her life in shame and sorrow at the treatment accorded by her father to Her Husband, Shiva took away the body, and, ever bearing it with Him, remained wholly distraught and spent with grief. To save the world from the forces of evil which arose and grew with the withdrawal of His Divine control, Vishnu with His discus (chakra) cut the dead body of Sati,

*which Shiva bore, into fifty-one fragments, which fell
to earth at the places thereafter known as the fifty-one
maha-pitha-sthana (referred to in the text), where Devi,
with Her Bhairava, is worshipped under various names.*

*Besides the forms of the Devi in the brahmanda there is
Her subtle form called Kundalini in the body (pindanda). These are but some only of Her endless forms. She
is seen as one and as many, as it were, but one moon
reflected in countless waters. She exists, too, in all animals and inorganic things, since the universe with all its
beauties is, as the Devi Purana says, but a part of Her.
All this diversity of form is but the infinite manifestations of the flowering beauty of the One Supreme Life,
a doctrine which is nowhere else taught with greater
wealth of illustration than in the Shakta Shastras, and
Tantras. The great Bharga in the bright Sun and all
Devatas, and, indeed, all life and being, are wonderful,
and are worshipful, but only as Her manifestations. And
he who worships them otherwise is, in the words of the
great Devi-bhagavata, "like unto a man who, with the
light of a clear lamp in his hands, yet falls into some waterless and terrible well." The highest worship for which
the sadhaka is qualified (adhikari) only after external
worship and that internal form known as sadhara, is
described as niradhara. Therein Pure Intelligence is the
Supreme Shakti who is worshipped as the Very Self, the*

Witness freed of the glamour of the manifold Universe.
By one's own direct experience of Maheshvari as the Self
She is with reverence made the object of that worship
which leads to liberation.

Guna.

It cannot be said that current explanations give a clear
understanding of this subject. Yet such is necessary, both
as affording one of the chief keys to Indian philosophy
and to the principles which govern Sadhana. The term
guna is generally translated "quality," a word which is
only accepted for default of a better. For it must not be
overlooked that the three guna (Sattva, rajas, and ta-
mas), which are of Prakriti, constitute Her very substan-
ce. This being so, all Nature which issues from Her, the
Maha-karana-svarupa., is called tri-gunatmaka, and is
composed of the same guna in different states of relation
to one another. The functions of sattva, rajas, and tamas
are to reveal, to make active, and to suppress respective-
ly. Rajas is the dynamic, as sattva and tamas are static
principles. That is to say, sattva and tamas can neither
reveal nor suppress without being first rendered active
by rajas. These gunas work by mutual suppression.

The unrevealed Prakriti (avyakta-prakriti) or Devi is
the state of stable equilibrium of these three guna. When

this state is disturbed the manifested universe appears, in every object of which one or other of the three guna is in the ascendant. Thus in Devas, as in those who approach the divya state, sattva predominates, and rajas and tamas are very much reduced. That is, their independent manifestation is reduced. They are in one sense still there, for where rajas is not independently active it is operating on sattva to suppress tamas, which appears or disappears to the extent to which it is, or is not, subject to suppression by the revealing principle. In the ordinary human jiva, considered as a class, tamas is less reduced than in the case of the Deva, but very much reduced when comparison is made with the animal jiva. Rajas has great independent activity, and sattva is also considerably active. In the animal creation sattva has considerably less activity. Rajas has less independent activity than in man, but is much more active than in the vegetable world. Tamas is greatly less preponderant than in the latter. In the vegetable kingdom tamas is more preponderant than in the case of animals, and both rajas and sattva less so. In the inorganic creation rajas makes tamas active to suppress both sattva and its own independent activity. It will thus be seen that the "upward" or revealing movement from the predominance of tamas to that of sattva represents the spiritual progress of the jivatma.

Again, as between each member of these classes one

or other of the three guna may be more or less in the ascendant.

Thus, in one man as compared with another, the sattva guna may predominate, in which case his temperament is sattvik, or, as the Tantra calls it, divyabhava. In another the rajoguna may prevail, and in the third the tamoguna, in which case the individual is described as rajasik, or tamasik, or, to use Tantrik phraseology, he is said to belong to virabhava, or is a pashu respectively. Again the vegetable creation is obviously less tamasik, and more rajasik and sattvik than the mineral, and even amongst these last there may be possibly some which are less tamasik than others.

Etymologically, sattva is derived from "sat," that which is eternally existent. The eternally existent is also chit, pure Intelligence or Spirit, and ananda or Bliss. In a secondary sense, sat is also used to denote the "good." And commonly (though such use obscures the original meaning), the word sattva guna is rendered "good quality." It is, however, "good" in the sense that it is productive of good and happiness. In such case, however, stress is laid rather on a necessary quality or effect (in the ethical sense) of "sat" than upon its original meaning. In the primary sense sat is that which reveals. Nature is a revelation of spirit (sat). Where Nature is such a revelation of spirit there it manifests as sattva guna. It is

*the shining forth from under the veil of the hidden spi-
ritual substance (sat). And that equality in things which
reveals this is sattva guna. So of a pregnant woman it
is said that she is antahsattva, or instinct with sattva;
she in whom sattva as jiva (whose characteristic guna is
sattva) is living in an hidden state.*

*But Nature not only reveals, but is also a dense covering
or veil of spirit, at times so dense that the ignorant fail to
discern the spirit which it veils. Where Nature is a veil of
spirit there it appears in its quality of tamoguna.*

*In this case the tamoguna is currently spoken of as
representative of inertia, because that is the effect of the
nature which veils. This quality, again, when translated
into the moral sphere, becomes ignorance, sloth, etc.*

*In a third sense nature is a bridge between spirit which
reveals and matter which veils. Where Nature is a
bridge of descent from spirit to matter, or of ascent from
matter to spirit, there it manifests itself as rajoguna.
This is generally referred to as the quality of activity,
and when transferred to the sphere of feeling it shows
itself as passion. Each thing in Nature then contains that
in which spirit is manifested or reflected as in a mirror
or sattvaguna; that by which spirit is covered, as it were,
by a veil of darkness or tamoguna, and that which is the
vehicle for the descent into matter or the return to spirit*

or rajoguna. Thus sattva is the light of Nature, as tamas is its shade. Rajas is, as it were, a blended tint oscillating between each of the extremes constituted by the other guna.

The object of Tantrik sadhana is to bring out and make preponderant the sattva guna by the aid of rajas, which operates to make the former guna active. The subtle body (lingasharira) of the jivatma comprises in it buddhi, ahangkara, manas, and the ten senses. This subtle body creates for itself gross bodies suited to the spiritual state of the jivatma. Under the influence of prarabdhda karmma, buddhi becomes tamasik, rajasik, or sattvik. In the first case the jivatma assumes inanimate bodies; in the second, active passionate bodies; and in the third, sattvik bodies of varying degrees of spiritual excellence, ranging from man to the Deva. The gross body is also trigunatmaka. This body conveys impressions to the jivatma through the subtle body and the buddhi in particular. When sattva is made active impressions of happiness result, and when rajas or tamas are active the impressions are those of sorrow and delusion. These impressions are the result of the predominance of these respective guna. The action of rajas on sattva produces happiness, as its own independent activity or operation on tamas produce sorrow and delusion respectively. Where sattva or happiness is predominant, there sorrow and delusion are suppressed. Where rajas or sorrow is

predominant, there happiness and delusion are suppres-
sed. And where tamas or delusion predominates there,
as in the case of the inorganic world, both happiness
and sorrow are suppressed. All objects share these three
states in different proportions. There is, however, always
in the jivatma an admixture of sorrow with happiness,
due to the operation of rajas. For happiness, which is the
fruit of righteous acts done to attain happiness, is after
all only a vikara. The natural state of the jivatma – that
is, the state of its own true nature – is that bliss (anan-
da) which arises from the pure knowledge of the Self, in
which both happiness and sorrow are equally objects of
indifference. The worldly enjoyment of a person involves
pain to self or others. This is the result of the pursuit of
happiness, whether by righteous or unrighteous acts. As
spiritual progress is made, the gross body becomes more
and more refined. In inanimate bodies karma operates
to the production of pure delusion. On the exhaustion
of such karma the jivatma assumes animate bodies for
the operation of such forms of karma as lead to sorrow
and happiness mixed with delusion. In the vegetable
world sattva is but little active, with a corresponding
lack of discrimination, for discrimination is the effect
of sattva in buddhi, and from discrimination arises the
recognition of pleasure and pain, conceptions of right
and wrong, of the transitory and intransitory, and so
forth, which are the fruit of a high degree of discrimina-

tion, or of activity of sattva. In the lower animal sattva in buddhi is not sufficiently active to lead to any degree of development of these conceptions. In man, however, the sattva in buddhi is considerably active, and in consequence these conceptions are natural in him. For this reason the human birth is, for spiritual purposes, so important. All men, however, are not capable of forming such conceptions in an equal degree. The degree of activity in an individual's buddhi depends on his prarabdha karma. However bad such karma may be in any particular case, the individual is yet gifted with that amount of discrimination which, if properly aroused and aided, will enable him to better his spiritual condition by inducing the rajoguna in him to give more and more activity to the sattva guna in his buddhi.

On this account proper guidance and spiritual direction are necessary. A good guru, by reason of his own nature and spiritual attainment and disinterested wisdom, will both mark out for the sishya the path which is proper for him, and aid him to follow it by the infusion of the tejas which is in the Guru himself. Whilst sadhana is, as stated, a process for the stimulation of the sattva guna, it is evident that one form of it is not suitable to all. It must be adapted to the spiritual condition of the sishya, otherwise it will cause injury instead of good. Therefore it is that the adoption of certain forms of sadhana by persons who are not competent (adhikari), may not only be fruitless of any good result, but may even lead to evils which sadhana as a general principle is designed to prevent. Therefore also is it said that it is better to follow one's own dharma than that, however exalted it be, of another.

The Worlds (Loka).

This earth, which is the object of the physical senses and of the knowledge based thereon, is but one of fourteen worlds or regions placed "above" and "below" it, of which (as the sutra says) knowledge may be obtained by meditation on the solar "nerve" (nada) sushumna in the merudanda. On this nadi six of the upper worlds are threaded, the seventh and highest overhanging it in the Sahasrara Padma, the thousand-petalled lotus. The sphere of earth (Bhurloka), with its continents, their mountains and rivers, and with its oceans, is the seventh or lowest of the upper worlds. Beneath it are the Hells and Nether Worlds, the names of which are given below. Above the terrestrial sphere is Bhuvarloka, or the atmospheric sphere known as the antariksha, extending "from the earth to the sun," in which the Siddhas and other celestial beings (devayoni) of the upper air dwell. "From the sun to the pole star" dhruva) is svarloka, or the heavenly sphere. Heaven (svarga) is that which delights the mind, as hell (naraka) is that which gives it pain. In the former is the abode of the Deva and the blest.

These three spheres are the region of the consequences of work, and are termed transitory as compared with the three highest spheres, and the fourth, which is of a mixed character. When the jiva has received his reward he is reborn again on earth. For it is not good action, but the knowledge of the atma which procures Liberation (moksha). Above Svarloka is Maharloka, and above it the three ascending regions known as the janarloka, ta-poloka, and satyaloka, each inhabited by various forms of celestial intelligence of higher and higher degree. Below the earth (Bhuh) and above the nether worlds are the Hells (commencing with Avichi), and of which, according to popular theology, there are thirty-four, though it is elsewhere said there are as many hells as there are offences for which particular punishments are meted out. Of these, six are known as the great at hells. Hinduism, however, even when popular, knows nothing of a hell of eternal torment. To it nothing is eternal but the Brahman. Issuing from the Hells the jiva is again reborn to make its future. Below the Hells are the seven nether worlds, Sutala, Vitala, Talatala, Mahatala, Rasatala, Atala, and Patala, where, according to the Puranas, dwell the Naga serpent divinities, brilliant with jewels, and where, too, the lovely daughters of the Daityas and Danavas wander, fascinating even the most austere. Yet

*below Patala is the form of Vishnu proceeding from the
dark quality (tamogunah), known as the Sesha serpent
or Ananta, bearing the entire world as a diadem, attended by his Shakti Varuni, his own embodied radiance.*

Inhabitants of the Worlds.

*The worlds are inhabited by countless grades of beings,
ranging from the highest Devas (of whom there are
many classes and degrees) to the lowest animal life. The
scale of beings runs from the shining manifestations of
Spirit to those in which it is so veiled that it would seem
almost to have disappeared in its material covering.
There is but one Light, one Spirit, whose manifestations
are many. A flame enclosed in a clear glass loses but
little of its brilliancy. If we substitute for the glass, paper,
or some other more opaque yet transparent substance,
the light is dimmer. A covering of metal may be so dense
as to exclude from sight the rays of light which yet burns
within with an equal brilliancy. As a fact, all such veiling forms are maya. They are none the less true for those
who live in and are themselves part of the mayik world.
Deva, or "heavenly and shining one" – for spirit is light
and self-manifestation – is applicable to those descending yet high manifestations of the Brahman, such
as the seven Shivas, including the Trinity (trimurtti),
Brahma, Vishnu, and Rudra. Devi, again, is the title of*

*the Supreme Mother Herself, and is again applied to the
manifold forms assumed by the one only Maya, such as
Kali, Sarasvati, Lakshmi, Gauri, Gayatri, Sandhya, and
others. In the sense also in which it is said, "Verily, in the
beginning there was the Brahman. It created the Devas,"
the latter term also includes lofty intelligencies belonging to the created world intermediate between Ishvara
(Himself a Purusha) and man, who in the person of the
Brahmana is known as Earth-deva (bhudeva). These
spirits are of varying degrees. For there are no breaks in
the creation which represents an apparent descent of the
Brahman in gradually lowered forms. Throughout these
forms play the divine currents of pravritti and nivritti,
the latter drawing to Itself that which the former has
sent forth.*

*Deva, jiva and jara (inorganic matter) are, in their real,
as opposed to their phenomenal and illusory, being,
the one Brahman, which appears thus to be other than
Itself through its connection with the upadhi or limiting
conditions with which ignorance (avidya) invests it.
Therefore all beings which are the object of worship are
each of them but the Brahman seen through the veil
of avidya. Though the worshippers of Devas may not
know it, their worship is in reality the worship of the
Brahman, and hence the Mahanirvana Tantra says that,
"as all streams flow to the ocean, so the worship given*

to any Deva is received by the Brahman." On the other hand, those who, knowing this, worship the Devas, do so as manifestations of the Brahman, and thus worship It mediately. The sun, the most glorious symbol in the physical world, is the mayik vesture of Her who is "clothed with the sun."

In the lower ranks of the celestial hierarchy are the Devayonis, some of whom are mentioned in the opening verses of the first chapter of the text. The Devas are of two classes: "unborn" (ajata) – that is, those which have not, and those which have (sadhya) evolved from humanity as in the case of King Nahusha, who became Indra. Opposed to the divine hosts are the Asura, Danava, Daitya, Rakshasa, who, with other spirits, represent the tamasik or demonic element in creation. All Devas, from the highest downwards, are subordinate to both time and karma. So it is said, "Salutation to Karma, over which not even Vidhi (Brahma) prevails" (Namastat karmmabhyovidhirapi na yebhyah prabhavati). The rendering of the term "Deva" by "God" has led to a misapprehension of Hindu thought. The use of the term "angel" may also mislead, for though the world of Devas has in some respects analogy to the angelic choirs, the Christian conception of these Beings, their origin and functions, does not include, but in fact excludes, other ideas connoted by the Sanskrit term.

The pitris, or "Fathers," are a creation (according to some) separate from the predecessors of humanity, and are, according to others, the lunar ancestry who are addressed in prayer with the Devas. From Brahma, who is known as the "Grandfather" Pita Maha of the human race, issued Marichi, Atri, and others, his "mental sons": the Agnishvattvah, Saumnyah, Havishmantah, Ushmapah, and other classes of Pitris, numbering, according to the Markandeya Purana, thirty-one. Tarpanam, or oblation, is daily offered to these pitris. The term is also applied to the human ancestors of the worshipper generally up to the seventh generation to whom in shraddha (the obsequial rites) pinda and water are offered with the mantra "svadha."

The Rishi are seers who know, and by their knowledge are the makers of shastra and "see" all mantras. The word comes from the root rish Rishati-prapnoti sarvvang mantrang jnanena pashyati sangsaraparangva, etc. The seven great Rishi or saptarshi of the first manvantara are Marichi, Atri, Angiras, Pulaha, Kratu, Pulastya, and Vashishtha. In other manvantara there are other sapta-rshi. In the present manvantara the seven are Kashyapa Atri, Vashishtha, Vishvamitra, Gautama, Jamadagni, Bharadvaja. To the Rishi the Vedas were revealed. Vyasa taught the Rigveda so revealed to Paila, the Yajurveda to Vaishampayana, the Samaveda to Jaimini, Atharvaveda to Samantu, and Itihasa and

Purana to Suta. The three chief classes of Rishi are the Brah-marshi, born of the mind of Brahma, the Devarshi of lower rank, and Rajarshi or Kings who became Rishis through their knowledge and austerities, such as Janaka, Ritaparna, etc. Thc Shrutarshi are makers of Shastras, as Sushruta. The Kandarshi are of the Karmakanda, such as Jaimini.

The Muni, who may be a Rishi, is a sage. Muni is so called on account of his mananam (mananat muni-ruchyate). Mananam is that thought, investigation, and discussion which marks the independent thinking mind. First there is shravanam listening; then mananam, which is the thinking or understanding, discussion upon, and testing of what is heard as opposed to the mere acceptance on trust of the lower intelligence. There two are followed by nididhyasanam, which is attention and profound meditation on the conclusions (siddhanta) drawn from what is so heard and reasoned upon. As the Mahabharata says, "The Veda differ, and so do the Sm-riti. No one is a muni who has no independent opinion of his own (nasau muniryasya matang na bhinnam).

The human being is called jiva – that is, the embodied Atma possessed by egoism and of the notion that it directs the puryashtaka, namely, the five organs of action (karmendriya), the five organs of perception (jnanend-riya), the fourfold antahkarana or mental self (Manas,

Buddhi, Ahangkara, Chitta), the five vital airs (Prana), the five elements, Kama (desire), Karma (action and its results), and Avidya (illusion). When these false notions are destroyed, the embodiment is destroyed, and the wearer of the mayik garment attains nirvana. When the jiva is absorbed in Brahman, there is no longer any jiva remaining as such.

Varna.

Ordinarily there are four chief divisions or castes (varna) of Hindu society – viz.: Brahmana (priesthood; teaching); Kshattriya (warrior); Vaishya (merchant); Shudra (servile) – said to have sprung respectively from the mouth, arm, thigh, and foot of Brahma. A man of the first three classes becomes an investiture, during the upanayana ceremony of the sacred thread, twice-born (dvija). It is said that by birth one is shudra, by sangs-kara (upanayana), dvija (twice-born); by study of the Vedas one attains the state of a vipra; and that he who has knowledge of the Brahman is a Brahmana. The present Tantra, however, speaks of a fifth or hybrid class (samanya), resulting from intermixture between the others. It is a peculiarity of Tantra that its worship is largely free of Vaidik exclusiveness, whether based on caste, sex, or otherwise. As the Gautamiya Tantra says, "The Tantra is for all men, of whatever caste, and for all

*women" (Sarvvavarnadhikaraschcha narinang yogya
eva cha).*

Ashrama.

*The four stages, conditions, or periods in the life of a
Brahman are: First, that of the chaste student, or brah-
machari; second, the period of secular life as a married
householder, or grihastha; third, that of the recluse, or
vanaprastha, when there is retirement from the world;
and lastly, that of the beggar, or bhikshu, who begs his
single daily meal, and meditates upon the Supreme
Spirit to which he is about to return. For the Kshattriya
there are the first three Ashramas; for the Vaishya, the
first two; and for the Shudra, the grihastha Ashrama
only. This Tantra states that in the Kali age there are
only two Ashrama. The second garhasthya and the last
bhikshuka or avadhuta. Neither the conditions of life,
nor the character, capacity, and powers of the people of
this age allow of the first and third. The two ashramas
prescribed for the Kali age are open to all castes indiscri-
minately.*

*There are, it is now commonly said, two main divisions
of avadhuta – namely, Shaivavadhuta and Brahmavad-
huta – of each of which there are, again, three divisions.
Of the first class the divisions are firstly Shaivavadhu-*

45

ta, who is apurna (imperfect). Though an ascetic, he is also a householder and like Shiva. Hence his name. The second is the wandering stage of the Shaiva (or the parivrajaka), who has now left the world, and passes his time doing puja, japa, etc., visiting the tirtha and pitha, or places of pilgrimage. In this stage, which, though higher, is still imperfect, the avadhuta is competent for ordinary sadhana with a shakti. The third is the perfect stage of a Shaiva. Wearing only the kaupina, he renounces all things and all rites, though within certain limits he may practise some yoga, and is permitted to meet the request of a woman who makes it of him. Of the second class the three divisions are, firstly, the Brahma-vadhuta, who, like the Shaivavadhuta, is imperfect (apurna) and a householder. He is not permitted, however, to have a Shaiva Shakti, and is restricted to sviya-shakti. The second-class Brahma-parivrajaka is similar to the Shaiva of the same class, except that ordinarily he is not permitted to have anything to do with any woman, though he may, under the guidance of his Guru, practise yoga accompanied by Shakti. The third or highest class – Hangsavadhuta – is similar to the third Shaiva degree, except that he must under no circumstances touch a woman or metals, nor may he practise any rites or keep any observances.

Correspondence Between Macrocosm and Microcosm

The universe consists of a Mahabrahmanda, or grand Kosmos, and of numerous Brihatbrahmanda, or macrocosms evolved from it. As is said by the Nirvana Tantra, all which is in the first is in the second. In the latter are heavenly bodies and beings, which are microcosms reflecting on a minor scale the greater worlds which evolve them. "As above, so below." This mystical maxim of the West is stated in the Vishvasara Tantra as follows: "What is here is elsewhere; what is not here is nowhere" (yadihasti tadanyatra yannehasti natatkvachit). The macrocosm has its meru, or vertebral column, extending from top to bottom. There are fourteen regions descending from Satyaloka, the highest. These are the seven upper and the seven nether worlds (vide ante). The meru of the human body is the spinal column, and within it are the chakra, in which the worlds are said to dwell. In the words of the Shaktananda-Tarangini, they are pindamadhyesthita. Satya has been said to be in the sahasrara, and Tapah, Janah, Mahah, Svah, Bhuvah, Bhuh in the ajna, vishuddha, anahata, manipura, svadishthana, and muladhara lotuses respectively. Below muladhara and in the joints, sides, anus, and organs of generation are the nether worlds. The bones near the spinal column are the kula-parvata. Such are the correspondences as to earth. Then as to water. The nadi are the rivers. The seven substances of the body (dhatu) are the seven islands. Sweat, tears, and the like are the oce-

ans. Fire exists in the muladhara, sushumna, navel, and elsewhere. As the worlds are supported by the pravaha-na and other vayu ("airs"), so is the body supported by the ten vayu prana, etc. There is the same akasha (ether) in both. The witness within is the purusha without, for the personal soul of the microcosm corresponds to the cosmic soul (hiranyagarbha) in the macrocosm.

The Ages.

The passage of time within a maha-yoga influences for the worse man and the world in which he lives. This passage is marked by the four ages (yuga), called Satya, Treta, Dvapara, and Kali-yuga, the last being that in which it is generally supposed the world now is. The yuga is a fraction of a kalpa, or day of Brahma of 4,320,000 human years. The kalpa is divided into fourteen manvantara, which are again subdivided into seventy-one maha.-yuga; the length of each of which is 4,320,000 human years. The maha-yuga (great age) is itself composed of four yuga (ages) – (a) Satya, (b) Treta, (c) Dvapara, (d) Kali. Official science teaches that man appeared on the earth in an imperfect state, from which he has since been gradually, though continually, raising himself. Such teaching is, however, in conflict with the traditions of all peoples – Jew, Babylonian, Egyptian, Hindu, Greek, Roman, and Christian – which speak of an age when man was both innocent and happy. From this state of primal perfection he fell, continuing his descent until such time as the great Avatara, Christ and others, descended to save his race and enable it to regain the righteous path. The Garden of Eden is the emblem of the paradisiacal body of man. There man was one with Nature. He was himself paradise, a privileged enclosure in a garden of delight – gan be Eden. Et eruditus est Moyse omni sapientia Ægyptiorum. The Satya Yuga is, according to Hindu belief, the Golden Age of righteousness, free of sin, marked by longevity, physical strength, beauty, and stature. "There were giants in those days" whose moral, mental, and physical strength enabled them to undergo long brahmacharyya (continence) and tapas (austerities). Longevity permitted lengthy spiritual exercises. Life then depended on the marrow, and lasted a lakh of years, men dying when they willed. Their stature was 21 cubits.

To this age belong the Avatara or incarnations of Vishnu, Matsya, Kurma, Varaha, Nri-singha, and Vamana. Its duration is computed to be 4,800 Divine years, which, when multiplied by 360 (a year of the Devas being equal to 360 human years) are the equivalent of 1,728,000 of the years of man. (b) The second age, or Treta (three-fourth) Yuga, is that in which righteousness (dharmma) decreased by one-fourth. The duration was

3,600 Divine years, or 1,296,000 human years. Longevity, strength, and stature decreased. Life was in the bone, and lasted 10,000 years. Man's stature was 14 cubits. Of sin there appeared one-quarter, and of virtue there remained three-quarters. Men were still attached to pious and charitable acts, penances, sacrifice, and pilgrimage, of which the chief was that to Naimisharanya. In this period appeared the avatars of Vishnu as Parashurama and Rama. (c) The third, or Dvapara (one-half) Yuga, is that in which righteousness decreased by one-half, and the duration of which was 2,400 Divine, or 864,000 human, years. A further decrease in longevity and strength, and increase of weakness and disease, mark this age. Life which lasted 1,000 years was centred in the blood. Stature was 7 cubits. Sin and virtue were of equal force. Men became restless, and, though eager to acquire knowledge, were deceitful, and followed both good and useful pursuits. The principal place of pilgrimage was Kurukshetra. To this age belongs (according to Vyasa, Anushtubhacharya and Jiya-deva) the avatara of Vishnu as Bala-rama, the elder brother of Krishna, who, according to other accounts, takes his place. In the sandhya, or intervening period of 1,000 years between this and the next yuga the Tantra was revealed, as it will be revealed at the dawn of every Kali-yuga. (d) Kali-yuga is the alleged present age, in which righteousness exists to the extent of one-fourth only, the duration of which is 1,200 Divine, or 432,000 human, years. According to some, this age commenced in 3120 B.C. on the date of Vishnu's return to heaven after the eighth incarnation. This is the periodwhich, according to the Puranas and Tantras, is characterized by the prevalence of viciousness, weakness, disease, and the general decline of all that is good. Humanlife, which lasts at most 120, or, as some say, 100, years,is dependent on food. Stature is 3½ cubits. The chief pilgrimage is now to the Ganges. In this age has appeared the Buddha Avatara. The last, or Kalki Avatara,the Destroyer of sin, has yet to come. It is He who will destroy iniquity and restore the age of righteousness. The Kalki Purana speaks of Him as One whose body is blue like that of the rain-charged cloud, who with sword in hand rides, as does the rider of the Apocalypse, a white horse swift as the wind, the Cherisher of the people, Destroyer of the race of the Kali-yuga, the Source of true religion. And Jayadeva, in his Ode to the Incarnations,addresses Him thus: "For the destruction of all the impure thou drawest thy cimeter like a blazing comet. O how tremendous! Oh, Keshava, assuming the body of Kalki! Be victorious. O Hari, Lord of the Universe!" With the Satya-yuga a new maha-yaga will commence, and the ages will continue to revolve with their rising and descending races until the close of the kalpa or day of Brahma.. Then a night of dissolution (pralaya) of equal duration follows, the Lord reposing in yoga-nidra (yoga sleep in pralaya) on the Serpent Shes ha, the Endless One, till day break, when the universe is created anew and the next kalpa follows.

The Scriptures of the Ages.

Each of these Ages has its appropriate Shastra or Scripture, designed to meet the characteristics and needs of the men who live in them The Hindu Shastra are classed into: (1) Shruti, which commonly includes the four Veda. (Rik, Yajuh, Sama, Atharva, and the Upanishads), the doctrine of which is philosophically exposed in the Vedanta-Darshana. (2) Smriti, such as the Dharma-Shastra of Manu and other works on family and social duty prescribing for pavritti-dhamia, as the Upanishads had revealed the nivritti-dharma. (3) The Puranas, of which, according to the Brahma-vai-vartta Purana, there were originally four lakhs, and of which eighteen are now regarded as the principal. (4) The Tantra.

For each of these ages a suitable Shastra is given. The Veda is the root of all Shastra (mula-shastra). All others are based on it. The Tantra is spoken of as a fifth Veda. Kulluka-Bhatta, the celebrated Commentator on Manu, says that Shruti is of two kinds, Vaidik and Tantrik (vaidiki-tantriiki chaiva dvi-vidha shrutih-kirttita). The various Shastras, however, are different presentments of shruti appropriate to the humanity of the age for which they are given. Thus the Tantra is that presentment of shruti which is modelled as regards its ritual to meet the characteristics and infirmities of the Kali-yuga. As men have no longer the capacity, longevity, and moral strength necessary for the application of the Vaidika Karma-kanda, the Tantra prescribes a special sadhana or means or practice of its own, for the attainment of that which is the ultimate and common end of all Shastra. The Kularnava Tantra says that in the Satya or Krita age the Shastra is Shruti (in the sense of the Veda and Upanishads); in Treta-yuga, Smriti (in the sense of the Dharma-Shastra and Shruti-jivika, etc.); in Dvapara Yuga the Purana; and in the last or Kali-yuga the Tantra, which should now be followed by all orthodox Hindu worshippers. The Maha-nirvana and other Tantras and Tantrik works lay down the same rule. The Tantra is also said to contain the very core of the Veda to which, it is described to bear the relation of the Paramatma to the Jivatma. In a similar way, Kaulachara is the central informing life of the gross body called vedachara, each of the achara which follow it up to kaulachara being more and more subtle sheaths.

The Human Body.

The human body is Brahma-para, the city of Brahman. Ishvara Himself enters into the universe as jiva. Where-

*fore the maha-vakya "That thou art" means that the ego
(which is regarded as jiva only from the standpoint of an
upadhi) is Brahman.*

The Five Sheaths.

*In the body there are five kosha or sheaths – an-
na-maya, prana-maya, mano-maya, vijñana-maya,
ananda-maya, or the physical and vital bodies, the two
mental bodies, and the body of bliss. In the first the Lord
is self-conscious as being dark or fair, short or tall, old
or youthful. In the vital body He feels alive, hungry, and
thirsty. In the mental bodies He thinks and understands.
And in the body of Bliss He resides in happiness. Thus
garmented with the five garments, the Lord, though all
pervading, appears as though He were limited by them.*

Anna-Maya Kosha.

*In the material body, which is called the "sheath of food"
(anna-maya kosha), reign the elements earth, water,
and fire, which are those presiding in the lowest Chakra,
the Muladhara, Svadhishthana, and mani-pura centres.
The two former produce food and drink, which is assimi-
lated by the fire of digestion, and converted into the body
of food. The indriya are both the faculty and organs of
sense. There are in this body the material organs, as
distinguished from the faculty of sense.*

In the gross body (sharira-kosha) there are six external kosha – viz., hair, blood, flesh, which come from the mother, and bone, muscle, marrow, from the father.

The organs of sense (indriya) are of two kinds – viz.: jnanendriya, or organs of sensation, through which knowledge of the external world is obtained (ear, skin, eyes, tongue, nose); and karmendriya, or organs of action – mouth, arms, legs, anus, penis, the functions of which are speech, holding, walking, excretion, and procreation.

Prana-Maya Kosha.

The second sheath is the prana-maya-kosha, or sheath of "breath" (prana), which manifests itself in air and ether, the presiding elements in the Anahata and Vishuddha chakra.

There are ten vayu (airs), or inner vital forces, of which the first five are the principal – namely, the sapphire prana; apana, the colour of an evening cloud; the silver vyana; udana, the colour of fire; and the milky samana. These are all aspects of the action of the one Prana-devata. Kundalini is the Mother of prana, which She the Mula-Prakriti, illumined by the light of the Supreme Atma, generates. Prana is vayu, or the universal force of activity, divided on entering each individual into fivefold function. Specifically considered, prana is inspiration, which with expiration is from and to a distance of eight and twelve inches respectively. Udana is the ascending vayu. Apana is the downward vayu, expelling wind, excrement, urine, and semen. The samana, or collective vayu, kindles the bodily fire, "conducting equally the food, etc., throughout the body." Vyana is the separate vayu, effecting division and diffusion. These forces cause respiration, excretion, digestion, circulation.

Mano-maya, Vijñana Kosha, and Ananda-maya Kosha.

The next two sheaths are the mano-maya and vijñana kosha. These constitute the antah-karana, which is fourfold – namely, mind in its twofold aspect of buddhi and manas, self-hood (ahankara), and chitta. The function of the first is doubt sangkalpa-vikalpatmaka, (uncertainty, certainty); of the second, determination (nishchaya-karini); of the third (egoity), consciousness (abhimana). Manas automatically registers the facts which the senses perceive. Buddhi, on attending to such registration, discriminates, determines, and cognizes the object registered, which is set over and against the subjective self by Ahangkara. The function of chitta is contemplation (chinta), the faculty whereby the mind in its widest sense raises for itself the subject of its thought and dwells thereon. For whilst buddhi has but three

*moments in which it is born, exists, and dies, chitta
endures.*

*The antah-karana is master of the ten senses, which
are the outer doors through which it looks forth upon
the external world. The faculties, as opposed to the
organs or instruments of sense, reside here. The centres
of the powers inherent in the last two sheaths are in the
Ajna Chakra and the region above this and below the
sahasrara lotus. In the latter the Atma of the last sheath
of bliss resides. The physical or gross body is called
sthula-sharira. The subtle body (sukshma-sharira, also
called linga-sharira and karana-shanra) comprises the
ten indriya, manas, ahangkara, buddhi, and the five
functions of prana. This subtle body contains in itself the
cause of rebirth into the gross body when the period of
reincarnation arrives.*

*The atma, by its association with the upadhis, has three
states of consciousness – namely, the jagrat, or waking
state, when through the sense organs are perceived
objects of sense through the operation of manas and
buddhi. It is explained in the Ishvara-pratya-bhijna as
follows – "the waking state dear to all is the source of
external action through the activity of the senses." The
jiva is called jagari – that is, he who takes upon himself
the gross body called Vishva. The second is svapna, the
dream state, when, the sense organs being withdrawn,*

Alma is conscious of mental images generated by the impressions of jagrat experience. Here manas ceases to record fresh sense impressions, and it and buddhi work on that which manas has registered in the waking state. The explanation of this state is also given in the work last cited. "The state of svapna is the objectification of visions perceived in the mind, due to the perception of ideas there latent." Jiva in the state of svapna is termed taijasa. Its individuality is merged in the subtle body. Hiranyagarbha is the collective form of these jiva, as Vaisvanara is such form of the jiva in the waking state. The third state is that of sushupti, or dreamless sleep, when manas itself is withdrawn, and buddhi, dominated by tamas, preserves only the notion: "Happily I slept; I was not conscious of anything" (Patanjala-yoga-sutra). In the Macrocosm the upadhi of these states are also called Virat, Hiranyagarbha, and Avyakta. The description of the state of sleep is given in the Shiva-sutra as that in which there is incapacity of discrimination or illusion. By the saying cited from the Patanjala-sutra three modifications of avidya are indicated – viz., ignorance, egoism, and happiness. Sound sleep is that state in which these three exist. The person in that state is termed prajna, his individuality being merged in the causal body (karana). Since in the sleeping state the prajna becomes Brahman, he is no longer jiva as before; but the jiva is then not the supreme one (Paramatma), because the state is associated with avidya. Hence, because the vehicle in the jiva

*in the sleeping state is Karana, the vehicle of the jiva in
the fourth is declared to be mahakarana. Ishvara is the
collective form of the prajna jiva.*

*Beyond sushupti is the turiya, and beyond turiya the
transcendent fifth state without name. In the fourth
state shuddha-vidya is acquired, and this is the only rea-
listic one for the yogi which he attains through, samadhi-yoga. Jiva in turiya is merged in the great causal body
(maha-karana). The fifth state arises from firmness
in the fourth. He who is in this state becomes equal to
Shiva, or, more strictly, tends to a close equality; for it is
only beyond that, that "the spotless one attains the highest equality," which is unity. Hence even in the fourth
and fifth states there is an absence of that full perfection
which constitutes the Supreme. Bhaskara-raya, in his
Commentary on the Lalita, when pointing out that the
Tantrik theory adds the fourth and fifth states to the
first three adopted by the followers of the Upanishads,
says that the latter states are not separately enumerated
by them owing to the absence in those two states of the
full perfection of Jiva or of Shiva.*

Nadi

*It is said that there are 3½ crores of nadi in the human
body, of which some are gross and some are subtle.*

*Nadi means a nerve or artery in the ordinary sense;
but all the nadis of which the books on Yoga speak are
not of this physical character, but are subtle channels of
energy. Of these nadi, the principal are fourteen; and
of these fourteen, ida, pingala, and sushumna are the
chief; and, again, of these three sushumna is the greatest,
and to it all others are subordinate. Sushumna is in the
hollow of the meru in the cerebro-spinal axis. It extends
from the Muladhara lotus, the Tattvik earth centre, to
the cerebral region. Sushumna is in the form of Fire
(vahni-svarupa), and has within it the vajrini-nadi in
the form of the sun (surya-svarupa). Within the latter is
the pale nectar-dropping chitra or chitrini-nadi, which
is also called Brahma-nadi, in the form of the moon
(chandra-svarupa,). Sushumna is thus triguna. The
various lotuses in the different Chakra of the body (vide
post) are all suspended from the chitra-nadi, the chakra
being described as knots in the nadi, which is as thin
as the thousandth part of a hair. Outside the meru and
on each side of sushumna are the nadi ida and pingala.
Ida is on the left side, and, coiling round sushumna, has
its exit in the left nostril. Pingala is on the right, and,
similarly coiling, enters the right nostril. The sushumna,
interlacing ida and pingala and the ajna-chakra round
which they pass, thus forms a representation of the ca-
duceus of Mercury. Ida is of a pale colour, is moon-like
(chandra-svarupa), and contains nectar. Pingala is red,
and is sun-like (suryya-svarupa), containing "venom,"*

*the fluid of mortality. These three "rivers," which are uni-
ted at the ajna-chakra, flow separately from that point,
and for this reason the ajna-chakra is called mukta
triveni. The muladhara is called Yukta (united)-tri-veni,
since it is the meeting-place of the three nadi, which are
also called Ganga (Ida), Yamuna (Pingala), and Sarasvati (sushumna), after the three sacred rivers of India.
The opening at the end of the sushumna in the muladhara is called brahma-dvara, which is closed by the coils
of the sleeping Devi Kundalini.*

Chakra

*There are six chakra, or dynamic Tattvik centres, in the
body – viz., the muladhara, svadhishthana, mani-pura,
anahata, vishuddha, and ajna – which are described in
the following notes. Over all there is the thousand-petalled lotus (sahasrara-padma).*

Muladhara

*Muladhara is a triangular space in the midmost portion
of the body, with the apex turned downwards like a
young girl's yoni. It is described as a red lotus of four
petals, situate between the base of the sexual organ and
the anus. "Earth" evolved from "water" is the Tattva
of this chakra. On the four petals are the four golden
varnas – "vang," "shang," "shang," and "sang," In the four*

petals pointed towards the four directions (Ishana, etc.) are the four forms of bliss – yogananda (yoga bliss), paramananda (supreme bliss), samaj-ananda (natural bliss), and virananda (vira bliss). In the centre of this lotus is Svayambhu-linga, ruddy brown, like the colour of a young leaf. Chitrini-nadi is figured as a tube, and the opening at its end at the base of the linga is called the door of Brahman (brahma-dvara), through which the Devi ascends. The lotus, linga and brahma-dvara, hang downwards. The Devi Kundalini, more subtle than the fibre of the lotus, and luminous as lightning, lies asleep coiled like a serpent around the linga, and closes with Her body the door of Brahman. The Devi has forms in the brahmanda. Her subtlest form in the pindanda, or body, is called Kundalini, a form of Prakriti pervading, supporting, and expressed in the form of the whole universe; ”the Glittering Dancer ”(as the Sarada-tilaka calls Her) ”in the lotus-like head of the yogi.” When awakened, it is She who gives birth to the world made of mantra. A red fiery triangle surrounds svayambhu-linga, and within the triangle is the red Kandarpa-vayu, or air, of Kama, a form of the apana vayu, for here is the seat of creative desire. Outside the triangle is a yellow square, called the prithivi-(earth)-mandala, to which is attached the ”eight thunders” (ashta-vajra). Here is the vija ”lang”, and with it prithivi on the back of an elephant. Here also are Brahma and Savitri, and the red four-handed Shakti Dakini.

Svadhisthana

*Svadhishthana is a six-petalled lotus at the base of the
sexual organ, above muladhara and below the navel. Its
pericarp is red, and its petals are like lightning. "Water" evolved from "fire" is the Tattva of this chakra. The
varnas on the petals are "bang," "bhang," "mang," "yang,"
"rang," and "lang." In the six petals are also the vritti
(states, qualities, functions, or inclinations) – namely,
prashraya (credulity), a-vishvasa (suspicion, mistrust),
avajna (disdain), murchchha (delusion, or, as some say,
disinclination), sarvva-nasha (false knowledge), and
krurata (pitilessness). Within a semicircular space in the
pericarp are the Devata, the dark blue Maha-vishnu,
Maha-lakshmi, and Sarasvati. In front is the blue
four-handed Rakini Shakti, and the vija of Varuna,
Lord of water or "vang." Inside the vija there is the region of Varuna., of the shape of an half-moon, and in it is
Varuna himself seated on a white alligator (makara).*

Mani-pura

*Mani-para-chakra is a ten-petalled golden lotus, situate
above the last in the region of the navel. "Fire" evolved
from "air" is the Tattva of this chakra. The ten petals are
of the colour of a cloud, and on them are the blue varnas
– "dang," "dhang," "nang," tang," "thang," "dang," "dhang,"*

*"nang," "pang," "phang," – and the ten vritti (vide ante),
namely, lajja (shame), pishunata (fickleness), irsha
(jealousy), trishna (desire), sushupti (laziness), vishada
(sadness), kashaya (dullness), moha (ignorance), ghrina
(aversion, disgust), bhaya (fear). Within the pericarp is
the vija of fire ("rang"), and a triangular figure (mandala) of Agni, Lord of Fire, to each side of which figure are
attached three auspicious signs or svastika. Agni, red,
four-handed, and seated on a ram, is within the figure.
In front of him are Rudra and his Shakti Bhadra-kali.
Rudra is of the colour of vermilion, and is old. His body
is smeared with ashes. He has three eyes and two hands.
With one of these he makes the sign which grants boons
and blessings, and with the other that which dispels
fear. Near him is the four-armed Lakini Shakti, of the
colour of molten gold (tapta-kanchana), wearing yellow
raiments and ornaments. Her mind is maddened with
passion (mada-matta-chitta). Above the lotus is the
abode and region of Suryya. The solar region drinks the
nectar which drops from the region of the Moon.*

Anahata

*Anahata-chakra is a deep red lotus of twelve petals,
situate above the last and in the region of the heart,
which is to be distinguished from the heart-lotus facing
upwards of eight petals, spoken of in the text, where the*

*patron deity (Ishta-devata) is meditated upon. "Air"
evolved from "ether" is the Tattva of the former lotus.
On the twelve petals are the vermilion varnas – "Kang"
"Khang," "Gang," "Ghang," "ngang," "chang", "Chhang,"
"Jang," "Jhang," "Nyang," "Tang," "Thang," and the
twelve vrittis (vide ante) – namely asha (hope), chinta
(care, anxiety), cheshta (endeavour), mamata (sense of
mineness), dambha (arrogance or hypocrisy), vikalata
(languor), ahangkara (conceit), viveka (discrimination),
lolata (covetousness), kapatata (duplicity), vitarka
(indecision), anutapa (regret). A triangular mandala
within the pericarp of this lotus of the lustre of lightning
is known as the Tri-kona Shakti. Within this mandala
is a red vana-linga, called Narayana or Hiranya-gar-
bha, and near it Ishvara and His Shakti Bhuvaneshvari.
Ishvara, who is the Overlord of the first three chakra,
is of the colour of molten gold, and with His two hands
grants blessings and dispels fear. Near him is the three-eyed Kakini Shakti, lustrous as lightning, with four
hands holding the noose and drinking-cup, and making
the sign of blessing, and that which dispels fear. She
wears a garland of human bones. She is excited, and her
heart is softened with wine. Here, also, are several other
Shakti, such as Kala-ratri, as also the vija of air (vayu)
or "vang." Inside the lotus is a six-cornered smoke-coloured mandala, and the circular region of smoke-coloured
Vayu, who is seated on a black antelope. Here, too, is the*

*embodied atma (jivatma), like the tapering flame of a
lamp.*

Vishuddha

*Vishuddha chakra or Bharatisthana, abode of the
Devi of speech, is above the last and at the lower end
of the throat (kantha-mula). The Tattva of this chakra
is "ether." The lotus is of a smoky colour, or the colour
of fire seen through smoke. It has sixteen petals, which
carry the red vowels – "ang," "ang" "ing," "ing," "ung,"
"ung"," "ring," "ring," "lring," "lring," "eng," "aing," "ong,"
"aung," "ang," "ah;" the seven musical notes (nishada,
rishabha, gandhara, shadaja, madhyama, dhaivata
and panchama): "venom" (in the eighth petal); the vija
"hung," "phat," "vaushat," "vashat," "svadha," "svaha,"
"namah," and in the sixteenth petal nectar (amrita). In
the pericarp is a triangular region, within which is the
androgyne Shiva, known as Arddha-narishvara. There
also are the region of the full moon and ether, with its
vija "hang." The akasha-mandala is transparent and
round in shape.*

*Akasha himself is here dressed in white, and mounted
on a white elephant. He has four hands, which hold the
noose (pasha), the elephant-hook (angkusha), and with
the other he makes the mudra which grant blessing and
dispel fear. Shiva is white, with five faces, three eyes, ten*

arms, and is dressed in tiger skins. Near Him is the white Shakti Shakini, dressed in yellow raiments, holding in Her four hands the bow, the arrow, the noose, and the hook.

Above the chakra, at the root of the palate (talumula) is a concealed chakra, called Lalana and, in some Tantras, Kala-chakra. It is a red lotus with twelve petals, bearing the following vritti – shraddha (faith), santosha (contentment), aparadha (sense of error), dana (self-command), mana (anger), sneha (affection), shoka (sorrow, grief), kheda (dejection), shuddhata (purity), arati (detachment), sambhrama (agitation), Urmmi (appetite, desire).

Ajna

Ajna chakra is also called parama-hula and muk-ta-tri-veni, since it is from here that the three nadis – Ida, Pingala, and Sushumna – go their separate ways. It is a two-petalled lotus, situate between the two eyebrows. In this Chakra there is no gross Tattva, but the subtle Tattva mind is here. Hakararddha, or half the letter La, is also there. On its two petals are the red varnas "hang "and "kshang."

In the pericarp is concealed the vija "ong." In the two

petals and the pericarp there are the three guna – sattva, rajas, and tamas. Within the triangular mandala in the pericarp there is the lustrous (tejo-maya) linga in the form of the pranava (pranavakriti), which is called Itara. Para-Shiva, in the form of hangsa (hangsa-rupa) is also there with his Shakti – Siddha-Kali. In the three corners of the triangle are Brahma, Vishnu, and Maheshvara, respectively. In this chakra there is the white Hakini-Shakti, with six heads and four hands, in which are jñana-mudra, a skull, a drum (damaru), and a rosary.

Sahasrara Padma

Above the ajna-chakra there is another secret chakra, called manas-chakra. It is a lotus of six petals, on which are shabda-jñana, sparsha-jñana, rupa-jñana, aghrano-palabdhi, rasopabhoga, and svapna, or the faculties of hearing, touch, sight, smell, taste, and sleep, or the absence of these. Above this, again, there is another secret chakra, called Soma-chakra. It is a lotus of sixteen petals, which are also called sixteen Kala. These Kala are called kripa (mercy), mriduta (gentleness), dhairyya (patience, composure), vairagya (dispassion), dhriti (constancy), sampat (prosperity), hasya (cheerfulness), romancha (rapture, thrill), vinaya (sense of propriety, humility), dhyana (meditation), susthirata (quietude, restfulness), gambhiryya (gravity), udyama (enterprise, effort), akshobha (emotionlessness), audarya (magnanimity), and ekagrata (concentration).

Above this last chakra is "the house without support" (niralamba-puri), where yogis see the radiant Ishvara. Above this is the pranava shining like a flame, and above pranava the white crescent Nada, and above this last the point Vindu. There is then a white lotus of twelve petals with its head upwards, and over this lotus there is the ocean of nectar (sudha-sagara), the island of gems (mani-dvipa), the altar of gems (mani-pitha), the forked lightning-like lines a, ka, tha, and therein Nada and Vindu. On Nada and Vindu, as an altar, there is the Paramahangsa, and the latter serves as an altar for the feet of the Guru; there the Guru of all should be meditated. The body of the Hangsa on which the feet of the Guru rest is jñana-maya, the wings Agama and Nigama, the two feet Shiva and Shakti, the beak Pranava, the eyes and throat Kama-Kala.

Close to the thousand-petalled lotus is the sixteenth digit of the moon, which is called ama-kala, which is pure red and lustrous like lightning, as fine as a fibre of the lotus, hanging downwards, receptacle of the lunar nectar. In it is the crescent nirvana-kala, luminous as the Sun, and finer than the thousandth part of a hair. This is the

Ishta-devata of all. Near nirvana-kala is parama-nirvana-Shakti, infinitely subtle, lustrous as the Sun, creatrix of tattva-jnana. Above it are Vindu and Visarga-Shakti, root and abode of all bliss.

Sahasrara-padma – or thousand petalled lotus of all colours – hangs with its head downwards from the brahma-randhra above all the chakra. This is the region of the first cause (Brahma-loka), the cause of the six proceeding causes. It is the great Sun both cosmically and individually, in whose effulgence Parama-Shiva and Adya-Shakti reside. The power is the vachaka-Shakti or saguna-brahman, holding potentially within itself, the gunas, powers, and planes. Parama-Shiva is in the form of the Great Ether (paramakasha-rupi), the Supreme Spirit (paramatma), the Sun of the darkness of ignorance. In each of the petals of the lotus are placed all the letters of the alphabet; and whatever there is in the lower chakra or in the universe (brahmanda) exist here in potential state (avyakta-bhava). Shaivas call this place Shiva-sthana, Vaishnavas, Parama-purusha, Shaktas, Devi-sthana, the Sankhya sages Prakriti-purusha-sthana. Others call it by other names, such as Hari-hara-sthana. Shakti-sthana, Parama-Brahma, Parama-hangsa, Parama-jyotih, Kula-sthana, and Parama-Shiva-Akula. But whatever the name, all speak of the same.

The Three Temperaments

*The Tantras speak of three temperaments, disposi-
tions, characters (bhava), or classes of men – namely,
the pashu-bhava (animal), vira-bhava (heroic), and
divya-bhava (deva-like or divine). These divisions are
based on various modifications of the guna (v. ante) as
they manifest in man (jiva). It has been pointed out that
the analogous Gnostic classification of men as material,
psychical, and spiritual, correspond to the three guna
of the Sankhya-darshana. In the pashu the rajo-guna
operates chiefy on tamas, producing such dark characteristics as error (bhranti), drowsiness (tandra), and
sloth (alasya). It is however, an error to suppose that the
pashu is as such a bad man; on the contrary, a jiva of
this class may prove superior to a jiva of the next. If the
former, who is greatly bound by matter, lacks enligh-
tenment, the latter may abuse the greater freedom he
has won. There are also numerous kinds of pashu, some
more some less tamasik than others. Some there are at
the lowest end of the scale, which marks the first advance upon the higher forms of animal life. Others approach
and gradually merge into the vira class. The term pashu
comes from the root pash, "to bind." The pashu is, in
fact, the man who is bound by the bonds (pasha), of
which the Kularnava Tantra enurnerates eight – namely, pity (daya), ignorance and delusion (moha), fear*

(bhaya), shame (lajja), disgust (ghrina), family (kula), custom (shila), and caste (varna). Other enumerations are given of the afflictions which, according to some, are sixty-two, but all such larger divisions are merely elaborations of the simpler enumerations. The pashu is also the worldly man, in ignorance and bondage, as opposed to the yogi and the tattva-jnani. Three divisions of pashsu are also spoken of – namely, sakala, who are bound by the three pasha, called anu (want of knowledge or erroneous knowledge of the self), bheda (the division also induced by maya of the one self into many), and karmma (action and its product. These are the three impurities (mala) called anava-mala, maya-mala, and Karmma-mala. Pratayakala are those bound by the first and last, and Vijnana-kevala are those bound by anava-mala only. He who frees himself of the remaining impurity of anu becomes Shiva Himself. The Devi bears the pasha, and is the cause of them, but She, too, is pashupasha-vimochini, Liberatrix of the pashu from his bondage.

What has been stated gives the root notion of the term pashu. Men of this class are also described in Tantra by exterior traits, which are manifestations of the interior disposition. So the Kubjika Tantra says: "Those who belong to pashu-bhava .re simply pashu. A pashu does not touch a yantra, nor make japa of mantra at night.

He entertains doubt about sacrifices and Tantra; regards a mantra as being merely letters only. He lacks faith in the guru, and thinks that the image is but a block of stone. He distinguishes one Deva from another, and worships without flesh and fish. He is always bathing, owing to his ignorance, and talks ill of others. Such an one is called pashu, and he is the worst kind of man." Similarly the Nitya Tantra describes the pashu as – "He who does not worship at night, nor in the evening, nor in the latter part of the day; who avoids sexual intercourse, except on the fifth day after the appearance of the courses (ritu-kalang vina devi ramanang parivarjayet); who do not eat meat, etc., even on the five auspicious days (parvvana)"; in short, those who, following Vedachara, Vaishnavachara, and Shaivachara, are bound by the Vaidik rules which govern all pashus.

In the case of vira-bhava, rajas more largely works on sattva, yet also largely (though in lessening degrees, until the highest stage of divya-bhava is reached) works independently towards the production of acts in which sorrow inheres. There are several classes of vira.

The third, or highest, class of man is he of the divya-bhava (of which, again, there are several degrees – some but a stage in advance of the highest form of vira-bhava, others completely realizing the deva-nature), in which rajas operate on sattva-guna to the confirmed preponderance of the latter.

The Nitya Tantra says that of the bhava the divya is the best, the vira the next best, and the pashu the lowest; and that devata-bhava must be awakened through vira-bhava. The Pichchhila Tantra says that the only difference between the vira and divya men is that the former are very uddhata, by which is probably meant excitable, through the greater prevalence of the independent working of the rajo-guna in them than in the calmer sattvik temperament. It is obvious that such statements must not be read with legal accuracy. There may be, in fact, a considerable difference between a low type of vira and the highest type of divya, though it seems to be true that this quality of uddhata which is referred to is the cause of such differences, whether great or small.

The Kubjika Tantra describes the marks of the divya as he "who daily does ablutions, sandhya; and wearing clean cloth, the tripundara mark in ashes, or red sandal, and ornaments of rudraksha beads, performs japa and archchana. He gives charity daily also. His faith is strong in Veda, Shastra, guru, and Deva. He worships the Pitri and Deva, and performs all the daily rites. He has a great knowledge of mantra. He avoids all food, except that which his guru offers him, and all cruelty

*and other bad actions, regarding both friend and foe
as one and the same. He himself ever speaks the truth,
and avoids the company of those who decry the Devata.
He worships thrice daily, and meditates upon his guru
daily, and, as a Bhairava, worships Parameshvari with
divya-bhava. All Devas he regards as beneficial. He
bows down at the feet of women, regarding them as his
guru (strinang pada-talang drishtva guru-vad bhavayet
sada). He worships the Devi at night, and makes japa at
night with his mouth full of pan, and makes obeisance
to the kula vriksha. He offers everything to the Supreme
Devi. He regards this universe as pervaded by stri (shakti), and as Devata. Shiva is in all men, and the whole
brahmanda is pervaded by Shiva-Shakti. He ever strives
for the attainment and maintenance of devata-bhava,
and is himself of the nature of a Devata.*

*Here, again, the Tantra only seeks to give a general
picture, the details of which are not applicable to all
men of the divya-bhava class. The passage shows that
it, or portions of it, refer to the ritual divya, for some of
the practices there referred to would not be performed
by the avadkuta, who is above all ritual acts, though he
would also share (possibly in intenser degree) the beliefs
of divya men of all classes – that he and all else are
but manifestations of the universe-pervading Supreme
Shakti.*

According to the temperament of the sadhaka, so is the form of worship and sadhana. In fact, the specific worship and sadhana of the other classes is strictly prohibited by the Tantra to the pashu.

It is said in this Tantra and elsewhere that, in the Kali-yuga, divya and pashu dispositions can scarcely be found. It may be thought difficult at first sight to reconcile this (so far as the pasha is concerned) with other statements as to the nature of these respective classes. The term pashu, in these and similar passages, would appear to be used in a good sense as referring to a man who, though tamasic, yet performs his functions with that obedience to nature which is shown by the still more tamasic animal creation free from the disturbing influences of rajas, which, if it may be the source of good, may also be, when operating independently, the source of evil.

The Commentator explains the passage cited from the Tantra as meaning that the conditions and character of the Kali-yuga are not such as to be productive of pasha-bhava (apparently in the sense stated), or to allow of its achara (that is, Vaidikachara). No one, he says, can fully perform the vedachara, vaishnavachara, and shavachara rites, without which the Vaidik, Pauranik mantra, and yajna are fruitless. No one now

*goes through the brahma-charya ashrama, or adopts
after the fiftieth year that called vana-prastha. Those
whom the Veda does not control cannot expect the fruit
of Vaidik observances. On the contrary, men have taken
to drink, associate with the low, and are fallen; as are
also those men who associate with them. There can
therefore be no pure pashu. Under these circumstances
the duties prescribed by the Vedas which are appropriate
for the pasha being incapable of performance, Shiva for
the liberation of men of the Kali Age has proclaimed the
Agama. "Now, there is no other way." The explanation
thus given, therefore, appears to amount to this. The
pure type of pashu for whom vedachara was designed
does not exist. For others who though pasha are not
purely so, the Tantra is the governing Shastra. This,
however, does not mean that all are now competent for
virachara.*

*It is to be noted, however, that the Prana-toshini cites
a passage purporting to come from the Mahanirvana
Tantra, which is apparently in direct opposition to the
foregoing:*

Divya-vira-mayo bhavah kalau nasti kada-chana

*Kevalang pasha-bhavena mantra-siddhirbhavennrin-
am.*

"In the Kali Age there is no divya or vira-bhava. It is only by the pashu-bhava that men may obtain mantra-siddhi."

This matter of the bhava prevalent in the Kali-yuga has been the subject of considerable discussion and difference of opinion, and is only touched upon here.

Guru and Shishya

The Guru is the religious teacher and spiritual guide to whose direction orthodox Hindus of all divisions of worshippers submit themselves. There is in reality but one Guru. The ordinary human Guru is but the manifestation on the phenomenal plane of the Adi-natha Maha-kala, the Supreme Guru abiding in Kailasa. He it is who enters into and speaks with the voice of the earthly Guru at the time of giving mantra. Guru is the root (mala) of diksha (imitation). Diksha is the root of mantra. Mantra is the root of Devata; and Devata is the root of siddhi. The Munda-mala Tantra says that mantra is born of Guru and Devata of mantra, so that the Guru occupies the position of a grandfather to the Ishta-devata.

It is the Guru who initiates and helps, and the relationship between him and the disciple (shishya) continues

*until the attainment of monistic siddhi. Manu says:
"Of him who gives natural birth and of him who gives
knowledge of the Veda the giver of sacred knowledge is
the more venerable father. Since second or divine birth
insures life to the twice-born in this world and the next."
The Shastra is, indeed, full of the greatness of Guru. The
Guru is not to be thought of as a mere man. There is no
difference between Guru, mantra, and Deva. Guru is
father, mother, and Brahman. Guru, it is said, can save
from the wrath of Shiva, but none can save from the
wrath of the Guru. Attached to this greatness there is,
however, responsibility; for the sins of the disciple recoil
upon him.*

*Three lines of Guru are worshipped: heavenly (divyang-
ga) siddha (siddhangga), and human (manavangga).
The kala-guru are four in number, viz.: the Guru,
Parama-guru, Parapara-guru, Parameshti-guru; each
of these being the guru of the preceding one. According
to the Tantra, woman with the necessary qualifications
may be a guru, and give initiation. Good qualities are
required in the disciple, and according to the Sara-san-
graha a guru should examine and test the intending
disciple for a year. The qualifications of a good disciple
are stated to be good birth, purity of soul (shuddhatma),
and capacity for enjoyment, combined with desire for
liberation (purushartha-parayanah). Those who are*

lewd (kamuka), adulterous (para-daratura), constantly addicted to sin (sada papa-kriya), ignorant, slothful, and devoid of religion, should be rejected.

The perfect sadhaka who is entitled to the knowledge of all Shastra is he who is pure-minded, whose senses are controlled (jitendriyah), who is ever engaged in doing good to all beings, free from false notions of dualism, attached to the speaking of, taking shelter with, and living in the supreme unity of the Brahman. So long as Shakti is not fully communicated (see next note) to the shishya's body from that of the guru, so long the conventional relation of guru and shishya exists. A man is shishya only so long as he is sadhaka. When, however, siddhi is attained, both Guru and Shishya are above this dualism. With the attainment of pure monism, natural-ly this relation, as all others, disappears.

Initiation

Diksha

Initiation is the giving of mantra by the guru. At the time of initiation the guru must first establish the life of the guru in his own body; that is the vital force (pra-na-shakti) of the Supreme Guru whose abode is in the thousand-petalled lotus. As an image is the instrument

*(yantra) in which divinity (devatva) inheres, so also is
the body of guru. The day prior thereto the guru should,
according to Tantra, seat the intending candidate on
a mat of kusha grass. He then makes japa of a "sleep
mantra" (supta-mantra) in his ear, and ties his crown
lock. The disciple, who should have fasted and observed
sexual continence, repeats the mantra thrice, prostrates
himself at the feet of the guru, and then retires to rest.
Initiation, which follows, gives spiritual knowledge and
destroys sin. As one lamp is lit at the flame of another, so
the divine shanti, consisting of mantra, is communicated
from the guru's body to that of the Shishya. Without
daksha, japa of the mantra, puja, and other ritual acts,
are said to be useless. Certain mantra are also said to be
forbidden to shudra and women. A note, however, in the
first Chalakshara Sutra, to the Lalita would, however,
show that even the shudra are not debarred the use even
of the Pranava, as is generally asserted. For, according
to the Kalika Purana (when dealing with svara or tone),
whilst the udatta, an-udatta, and prachita are appropriate to the first of these castes, the svara, called aukara,
with anusvara and nada, is appropriate to shudra, who
may use the Pranava, either at the beginning or end
of mantra, but not, as the dvija may, at both places.
The mantra chosen for initiation should be suitable
(anukala). Whether a mantra is sva-kula or a-kula
to the person about to be initiated is ascertained by*

*the kula-chakra, the zodiacal circle called rashichakra
and other chakra which may be found described in the
Tantra-sara. Initiation by a woman is efficacious; that
by a mother is eight-fold so. Certain special forms of initiation, called abhisheka, are described in the next note.*

Abhisheka

*Abhisheka is of eight kinds, and the forms of abhisheka
which follow the first at later stages, mark greater and
greater degrees of initiation. The first shaktabhisheka
is given on entrance into the path of sadhana. It is so
called because the guru then reveals to the shishya the
preliminery mysteries of shakti-tattva. By it the shishya
is cleansed of all sinful or evil shakti or proclivities, and
acquires a wonderful new shakti. The next purnabhisheka is given in the stage beyond dakshinachara, when the
disciple has qualified himself by purascharana and other
practices to receive it. Here the real work of sadhana
begins. Asana, yama, etc., strengthen the disciple's deter-
mina,tion (pratijna) to persevere along the higher stages
of sadhana. The third is the difficult stage commenced
by krama-dikshabhisheka, in which it is said the great
Vashishtha became involved, and in which the Rishi
Vishvamitra acquired brahma-jnana, and so became a
Brahmana. The sacred thread is now worn round the
neck like a garland. The shishya, then undergoing va-*

rious ordeals (pariksha), receives samrajyabhisheka and maha-samrajyabhisheka, and at length arrives at the most dificult of all stages introduced by yoga-dikshabhisheka. In previous stages the sadhaka has performed the panchanga-puraschharana, and, with the assistance of his guru (with whom he must constantly reside, and whose instructions he must receive direct), he does the panchanga-yoga – that is, the last five limbs of the ashtanga. He is thereafter qualified for purna-dikshabhisheka, and, following that, maha-purna-diksha-bhisheka, sometimes called viraja-grahanabhisheka. On the attainment of perfection in this last grade, the sadhaka performs his own funeral rite (shraddha), makes purnahuti with his sacred thread and crown lock. The relation of guru and shishya now ceases. From this point he ascends by himself until he realizes the great saying, So'ham ("I am He"). At this stage, which the Tantra calls jivan-mukta (liberated whilst yet living), he is called parama-hangsa.

Sadhana

Sadhana is that which produces siddhi (q.v.). It is the means, or practice, by which the desired end may be attained, and consists in the exercise and training of the body and psychic faculties, upon the gradual perfection of which siddhi follows; the nature and degree of which, again, depends upon the progress made towards the realization of the atma, whose veiling vesture the body is. The means employed are various, such as worship (puja), exterior or mental; shastric learning; austerities (tapas); the pancha-tattva, mantra, and so forth. Sadhana takes on a special character, according to the end sought. Thus, sadhana for brahma-jñana, which consists in the acquisition of internal control (shama) over buddhi, manas, and ahangkara; external control (dama) over the ten indriya, discrimination between the transitory and the external, and renunciation both of the world and heaven (svarga), is obviously different from that prescribed for, say, the purposes of the lower magic. The sadhaka and sadhika are respectively the man or woman who perform sadhana. They are, according to their physical, mental, and moral qualities, divided into four classes – mridu, madhya, adhimatraka, and the highest adhimatrama, who is qualified (adhikari) for all forms of yoga. In a similar way the Kaula division of worshippers are divided into the prakriti, or common Kaula following virachara, addicted to ritual practice, and sadhana, with pancha-tattva; the madhyama-kaulika, or middling Kaula, accomplishing the same sadhana, but with a mind more turned towards meditation, knowledge, and samadhi; and the highest type of Kaula (kaulikottama), who, having surpassed all ritualism, meditates upon the Universal Self.

Worship Generally

There are four different forms of worship corresponding with four states (bhava). The realization that the jivat-ma and paramatma are one, that everything is Brahman, and that nothing but the Brahman exists, is the highest state, or brahma-bhava. Constant meditation by the yoga process upon the Devata in the heart is the lower and middlemost (dhyana-bhava) japa (q.v.) and stava (hymns and prayer) is still lower and the lowest of all is mere external worship (puja) (q.v.). Puja-bhava is that which arises out of the dualistic notions of worshipper and worshipped; the servant and the Lord. This dualism exists in greater or less degree in all the states except the highest. But for him who, having realized the advaita-tattva, knows that all is Brahman, there is neither worshipper nor worshipped, neither yoga nor puja, nor dharana, dhyana, stava, japa, vrata, or other ritual or process of sadhana.

In external worship there is worship either of an image (pratima), or of a yantra (q.v.), which takes its place. The sadhaka should first worship inwardly the mental image of the form assumed by the Devi, and then by the life-giving (prana-pratishtha) ceremony infuse the image with Her life by the communication to it of the light and energy (tejas) of the Brahman which is within him to the image without, from which there bursts the lustre of Her whose substance is consciousness itself (chaitanya-mayi). She exists as Shakti in stone or metal, or elsewhere, but is there veiled and seemingly inert. Chaitanya (consciousness) is aroused by the worshipper through the prana-pratishtha mantra.

Rites (karma) are of two kinds. Karma is either nitya nr naimittika. The first is both daily and obligatory, and is done because so ordained. Such as the sandhya (v. post), which in the case of Shudras is in the Tantrik form; and daily puja (v. post) of the Ishta- and Kula-Devata (v. post); and for Brahmamas the pancha-maha-yajna (v. post). The second or conditional karma is occasional and voluntary, and is kamya when done to gain some particular end, such as yajna for a particular object; tapas with the same end (for certain forms of tapas are also nitya); and vrata (v. post).

The Shudra is precluded from the performance of Vaidik rites, or the reading of the Vedas, or the recital of the Vaidik mantra. His worship is practically limited to that of the Ishta-Devata and the Bana-linga-puja, with Tantrik and Pauranik mantra and such vrata as consist in penance and charity. In other cases the vrata is performed through a Brahmana. The Tantra makes no caste distinctions as regards worship. All may read the Tantras, perform the Tantrik worship, such as the sandhya (v. post), and recite the Tantrik mantra, such as the Tantrik Gayatri. All castes, and even the lowest chandala, may be a member of a chakra, or Tantrik circle of worship. In the chakra all its members partake of food and drink together, and are deemed to be greater than Brahmanas; though upon the break-up of the chakras the ordinary caste and social relations are re-established. All are competent for the specially Tantrik worship, for, in the words of the Gautamiya Tantra, the Tantra Shastra is for all castes and for all women. The latter are also excluded under the present Vaidik system, though it is said by Shankha Dharma-shastra-kara that the wife may, with the consent of her husband, fast, take vows, perform homa and vrata, etc. According to the Tantra, a woman may not only receive mantra, but may, as a Guru, initiate and give it. She is worshipful as Guru, and as wife of Guru. The Devi is Herself Guru of all Shastras and woman, as, indeed, all females who are Her embodiments are, in a peculiar sense, Her earthly representatives.

Forms of Achara

There are seven, or, as some say, nine, divisions of worshippers. The extra divisions are bracketed in the following quotation. The Kularnava Tantra mentions *seven, which are given in their order of superiority, the first being the lowest: Vedachara, Vaishnavachara, Shaivachara, Dakshinachara, Vamachara, Siddhantachara (Aghorachara, Yogachara), and Kaulachara, the highest of all. The achara is the way, custom, and practice of a particular class of sadhaka. They are not, as sometimes supposed, different sects, but stages through which the worshipper in this or other births has to pass before he reaches the supreme stage of the Kaula. Vedachara, which consists in the daily practice of the Vaidik rites, is the gross body (sthula-deha), which comprises within it all other acharas, which are, as it were, its subtle bodies (sukshma-deha) of various degrees. The worship is largely of an external and ritual character, the object of which is to strengthen dharma. This is the path of action (kriya-marga). In the second stage the worshipper passes from blind faith to an understanding of the supreme protecting energy of the Brahman, towards which he has feelings of devotion. This is the path of devotion (bhakti-marga), and the aim at this stage is the union of it and faith previously acquired. With an increasing determination to protect dharma and destroy a-dharma, the sadhaka passes into Shaivachara, the warrior (kshatriya) stage, wherein to love and mercy are added strenuous striving and the cultivation of power. There is union of faith, devotion (bhakti), and inward determination (antar-laksha). Entrance is made*

*upon the path of knowledge (jnana-marga). Following
this is Dakshinachara, which in Tantra does not mean
"right-hand worship," but "favourable" – that is, that
achara which is favourable to the accomplishment of the
higher sadhana, and whereof the Devi is the Dakshina
Kalika. This stage commences when the worshipper can
make dhyana and dharana of the threefold shakti of
the Brahman (kriya, ichchha, jñana), and understands
the mutual connection (samanvaya) of the three guna
until he receives purnabhisheka (q.v.). At this stage the
sadhaka is Shakta, and qualified for the worship of the
threefold shakti of Brahma, Vishnu, Maheshvara. He
is fully initiated in the Gayatri-mantra, and worships
the Devi Gayatri, the Dakshina Kalika, or Adya Shakti
– the union of the three Shakti. This is the stage of indi-
vidualistic Brahmana-tattva, and its aim is the union
of faith, devotion, and determination, with a knowledge
of the threefold energies. After this a change of great importance occurs, marking, as it does, the entry upon the
path of return (nivritti). This it is which has led some
to divide the achara into the two broad divisions of
Dakshinachara (including the first four) and Vamachara (including the last three), it being said that men are
born into Dakshinachara, but are received by initiation
into Vamachara. The latter term does not mean, as is
vulgarly supposed, "left-hand worship," but the worship
in which woman (vama) enters that is lata-sadhana. In*

this achara there is also worship of the Vama Devi. Vija is here "adverse," in that the stage is adverse to pravritti, which governed in varying degrees the preceding achara, and entry is here made upon the path of nivritti, or return to the source whence the world sprung. Up to the fourth stage the sadhaka followed pravrittimarga, the outgoing path which led from the source, the path of worldly enjoyment, albeit curved by dharma. At first unconsciously, and later consciously, sadhana sought to induce nivrittt, which, however, can only fully appear after the exhaustion of the forces of the outward current. In Vamachara, however, the sadhaka commences to directly destroy pravritti, and with the help of the Guru (whose help throughout is in this necessary) to cultivate nivritti. The method at this stage is to use the force of pravritti in such a way as to render them self-destructive. The passions which bind may be so employed as to act as forces whereby the particular life of which they are the strongest manifestation is raised to the universal life. Passion, which has hitherto run downwards and outwards to waste, is directed inwards and upwards, and transformed to power. But it is not only the lower physical desires of eating, drinking, and sexual intercourse which must be subjugated. The sadhaka must at this stage commence to cut off all the eight bonds (pasha) which mark the pashu which the Kularnava Tantra enumerates as pity (daya), ignorance (moha), shame (lajja), family (kula), custom (shila), and caste (varna). When Shri Krishna stole the clothes of the bathing Gopi, and made them approach him naked, he removed the artificial coverings which are imposed on man in the sangsara. The Gopi were eight, as are the bonds (pasha), and the errors by which the jiva is misled are the clothes which Shri Krishna stole. Freed of these, the jiva is liberated from all bonds arising from his desires, family, and society. He then reaches the stage of Shiva (shivatva). It is the aim of Vamachara to liberate from the bonds which bind men to the sangsara, and to qualify the sadhaka for the highest grades of sadhana in which the sattvika guna predominates. To the truly sattvik there is neither attachment, fear, or disgust. That which has been commenced in these stages is by degrees completed in those which follow – viz.: Siddhantachara, and according to some, Aghorachara and Yogachara. The sadhaka becomes more and more freed from the darkness of the sangsara, and is attached to nothing, hates nothing, and is ashamed of nothing, having freed himself of the artificial bonds of family, caste, and socie-ty. The sadhaka becomes, like Shiva himself, a dweller in the cremation ground (smashana). He learns to reach the upper heights of sadhana and the mysteries of yoga. He learns the movements of the different vayu in the microcosm the Kshudra-brahmanda, the regulation of which controls the inclinations and propensities (vritti). He learns also the truth which concern the macrocosm (brahmanda). Here also the Guru teaches him the inner

core of Vedachara. Initiation by yoga-diksha fully qualifies him for yogachara. On attainment of perfection
in ashtanga-yoga, he is fit to enter the highest stage of
Kaulachara.

Kaula-dharma is in no wise sectarian, but, on the contrary, is the heart of all sects. This is the true meaning
of the phrase which, like many another touching the
Tantra, is misunderstood, and used to fix the kaula with
hypocrisy – antah-shaktah, vahih-shaivah sabhayang
vaishnavahmatah nana – rupadharah kaulah vicharan-
ti mahitale (outwardly Shaivas; in gatherings, Vaishnavas; at heart, Shaktas; under various forms the Kaulas
wander on earth). A Kaula is one who has passed
through these and other stages, which have as their own
inmost doctrine (whether these worshippers know it or
not) that of Kaulachara. It is indifferent what the Kaula's apparent sect may be. The form is nothing and everything. It is nothing in the sense that it has no power to
narrow the Kaula's own inner life; it is everything in the
sense that knowledge may infuse its apparent limitations with an universal meaning. So understood, form is
never a bond. The Vishva-sara Tantra, says of the Kaula
that "for him there is neither rule of time; nor place. His
actions are unaffected either by the phases of the moon
or the position of the stars. The Kaula roams the earth
in differing forms. At times adhering to social rules

(shishta), he at others appears, according to their standard, to be fallen (bhrashta). At times, again, he seems to be as unearthly as a ghost (bhuta or pishacha) To him no difference is there between mud and sandal paste, his son and an enemy, home and the cremation ground."

At this stage the sadhaka attains to Brahma-jnana, which is the true gnosis in its perfect form. On receiving mahapurna-daksha he performs his own funeral rites and is dead to the sangsara. Seated alone in some quiet place, he remains in constant samadhi, and attains its nir-vikalpa form. The Great Mother, the Supreme Prakriti Maha-shakti, dwells in the heart of the sadhaka, which is now the cremation ground wherein all passions have been burnt away. He becomes a Parama-hangsa, who is liberated whilst yet living (javan-mukta).

It must not, however, be supposed that each of these stages must necessarily be passed through by each jiva in a single life. On the contrary, they are ordinarily traversed in the course of a multitude of births. The weaving of the spiritual garment is recommenced where in a previous birth, it was dropped on death. In the present life a sadhaka may commence at any stage. If he is born into Kaulachara, and so is a Kaula in its fullest sense, it is because in previous births he has by sadhana, in the preliminary stages, won his entrance into it. Knowled-

ge of Shakti is, as the Niruttara Tantra says, acquired after many births; and, according to the Mahanirvana Tantra, it is by merit acquired in previous births that the mind is inclined to Kaulachara.

Mantra

Shabda, or sound, which is of the Brahman, and as such the cause of the Brahmanda, is the manifestation of the Chit-shakti Itself. The Vishva-sara Tantra says that tha Para-brahman, as Shabda-brahman, whose substance is all mantra, exists in the body of the jivatma. It is either unlettered (dhvani) or lettered (varna). The former, which produces the latter, is the subtle aspect of the jiva's vital shakti. As the Prapancha-sara states, the brahmanda is pervaded by shakti, consisting of dhvani, also called nada, prana, and the like. The manifestation of the gross form (sthula) of shabda is not possible unless shabda exists in a subtle (sukshma) form. Mantras are all aspects of the Brahman and manifestations of Kula-kundalini. Philosophically shabda is the guna of akasha, or ethereal space. It is not, however, produced by akasha, but manifests in it. Shabda is itself the Brahman. In the same way, however, as in outer space, waves of sound are produced by movements of air (vayu); so in the space within the jiva's body waves of sound are produced according to the movements of the vital air

*(prana-vayu) and the process of inhalation and exha-
lation. Shabda first appears at the muladhara, and that
which is known to us as such is, in fact, the shakti which
gives life to the jiva. She it is who, in the muladhara, is
the cause of the sweet indistinct and murmuring dhvani,
which sounds like the humming of a black bee.*

*The extremely subtle aspect of sound which first appears
in the Muladhara is called para; less subtle when it
has reached the heart, it is known as pashyanti. When
connected with buddhi it becomes more gross, and is
called madhyama. Lastly, in its fully gross form, it issues
from the mouth as vaikhari. As Kula-Kundalini, whose
substance is all varna and dhvani, is but the manifestation of, and Herself the Paramatma; so the substance
of all mantra is chit, notwithstanding their external
manifestation, as sound, letters, or words; in fact, the
letters of the alphabet, which are known as akshara, are
nothing but the yantra of the akshara, or imperishable
Brahman. This, however, is only realized by the sadhaka
when his shakti, generated by sadhana, is united with
the mantra-shakti.*

*It is the sthula or gross form of Kulakundalini, ap-
pearing in different aspects as different Devata, which
is the presiding Devata (adhishthatri) of all mantra,
though it is the subtle or sukshma form at which all*

sadhakas aim. When the mantrashakti is awakened by sadhana the Presiding Devata appears, and when perfect mantra-siddhi is acquired, the Devata, who is sachchidananda, is revealed. The relations of varna, nada, vindu, vowel and consonant in a mantra, indicate the appearance of Devata in different forms. Certain vibhuti, or aspects, of the Devata are inherent in certain varna, but perfect Shakti does not appear in any but a whole mantra. Any word or letter of the mantra cannot be a mantra. Only that mantra in which the playful Devata has revealed any of Her particular aspects can reveal that aspect, and is therefore called the individual mantra of that one of Her particular aspects. The form of a particular Devata, therefore, appears out of the particular mantra of which that Devata is the adhishthatri Devata.

A mantra is composed of certain letters arranged in definite sequence of sounds of which the letters are the representative signs. To produce the designed effect mantra must be intoned in the proper way, according to svara (rhythm), and varna (sound). Their textual source is to be found in Veda, Purana, and Tantra. The latter is essentially the mantra-shastra, and so it is said of the embodied shastra, that Tantra, which consists of mantra, is the paramatma, the Vedas are the jivatma, Darshana (systems of philosophy) are the senses, Pura-

*nas are the body, and Smriti are the limbs. Tantra is
thus the shakti of consciousness, consisting of mantra. A
mantra is not the same thing as prayer or self-dedication
(atma-nivedana). Prayer is conveyed in what words the
worshipper chooses, and bears its meaning on its face.
It is only ignorance of shastrik principle which supposes
that mantra is merely the name for the words in which
one expresses what one has to say to the Divinity. If
it were, the sadhaka might choose his own language
without recourse to the eternal and determined sounds
of Shastra.*

*A mantra may, or may not, convey on its face its mea-
ning. Vija (seed) mantra, such as Aing, Kling, Hring,
have no meaning, according to the ordinary use of language. The initiate, however, knows that their meaning is
the own form (sva-rupa) of the particular Devata, whose mantra they are, and that they are the dhvani which
makes all letters sound and which exists in all which we
say or hear. Every mantra is, then, a form (rupa) of the
Brahman. Though, therefore, manifesting in the form
and sound of the letters of the alphabet, Shastra says
that they go to Hell who think that the Guru is but a stone, and the mantra but letters of the alphabet.*

*From manana, or thinking, arises the real understan-
ding of the monistic truth, that the substance of the*

Brahman and the brahmanda are one and the same. Man- of mantra comes from the first syllable of mana-na, and -tra from trana, or liberation from the bondage of the sangsara or phenomenal world. By the combination of man- and -tra, that is called mantra which calls forth (amantrana), the chatur-varga (vide post), or four aims of sentient being. Whilst, therefore, mere prayer often ends in nothing but physical sound, mantra is a potent compelling force, a word of power (the fruit of which is mantra-siddhi), and is thus effective to produce the chatur-varga, advaitic perception, and mukti. Thus it is said that siddhi is the certain result of japa (q.v.). By Mantra the sought for (sadhya) Devata, is attained and compelled. By siddhi in mantra is opened the vision of the three worlds. Though the purpose of worship (puja), reading (patha), hymn (stava), sacrifice (homa), dhyana, dharana, and samadhi (vide post), and that of the diksha-mantra are the same, yet the latter is far more powerful, and this for the reason that, in the first, the sadhaka's sadhana-shakti only operates, whilst in the case of mantra that sadhana-shakti works, in conjunction with mantra-shakti, which has the revelation and force of fire, and than which nothing is more powerful. The special mantra which is received at initiation (diksha) is the vija, or seed mantra, sown in the field of the sadhaka's heart, and the Tantrik sandhya, nyasa, puja, and the like are the stem and branches upon which hymns of praise (stuti) and prayer and homage (vandana) are the leaves and flower, and the kavacha, consisting of mantra, the fruit.

Mantra are solar (saura) and lunar (saumya), and are masculine, feminine, or neuter. The solar are masculine and lunar feminine. The masculine and neuter forms are called mantra. The feminine mantra is known as vidya. The neuter mantra, such as the Pauranik-mantra, ending with namah, are said to lack the force and vitality of the others. The masculine and feminine mantra end differently. Thus, Hung, Phat, are masculine terminations, and "thang," or svaha, are feminine ones.

The Nitya Tantra gives various names to mantra. according to the number of their syllables, a one-syllabled mantra being called pinda, a three-syllabled one kartari, a mantra with four to nine syllables vija, with ten to twenty syllables mantra, and mantra with more than twenty syllables mala. Commonly, however, the term vija is applied to monosyllabic mantra. The Tantrik mantras called vija (seed) are so named because they are the seed of the fruit, which is siddhi, and because they are the very quintessence of mantra. They are short, unetymological vocables, such as Hring, Shring, Kring, Hung, Aing, Phat, etc., which will be found throughout the text. Each Devata has His or Her vija.

The primary mantra of a Devata is known as the root mantra (mula-mantra). It is also said that the word mula denotes the subtle body of the Devata called Kama-kala. The utterance of a mantra without knowledge of its meaning or of the mantra method is a mere movement of the lips and nothing more. The mantra sleeps. There are various processes preliminary to, and involved in, its right utterance, which processes again consist of mantra, such as, purification of the mouth (mukha-shodhana), purification of the tongue (jihva-shodhana), and of the mantra (ashaucha-bhanga), kulluka, nirvvana, setu, nidra-bhanga, awakening of mantra, mantra-chaitanya, or giving of life or vitality to the mantra. Mantrarthabhavana, forming of mental image of the Divinity. There are also ten sangskara of the mantra. Dipani is seven japa of the vija, preceded and followed by one. Where hring is employed instead of Ong it is prana-yoga. Yoni-mudra is meditation on the Guru in the head and on the Ishta-devata in the heart, and then on the Yoni-rupa Bhagavati from the head to the muladhara, and from the muladhara to the head, making japa of the yoni vija (eng) ten times. The mantra itself is Devata. The worshipper awakens and vitalizes it by chit-shakti, putting away all thought of the letter, piercing the six Chakra, and contemplating the Spotless One. The shakti of the mantra is the vachaka-shakti, or the means by which the vachya-shakti or *object of the mantra is attained. The mantra lives by the energy of the former. The saguna-shanti is awakened by sadhana and worshipped, and She it is who opens the portals whereby the vachya-shakti is reached. Thus the Mother in Her saguna form is the presiding deity (adhishthatri Devata) of the Gayatri-mantra. As the nirguna (formless) One, She is its vachya-shakti. Both are in reality one and the same; but the jiva, by the laws of his nature and its three guna, must first meditate on the gross (sthula) form before he can realize the subtle (sukshma) form, which is his liberator.*

The mantra of a Devata is the Devata. The rhythmical vibrations of its sounds not merely regulate the unsteady vibrations of the sheaths of the worshipper, thus transforming him, but from it arises the form of the Devata, which it is. Mantra-siddhi is the ability to make a mantra efficacious and to gather its fruit in which case the mantra is called mantra-siddha. Mantra are classified as siddha, sadhya, susiddha, and ari, according as they are friends, servers, supporters, or destroyers – a matter which is determined for each sadhaka by means of chakra calculations.

The Gayatri Mantra

The Gayatri is the most sacred of all Vaidik mantras. In it the Veda lies embodied as in its seed. It runs: Ong bhur bhuvah svah: tat savitur varenyam bhargo devasya dhimahi: dhiyo yo nah prachodayat. Om. "Ong. Let us contemplate the wondrous spirit of the Divine Creator (Savitri) of the earthly, atmospheric, and celestial spheres. May He direct our minds (that is, 'towards' the attainment of dharmma., artha, kama, and moksha), Om."

The Gayatrt-Vyakarana of Yogi Yajnavalkya thus explains the following words: Tat, that. The word yat (which) is understood. Savituh is the possessive case of Savitri, derived from the root su, "to bring forth." Savitri is, therefore, the Bringer-forth of all that exists. The Sun (Suryya) is the cause of all that exists, and of the state in which they exist. Bringing forth and creating all things, it is called Savitri. The Bhavishya Purana says Suryya is the visible Devata. He is the Eye of the world and the Maker of the day. There is no other Devata eternal like unto Him. This universe has emanated from, and will be again absorbed into, Him. Time is of and in Him. The planets, sta.rs, the Vasus. Rudras, Vayu, Agni, and the rest are but parts of Him. By Bhargah is meant the Aditya-devata, dwelling in the region of the Sun (suryya-mandala) in all His might and glory. He is to the Sun what our spirit (atma) is to our body. Though He is in the region of the sun in the outer or material sphere He also dwells in our inner selves. He is the light

*of the light in the solar circle, and is the light of the lives
of all beings. As He is in the outer ether, so also is He in
the ethereal region of the heart. In the outer ether He
is Suryya, and in the inner ether He is the wonderful
Light which is the Smokeless Fire. In short, that Being
whom the sadhaka realizes in the region of his heart
is the Aditya in the heavenly firmament. The two are
one. The word is derived in two ways: (1) from the root
bhrij, "to ripen, mature, destroy, reveal, shine." In this
derivation Suryya is He who matures and transforms all
things. He Himself shines and reveals all things by His
light. And it is He who at the final Dissolution (pralaya)
will in His image of destructive Fire (kalagni) destroy all
things. (2) From bha = dividing all things into different
classes; ra = colour; for He produces the colour of all
created objects; ga, constantly going and returning. The
sun divides all things, produces the different colours of
all things, and is constantly going and returning. As the
Brahmana-sarvasva says: "The Bhargah is the Atma
of all that exists, whether moving or motionless, in the
three loka (Bhur bhuvah svah). There is nothing which
exists apart from it."*

*Devasya is the genitive of Deva, agreeing with Savituh.
Deva is the radiant and playful (lilamaya) one. Suryya
is in constant play with creation (srishti), existence
(sthiti), and destruction (pralaya), and by His radian-*

ce pleases all. (Lila, as applied to the Brahman, is the equivalent of maya.) Varenyam = varaniya, or adorable. He should be meditated upon and adored that we may be relieved of the misery of birth and death. Those who fear rebirth, who desire freedom from death and liberation and who strive to escape the three kinds of pain (tapa-traya), which are adhyatmika, adhidaivika, and adhibhautika, meditate upon and adore the Bharga, who, dwelling in the region of the Sun, is Himself the three regions called Bhur-loka, Bhuvar-loka, and Svar-loka. Dhimahi = dhya-yema, from the root dhyai. We meditate upon, or let us meditate upon.

Prachodayat = may He direct. The Gayatri does not so expressly state, but it is understood that such direction is along the chatur-varga, or four-fold path, which is dharmma, artha, kama, and moksha (piety, wealth, desire and its fulfilment, and liberation, vide post). The Bhargah is ever directing our inner faculties (buddhi-vritti) along these paths.

The above is the Vaidika Gayatri, which, according to the Vaidik system, none but the twice-born may utter. To the Shudra whether man or woman, and to women of all other castes it is forbidden. The Tantra, which has Gayatri-Mantra of its own, shows no such exclusiveness; Chapter III., verses 109-111, gives the Brahma-gayatri

*for worshippers of the Brahman: "Parameshva-raya
vidmahe para-tattvaya dhimahi: tan no Brahma
prachodayat "(May we know the supreme Lord. Let us
contemplate the Supreme essence. And may that Brahman direct us).*

Yantra

*This word in its most general sense means an instru-
ment, or that by which anything is accomplished. In
worship it is that by which the mind is fixed on its
object. The Yogini Tantra says that the Devi should
be worshipped either in pratima (image), mandala,
or yantra. At a certain stage of spiritual progress the
sadhaka is qualified to worship yantra. The siddha-yogi
in inward worship (antar-puja) commences with the
worship of yantra, which is the sign (sangketa) of brah-
ma-vijnana as the mantra is the sangketa of the Devata.
It is also said that yantra is so called because it subdues
(niyantrana) lust, anger, and the other sins of jiva and
the sufferings caused thereby.*

*This yantra is a diagram engraved or drawn on metal,
paper, or other substances, which is worshipped in
the same manner as an image (pratima). As different
mantra are prescribed for different worships, so are
different yantra. The yantras are therefore of various*

designs, according to the object of worship. The cover of this work shows a silver Gayatri yantra belonging to the author. In the centre triangle are engraved in the middle the words, Shri Shri Gayatri sva-prasada siddhing kuru ("Shri Shri Gayatri Devi: grant me success"), and at each inner corner there are the vija Hring and Hrah. In the spaces formed by the intersections of the outer ovoid circles is the vija "Hring." The outside circular band contains the vija "Tha" which indicates "Svaha," commonly employed to terminate the feminine mantra or vidya. The eight lotus petals which spring from the band are inscribed with the vija, "Hring, Ing, Hrah." The outermost band contains all the matrika, or letters of the alphabet, from ankara to laksha. The whole is enclosed in the way common to all yantra by a bhupura, by which, as it were, the yantra is enclosed from the outer world. The yantra when inscribed with mantra, serves (so far as these are concerned) the purpose of a mnemonic chart of the mantra appropriate to the particular Devata whose presence is to be invoked into the yantra. Certain preliminaries precede, as in the case of a pratima, the worship of a yantra. The worshipper first meditates upon the Devata, and then arouses Him or Her in himself. He then communicates the divine presence thus aroused to the yantra. When the Devata has by the appropriate mantra been invoked into the yantra, the vital airs (prana) of the Devata are infused therein by the prana-pratishtha ceremony, mantra, and mudra.

*The Devata is thereby installed in the yantra, which is
no longer mere gross matter veiling the spirit which has
been always there, but instinct with its aroused presence, which the sadhaka first welcomes and then worships.
Mantra in itself is Devata, and yantra is mantra in that
it is the body of the Devata who is mantra.*

Mudra

*The term mudra is derived from the root mud, "to
please," and in its upasana form is so called because it
gives pleasure to the Devas. Devanang moda-da mudra
tasmat tang yatnatashcharet. It is said that there are
108, of which 55 are commonly used. The term means
ritual gestures made with the hands in worship or
positions of the body in yoga practice. Thus of the first
class the matsya – (fish) mudra is formed in offering
arghya by placing the right hand on the back of the left
and extending, fin-like, on each side the two thumbs,
with the object that the conch which contains water
may be regarded as an ocean with aquatic animals; and
the yoni-mudra which presents that organ as a triangle
formed by the thumbs, the two first fingers, and the two
little fingers is shown with the object of invoking the
Devi to come and take Her place before the worshipper,
the yoni being considered to be Her pitha or yantra.
The upasana mudra is thus nothing but the outward*

expression of inner resolve which it at the same time intensifies. Mudra are employed in worship (archchana) japa, dhyana (q.v.), kamya-karma (rites done to effect particular objects), pratishtha (q.v.), snana (bathing), avahana (welcoming), naivedya (offering of food), and visarjana, or dismissal of the Devata. Some mudra of hatha yoga are described sub voc. "Yoga." The Gheranda Sanghita says that knowledge of the yoga mudras grants all siddhi, and that their performance produces physical benefits such as stability, firmness and cure of disease.

Sandhya

The Vaidika sandhya is the rite performed by the twice-born castes thrice a day, at morning, midday, and evening. The morning sandhya is preceded by the following acts. On awakening, a mantra is said in invocation of the Tri-murtti and the sun, moon, and planets, and salutation is made to the Guru. The Hindu dvi-ja then recites the miantra: "I am a Deva. I am indeed the sorrowless Brahman. By nature I am eternally free, and in the form of existence, intelligence, and Bliss." He then offers the actions of the day to the Deity, confesses his inherent frailty, and prays that he may do right. Then, leaving his bed and touching the earth with his right foot, the dvi-ja says, "Om, 0 Earth! salutation to Thee, the Guru of all that is good." After attending to natural calls, the twice-born does achamana (sipping of water) *with mantra, cleanses his teeth, and takes his early morning bath to the accompaniment of mantra. He then puts on his caste-mark (tilaka) and makes tarpanam, or oblation of water, to the Deva, Rishi, and Pitri. The sandhya follows, which consists of achamana (sipping of water), marjjana-snanam (sprinkling of the whole body with water taken with the hand or kasha-grass), pra-nayama (regulation of prana through its manifestation in breath), agha-marshana (expulsion of the person of sin from the body; the prayer to the sun, and then (the canon of the sandhya) the silent recitation (japa) of the Gayatn mantra, which consists of invocation (avahana) of the Gayatri-Devi; rishi-nyasa and shadanga-nya-sa (vide post), meditation on the Devi-Gayatri in the morning as Brahmani; at midday as Vaishnavi; and in the evening as Rudrani; japa of the Gayatri a specified number of times; dismissal (visarjana) of the Devi, followed by other mantra.*

Besides the Brahmanical Vaidiki-sandhya from which the Shudras are debarred, there is the Tantriki-sandhya, which may be performed by all. The general outline is similar; the rite is simpler; the mantra vary; and the Tantrika-vijas or "seed" mantras are employed.

Puja

This word is the common term for worship of which there are numerous synonyms in the Sanskrit language. Puja is done daily of the Ishta-devata or the particular Deity worshipped by the sadhaka – the Devi in the case of a Shakti, Vishnu in the case of a Vaishnava, and so forth. But though the Ishta-devata is the principal object of worship, yet in puju all worship the Pancha-devata, or the Five Deva – Aditya (the Sun), Ganesha, the Devi, Shiva, and Vishnu, or Narayana. After worship of the Pancha-devata, the family Deity (Kula-devata), who is generally the same as the Ishta-devata, is worshipped. Puja, which is kamya, or done to gain a particular end as also vrata, are preceded by the sangkalpa; that is, a statement of the resolution to do the worship, as also of the particular object, if any, with which it is done.

There are sixteen upachara, or things done or used in puja: (1) asana (seat of the image); (2) svagata (welco-me); (3) padya (water for washing the feet); (4) arghya (offering of unboiled rice, flowers, sandal paste, durva grass, etc., to the Devata in the kushi) (vessel); (5 and 6) achamana (water for sipping, which is offered twice); (7) madhuparka (honey, ghee, milk, and curd offered in a silver or brass vessel); (8) snana (water for bathing); (9) vasana (cloth); (10) abharana (jewels); (11) gandha (scent and sandal paste is given); (12) pushpa (flowers); (13) dhupa (incense stick); (14) dipa (light); (15) nai-

vedya (food); (16) vandana or namas-kara (prayer). Other articles are used which vary with the puja, such as Tulasi leaf in the Vishnu-puju and bael-(bilva) leaf in the Shiva-puja. The mantras said also vary according to the worship. The seat (asana) of the worshipper is purified. Salutation being made to the Shakti of support or the sustaining force (adhara-shakti); the water, flowers, etc., are purified. All obstructive spirits are driven away (Bhutapasarpana), and the ten quarters are fenced from their attack by striking the earth three times with the left foot, uttering the Astra vija "phat," and by snapping the fingers (twice) round the head. Pranayama (regulation of breath) is performed and (vide post) the elements of the body are purified (bhuta-shuddhi). There is nyasa (vide post); dhyana (meditation) offering of the upachara; japa (vide post), prayer and obeisance (pranama). In the ashta-murti-puja of Shiva the Deva is worshipped under the eight forms: Sharvva (Earth), Bhava (Water), Rudra (Fire), Ugra (Air), Bhima (Ether), Pashupati (yajamana – the Sacrificer man), Ishana (Sun), Mahadeva (Moon).

Yajna

This word, which comes from the root yaj (to worship), is commonly translated "sacrifice." The Sanskrit word is, however, retained in the translation, since Yajna

*means other things also than those which come within
the meaning of the word "sacrifice," as understood
by an English reader. Thus the "five great sacrifices"
(pancha-maha-yajna) which should be performed daily
by the Brahmana are: The homa sacrifice, including
Vaishva-deva offering, "bhuta-yajna or vali, in which
offerings are made to Deva, Bhuta, and other Spirits
and to animals; pitri-yajna or tarpana, oblations to the
pitri; Brahma-yajna, or study of the Vedas and Manus-
hyayajna, or entertainment of guests (atithisaparyya).
By these five yajna the worshipper places himself in right
relations with all being, affirming such relation between
Deva, Pitri, Spirits, men, the organic creation, and
himself.*

*Homa, or Deva-yajna, is the making of offerings to Fire.
which is the carrier thereof to the Deva. A firepit (kunda) is prepared and fire when brought from the house
of a Brahmana is consecrated with mantra. The fire is
made conscious with the mantra – Vang vahni-chaita-
nyaya namah, and then saluted and named. Meditation is then made on the three nadis (vide ante) – Ida,
Pingala, and Sushumna – and on Agni, the Lord of Fire.
Offerings are made to the Ishta-devata in the fire. After
the puja of fire, salutation is given as in Shadanga-nyasa, and then clarified butter (ghee) is poured with a
wooden spoon into the fire with mantra, commencing*

*with Om and ending with Svaha. Homa is of various
kinds, several of which are referred to in the text, and
is performed either daily, as in the case of the ordinary
nitya-vaishva-deva-homa, or on special occasions, such
as the upanayana or sacred thread ceremony, marriage, vrata, and the like. It is of various kinds, such as
prayashchitta-homa, srishtikrit-homa, janu homa,
dhara-homa, and others, some of which will be found in
the text.*

*Besides the yajna mentioned there are others. Manu
speaks of four kinds: deva, bhauta (where articles and
ingredients are employed, as in the case of homa, daiva,
vali), nriyajna, and pitri-yajna. Others are spoken of,
such as japa-yajna, dhyana-yajna, etc. Yajna are also
classified according to the dispositions and intentions
of the worshipper into sattvika, rajasika, and tamasika
yajna.*

Vrata

*Vrata is a part of Naimittika, or voluntary karma. It is
that which is the cause of virtue (punya), and is done
to achieve its fruit. Vrata are of various kinds. Some
of the chief are Janmashtami on Krishna's birthday;
Shiva-ratri in honour of Shiva; and the Shat-pancha-
mi, Durvashtami, Tala-navami. Ananta-chaturdashi*

performed at specified times in honour of Lakshmi, Narayana, and Ananta. Others may be performed at any time, such as the Savitri vrata by women only, and the Karttikeya-puja by men only. The great vrata is the celebrated Durga-puja, maha-vrata in honour of the Devi as Durga, which will continue as long as the sun and moon endure, and which, if once commenced, must always be continued. There are numerous other vrata which have developed to a great extent in Bengal, and for which there is no Shastric authority such as Madhu-sankranti-vrata, Jala-sankranti-vrata, and others. While each vrata has its peculiarities, certain features are common to vrata of differing kinds. There is both in preparation and performance sangyama, such as sexual continence, eating of particular food, such as havishyanna, fasting, bathing. No flesh or fish are taken. The mind is concentrated to its purposes, and the vow or resolution (niyama) is taken. Before the vrata the Sun, Planets, and Kula-devata are worshipped, and by the "suryahsomoyamahkala" mantra all Deva and Beings are invoked to the side of the worshipper. In the vaidika vrata the sangkalpa is made in the morning, and the vrata is done before midday.

Tapas

This term is generally translated as meaning penan-

ce or austerities. It includes these, such as the four monthly fast (chatur-masya), the sitting between five fires (pancha-gnitapah), and the like. It has, however, also a wider meaning, and in this wider sense is of three kinds, namely, sharira, or bodily; vachika, by speech; manasa, in mind. The first includes external worship, reverence, and support given to the Guru, Brahmanas, and the wise (prajna), bodily cleanliness, continence, simplicity of life and avoidance of hurt to any being (a-hingsa). The second form includes truth, good, gentle, and affectionate speech, and the study of the Vedas. The third or mental tapas in-cludes self-restraint, purity of disposition, silence, tranquillity, and silence. Each of these classes has three subdivisions, for tapas may be sattvika, rajasika, or tamasika, according as it is done with faith, and without regard to its fruit; or for its fruit; or is done through pride and to gain honour and res-pect; or, lastly, which is done ignorantly or with a view to injure and destroy others, such as the sadhana of the Tantrika-shat-karma, when performed for a malevolent purpose (abhichara).

Japa

Japa is defined as "vidhanena mantrochcharanam," or the repeated utterance or recitation of mantra according to certain rules. It is according to the Tantra-sara of three kinds: Vachika or verbal japa, in which the mantra is audibly recited, the fifty matrika being sounded nasally with vindu; Upangshu-japa, which is superior to the last kind, and in which the tongue and lips are moved, but no sound, or only a slight whisper, is heard; and, lastly, the highest form which is called manasa-japa, or mental utterance. In this there is neither sound nor movement of the external organs, but a repetition in the mind which is fixed on the meaning of the mantra. One reason given for the differing values attributed to the several forms is that where there is audible utterance the mind thinks of the words and the process of correct utterance, and is therefore to a greater (as in the case of vachika-japa), or to a less degree (as in the case of upangshu-japa), distracted from a fixed attention to the meaning of the mantra. The japa of different kinds have also the relative values attachable to thought and its materialization in sound and word. Certain conditions are prescribed as those under which japa should be done, relating to physical cleanliness, the dressing of the hair, and wearing of silk garments, the seat (asana), the avoidance of certain conditions of mind and actions, and the nature of the recitation. The japa is useless unless done a specified number of times – of which 108 is esteemed to be excellent. The counting is done either with a mala or rosary (mala-japa), or with the thumb of the right hand upon the joints of the fingers of that hand (kara-japa).

The method of counting in the latter case may differ according to the mantra.

Sangskara

There are ten (or, in the case of Shudras, nine) purificatory ceremonies, or "sacraments," called sangskara, which are done to aid and purify the jiva in the important events of his life. These are jiva-sheka, also called garbhadhana-ritu-sangskara, performed after menstruation, with the object of insuring and sanctifying conception. The garbhadhana ceremony takes place in the daytime on the fifth day, and qualifies for the real garbhadhana at night – that is, the placing of the seed in the womb. It is preceded on the first day by the ritu-sangskara which is mentioned in Chapter IX. of the text. After conception and during pregnancy, the pung-savana and simantonnayana rites are performed; the first upon the wife perceiving the signs of conception, and the second during the fourth, sixth, or eighth month of pregnancy.

In the ante-natal life there are three main stages, whether viewed from the objective (physical) standpoint, or from the subjective (super-physical) standpoint. The first period includes on the physical side all the structural and physiological changes which occur in the fertilized ovum from the moment of fertilization until the period when the embryonic body, by the formation of trunk, limbs, and organs, is fit for the entrance of the individualized life, or jivatma. When the pronuclear activity and differentiation are completed, the jivatma, whose connection with the pronuclei initiated the pro-nuclear or formative activity, enters the miniature human form, and the second stage of growth and de-velopment begins. The second stage is the fixing of the connection between the jiva and the body, or the rendering of the latter viable. This period includes all the anatomical and physiological modifications by which the embryonic body becomes a viable fœtus. With the attainment of viability, the stay of the jiva has been assured; physical life is possible for the child, and the third stage in ante-natal life is entered. Thus, on the form side, if the language of comparative embryology is used, the first sangskara denotes the impulse to development, from the "fertilization of the ovum" to the "critical period." The second sangskara denotes the impulse to development from the "critical period" to that of the "viability stage of the fœtus"; and the third sangskara denotes the development from "viability" to "full term."

On the birth of the child there is the jata-karma, performed for the continued life of the new-born child. Then follows the nama-karana, or naming ceremony, and nishkramana in the fourth month after delivery, when the child is taken out of doors for the first time and shown the sun, the vivifying source of life, the material embodiment of the Divine Savita. Between the fifth and eighth month after birth the annaprasana ceremony is observed, when rice is put in the child's mouth for the first time. Then follows the chuda-karana, or tonsure ceremony; and in the case of the first three, or "twice-born" classes, upanayana, or investiture with the sacred thread. Herein the jiva is reborn into spiritual life. There is, lastly, udvaha, or marriage, whereby the unperfected jiva insures through offspring that continued human life which is the condition of its progress and ultimate return to its Divine Source. These are all described in the Ninth Chapter of this Tantra. There are also ten sangskara of the mantra (q.v.). The sangskara are intended to be performed at certain stages in the development of the human body, with the view to effect results beneficial to the human organism. Medical science of to-day seeks to reach the same results, but uses for this purpose the physical methods of modern Western science, suited to an age of materiality; whereas in the sangskara the super-physical (psychic, or occult, or metaphysical and subjective) methods of ancient Eastern science are employed. The sacraments of the Catholic Church and other of its ceremonies, some of which have now fallen into disuse, are Western examples of the same psychic method.

Purashcharana

This form of sadhana consists in the repetition (after certain preparations and under certain conditions) of a mantra a large number of times. The ritual deals with the time and place of performance, the measurements and decoration of the mandapa, or pandal, and of the altar and similar matters. There are certain rules as to food both prior to, and during, its performance. The sadhaka should eat havishyanna, or alternately boiled milk (kshira), fruits, or Indian vegetables, or anything obtained by begging, and avoid all food calculated to influence the passions. Certain conditions and practices are enjoined for the destruction of sin, such as continence, bathing, japa (q.v.) of the Savitri-mantra 5,008, 3,008, or 1,008 times, the entertainment of Brahmamas, and so forth. Three days before puja there is worship of Ganesha and Kshetra-pala, Lord of the Place. Pancha-gavya, or the five products of the cow, are eaten. The Sun, Moon, and Devas are invoked. Then follows the sangkalpa. The ghata, or kalasa (jar), is then placed into which the Devi is to be invoked. A mandala, or figure of a particular design, is marked on the ground, and on it the ghata is placed. Then the five or nine gems are placed on the kalasa, which is painted with red and covered with leaves. The ritual then prescribes for the tying of the crown lock (shikha), the posture (asana) of the sadhaka; japa (q.v.) nyasa (q.v.), and the mantra ritual or process. There is meditation, as directed. Kulluka is said, and the mantra "awakened" (mantra-chaitanya), and recited the number of times for which the vow has been taken.

Bhuta-shuddhi

The object of this ritual, which is described in Chapter V., verses 93 et seq., is the purification of the elements of which the body is composed.

The Mantra-mahodadhi speaks of it as a rite which is preliminary to the worship of a Deva. The process of evolution from the Para-brahman has been described. By this ritual a mental process of involution takes place whereby the body is in thought resolved into the source from whence it has come. Earth is associated with the sense of smell, water, with taste, fire, with sight, air, with touch, and ether, with sound. Kundalini is roused, and led to the svadhishthana Chakra. The "earth" element is dissolved by that of "water," as "water" is by "fire," "fire" by "air," and "air" by "ether." This is absorbed by a higher emanation, and that by a higher, and so on, until the Source of all is reached. Having dissolved each gross element (maha-bhuta), together with the subtle element (tan-matra) from which it proceeds, and the connected organ of sense (indriya) by another, the worshipper absorbs the last element, "ether," with the tan-matra sound into self-hood (ahangkara), the latter into Mahat, and that, again, into Prakriti, thus retracing the steps of evolution. Then, in accordance with the monistic teaching of the Vedanta, Prakriti is Herself thought of as the Brahman, of which She is the energy, and with which, therefore, She is already one. Thinking then of the black Purusha, which is the image of all sin, the body is purified by mantra, accompanied by kumbhaka and rechaka, and the sadhaka meditates upon the new celestial (deva) body, which has thus been made and which is then strengthened by a "celestial gaze."

Nyasa

This word, which comes from the root "to place," means placing the tips of the fingers and palm of the right hand on various parts of the body, accompanied by particular mantra. The nyasa are of various kinds. Jiva-nyasa follows upon bhuta-shuddhi. After the purification of the old, and the formation of the celestial body, the sadhaka proceeds by jiva-nyasa to infuse the body with the life of the Devi. Placing his hand on his heart, he says the "so'hang" mantra ("I am He"), thereby identifying himself with the Devi. Then, placing the eight Kula-kunda-lini in their several places he says the following mantra:

*Ang, Kring, Kring, Yang, Rang, Lang, Vang, Shang,
Shang, Sang, Hong, Haung, Hangsah: the vital airs of
the highly blessed and auspicious Primordial Kalika are
here. "Ang, etc., the embodied spirit of the highly blessed
and auspicious Kalika is placed here." "Ang, etc., here
are all the senses of the highly auspicious and blessed
Kalika," and, lastly, "Ang, etc., may the speech, mind,
sight, hearing, smell, and vital airs of the highly blessed
and auspicious Kalika coming here always abide here in
peace and happiness Svaha." The sadhaka then becomes
devata-maya. After having thus dissolved the sinful
body, made a new Deva body, and infused it with the
life of the Devi, he proceeds to matrika-nyasa. Mahika
are the fifty letters of the Sanskrit alphabet; for as from
a mother comes birth, so from matrika, or sound, the
world proceeds. Shabda-brahman, the "Sound," "Logos,"
or "Word," is the Creator of the worlds of name and of
form.*

*The bodies of the Devata are composed of the fifty
matrika. The sadhaka, therefore, first sets mentally
(antar-matrika-nyasa) in their several places in the
six chakra, and then externally by physical action
(Vahy-amatrika-nyasa) the letters of the alphabet which
form the different parts of the body of the Devata, which
is thus built up in the sadhaka himself. He places his
hand on different parts of his body, uttering distinctly at
the same time the appropriate matrika for that part.*

The mental disposition in the chakra is as follows: In the Ajna Lotus, Hang, Kshang (each letter in this and the succeeding cases is said, followed by the mantra namah); in the Vishuddha Lotus Ang, Ang, and the rest of the vowels; in the Anahata Lotus kang, khang to thang; in the Manipura Lotus, dang dhang, etc., to Phang; in the Svadisthana Lotus bang, bhang to lang; and, lastly, in the Muladhara Lotus, vang, shang, shang, sang. The external disposition then follows. The vowels in their order with anusvara and visarga are placed on the forehead, face, right and left eye, right and left ear, right and left nostril, right and left cheek, upper and lower lip, upper and lower teeth, head, and hollow of the mouth. The consonants kang to vang are placed on base of right arm and the elbow, wrist, base and tips of fingers, left arm, right and left leg, right and left side, back, navel, belly, heart, right and left shoulder, space between the shoulders (kakuda), and then from the heart to the right palm shang is placed; and from the heart to the left palm the (second) shang; from the heart to the right foot, sang; from the heart to the left foot, hang; and, lastly, from the heart to the belly, and from the heart to the mouth, kshang. In each case ong is said at the beginning and namah at the end. According to the Tantra-sara, matrika-nyasa is also classified into four kinds, performed with different aims – viz.: kevala where the matrika is pronounced without vindu; vindu-sangyuta with vindu; sangsarga with visarga; and sobhya with visarga and vindu.

Rishi-nyasa then follows for the attainment of the chatur-varga. The assignment of the mantra is to the head, mouth, heart, anus, the two feet, and all the body generally. The mantra commonly employed are: "In the head, salutation to the Rishi (Revealer) Brahma; in the mouth, salutation to the mantra Gayatri, in the heart, salutation to the Devi Mother Sarasvati; in the hidden part, salutation to the vija, the consonants; salutation to the shakti, the vowels in the feet, salutation to visargah, the kilaka in the whole body." Another form in which the vija employed is that of the Aiya: it is referred to but not given in Chap. V., verse 123, and is: "In the head, salutation to Brahma and the Brahmarshis, in the mouth, salutation to Gayatri and the other forms of verse; in the heart, salutation to the primordial Devata Kali, in the hidden part, salutation to the vija, kring; in the two feet, salutation to the shakti, Hring; in all the body, salutation to the Kalika Shring."

Then follows anga-nyasa and kara-nyasa. These are both forms of shad-anga-nyasa. When shad-anga-nyasa is performed on the body, it is called hridayadi-shad-anga-nyasa; and when done with the five fingers and palms of the hands only, angushthadi-shad-anga-nyasa.

*The former kind is done as follows: The short vowel
a, the consonants of the ka-varga group, and the long
vowel a, are recited with "hridayaya namah" (namah
salutation to the heart). The short vowel i, the consonants of the cha-varga group, and the long vowel i, are
said with "shirasi svaha" (svaha to the head). The hard
ta-varga consonants set between the two vowels u are
recited with "shikhayai vashat" (vashat to the crown
lock); similarly the soft ta-varga between the vowels
e and ai are said with "kavachaya hung." The short
vowel o, the pavarga, and the long vowel o are recited
with netra-trayaya vaushat (vaushat to the three eyes).
Lastly, between vindu and visargah the consonants ya
to ksha with "kara-tala-prishthabhyang astraya phat"
(phat to the front and back of the palm).*

*The mantras of shadanga-nyasa on the body are used
for Kara-nyasa, in which they are assigned to the thumbs, the "threatening" or index fingers, the middle fingers,
the fourth, little fingers, and the front and back of the
palm.*

*These actions on the body, fingers, and palms also sti-
mulate the nerve centres and nerves therein.*

*In pitha-nyasa the pitha are established in place of the
matrika. The pitha, in their ordinary sense, are Ka-*

ma-rupa and the other places, a list of which is given in the Yogini-hridaya.

For the attainment of that state in which the sadhaka feels that the bhava (nature, disposition) of the Devata has come upon him nyasa is a great auxiliary. It is, as it were, the wearing of jewels on different parts of the body. The vija of the Devata are the jewels which the sudkaka places on the different parts of his body. By nyasa he places his Abhishta-devata in such parts, and by vyapaka-nyasa he spreads Its presence throughout himself. He becomes permeated by it losing himself in the divine Self.

Nyasa is also of use in effecting the proper distribution of the shaktis of the human frame in their proper positions so as to avoid the production of discord and distraction in worship. Nyasa as well as Asana are necessary for the production of the desired state of mind and of chitta-shuddhi (its purification). "Das denken ist der mass der Dinge." Transformation of thought is Transformation of being. This is the essential principle and rational basis of all this and similar Tantrik sadhana.

Panchatattva

There are, as already stated, three classes of men – pashu, Vira, and Divya. The operation of the guna which produce these types affect, on the gross material plane, the animal tendencies, manifesting in the three chief physical functions – eating and drinking, whereby the annamayakosha is maintained; and sexual intercourse, by which it is reproduced. These functions are the subject of the panchatattva or panchamakara ("five m's"), as they are vulgarly called – viz.: madya (wine), mangsa (meat), matsya (fish), mudra (parched grain), and maithuna (coition). In ordinary parlance, mudra means ritual gestures or positions of the body in worship and hathayoga, but as one of the five elements it is parched cereal, and is defined as Bhrishtadanyadikang yadyad chavyaniyam prachakshate, sa mudra kathita devi sarvveshang naganam-dini. The Tantras speak of the five elements as pancha-tattva, kuladravya, kulatattva, and certain of the elements have esoteric names, such as Karanavari or tirtha-vari, for wine, the fifth element being usually called lata-sadhana (sadhana with woman, or shakti). The five elements, moreover have various meanings, according as they form part of the tamasika (pashvachara), rajasika (virachara), or divya or sattvika sadhanas respectively.

All the elements or their substitutes are purified and consecrated, and then, with the appropriate ritual,

*the first four are consumed, such consumption being
followed by lata-sadhana or its symbolic equivalent.
The Tantra prohibits indiscriminate use of the elements, which may be consumed or employed only after
purification (sho-dhana) and during worship according
to the Tantric ritual. Then, also, all excess is forbidden.
The Shyama-rahasya says that intemperance leads
to Hell, and this Tantra condemns it in Chapter V. A
well-known saying in Tantra describes the true "hero"
(vira) to be, not he who is of great physical strength and
prowess, the great eater and drinker, or man of powerful
sexual energy, but he who has controlled his senses, is
a truth-seeker, ever engaged in worship, and who has
sacrificed lust and all other passions. (Jitendriyah satya-
vadi nityanushthanatatparah kamadi-validanashcha sa
vira iti giyate.)*

*The elements in their literal sense are not available in
sadhana for all. The nature of the Pashu requires strict
adherence to Vaidik rule in the matter of these physical
functions even in worship. This rule prohibits the drinking of wine, a substance subject to the three curses of*

*Brahma, Kacha, and Krishna, in the following terms:
Madyamapeyamadeyamagrahyam ("Wine must not be
drunk, given, or taken"). The drinking of wine in ordinary life for satisfaction of the sensual appetite is, in fact,*

*a sin, involving prayaschiyta, and entailing, according
to the Vishnu Purama, punishment in the same Hell as
that to which a killer of a Brahmana goes. As regards
flesh and fish, the higher castes (outside Bengal) who
submit to the orthodox Smarta discipline eat neither.
Nor do high and strict Brahmanas even in that Pro-
vince. But the bulk of the people there, both men and
women, eat fish, and men consume the flesh of male goats which have been previously offered to the Deity. The
Vaidika dharmma is equally strict upon the subject of
sexual intercourse. Maithuna other than with the householder's own wife is condemned. And this is not only in
its literal sense, but in that of which is known as Ashtanga (eight-fold) maithuna – viz., smaranam (thinking
upon it), kirttanam (talking of it), keli (play with women), prekshanam (looking upon women), guhyabhas-
hanan (talk in private with women), sangkalpa (wish
or resolve for maithuua), adhyavasaya (determination
towards it), kriyanishpati (actual accomplishment of the
sexual act). In short, the pashu (and except for ritual
purposes those who are not pashu) should, in the words
of the Shaktakramya, avoid maithuna, conversation
on the subject, and assemblies of women (maithunam
tatkathalapang tadgoshthing parivarjjayet). Even in the
case of the householder's own wife marital continency is
enjoined. The divinity in woman, which the Tantra in
particular proclaims, is also recognized in the ordinary*

Vaidik teaching, as must obviously be the case given the common foundation upon which all the Shastra rest. Woman is not to be regarded merely as an object of enjoyment, but as a house-goddess (grihadevata). According to the sublime notions of Shruti, the union of man and wife is a veritable sacrificial rite – a sacrifice in fire (homa), wherein she is both hearth (kunda) and flame – and he who knows this as homa attains liberation. Similarly the Tantrika Mantra for the Shivashakti Yoga runs: "This is the in-ternal homa in which, by the path of sushumna, sacrifice is made of the functions of sense to the spirit as fire kindled with the ghee of merit and demerit taken from the mind as the ghee-pot Svaha." It is not only thus that wife and husband are associated, for the Vaidika dharmma (in this now neglected) prescribes that the householder should worship in company with his wife. Brahmacharyya, or continency, is not as is sometimes supposed, a requisite of the student ashrama only, but is a rule which governs the married householder (grihastha) also. According to Vaidika injunctions, union of man and wife must take place once a month on the fifth day after the cessation of the menses, and then only. Hence it is that the Nitya Tantra, when giving the characteristics of a pashu, says that he is one who avoids sexual union except on the fifth day (ritukalangvina devi rama-nang parivarjjayet). In other words, the pashu is he who in this case, as in other matters, follows for

*all purposes, ritual or otherwise, the Vaidik injunctions
which govern the ordinary life of all.*

*The above-mentioned rules govern the life of all men.
The only exception which the Tantra makes is for purpose of sudhana in the case of those who are competent
(adhikari) for virachara. It is held, indeed, that the exception is not strictly an exception to Vaidik teaching at
all, and that it is an error to suppose that the Tantrika
rahasya-puja is opposed to the Vedas. Thus, whilst the
vaidik rule prohibits the use of wine in ordinary life, and
for purpose of mere sensual gratification it prescribes the
religious yajna with wine. This ritual use the Tantra also
allows, provided that the sadhaka is competent for the
sadhana, in which its consumption is part of its ritual
and method.*

*The Tantra enforces the Vaidik rule in all cases, ritual or
otherwise, for those who are governed by the vaidikachara. The Nitya Tantra says: "They (pashu) should
never worship the Devi during the latter part of the
day in the evening or at night" (ratrau naiva yajedde-
ving sandhyayang vaparanhake); for all such worship
connotes maithuna prohibited to the pashu. In lieu of
it, varying substitutes are prescribed, such as either an
offering of flowers with the hands formed into the kach-
chchapa mudra, or union with the worshipper's own*

*wife. In the same way, in lieu of wine, the pashu should
(if a Brahmana) take milk, (if a Kshattriya) ghee, (if a
vaishya) honey, and (if a shudra) a liquor made from
rice. Salt, ginger, sesamum, wheat, mashkalai (beans),
and garlic are various substitutes for meat; and the white brinjal vegetable, red radish, masur (a kind of gram),
red sesamum, and paniphala (an aquatic plant), take
the place of fish. Paddy, rice, wheat, and gram geneally
are mudra.*

*The vira, or rather he who is qualified (adhikari) for
virachara – since the true vira is its finished product –
commences sadhana with the rajasika panchatattva first
stated, which are employed for the destruction of the
sensual tendencies which they connote. For the worship
of Shakti the panchatattva are declared to be essential.
This Tantra declares that such worship without their use
is but the practice of evil magic.*

*Upon this passage the commentator Jaganmohana
Tarkalangkara observes as follows: "Let us consider
what most contributes to the fall of a man, making him
forget his duty, sink into sin, and die an early death.
First among these are wine and women, fish, meat and
mudra, and accessories. By these things men have lost
their manhood. Shiva then desires to employ these very
poisons in order to eradicate the poison in the human*

system. Poison is the antidote for poison. This is the right treatment for those who long for drink or lust for women. The physician must, however, be an experienced one. If there be a mistake as to the application, the patient is like to die. Shiva has said that the way of Kulachara is as difficult as it is to walk on the edge of a sword or to hold a wild tiger. There is a secret argument in favour of the panchatattva, and those tattva so understood should be followed by all. None, however, but the initiate can grasp this argument, and therefore Shiva has directed that it should not be revealed before anybody and everybody. An initiate, when he sees a woman, will worship her as his own mother or goddess (Ishtadevata), and bow before her. The Vishnu Purana says that by feeding your desires you cannot satisfy them. It is like pouring ghee on fire. Though this is true, an experienced spiritual teacher (guru) will know how, by the application of this poisonous medicine, to kill the poison of sangsara. Shiva has, however, prohibited the indiscriminate publication of this. The meaning of this passage would therefore appear to be this: "The object of Tantrika worship is brahmasayujya, or union with Brahman. If that is not attained, nothing is attained. And, with men's propensities as they are, this can only be attained through the special treatment prescribed by the Tantras. If this is not followed, then the sensual pro-pensities are not eradicated, and the work is for the desired end of Tantra as useless as magic which, worked by such a man, leads only to the injury of others." The other secret argument here referred to is that by which it is shown that the particular may be raised to the universal life by the vehicle of those same passions, which, when flowing only in an outward and downward current, are the most powerful bonds to bind him to the former. The passage cited refers to the necessity for the spiritual direction of the Guru. To the want of such is accredited the abuses of the system. When the patient (sishya) and the disease are working together, there is poor hope for the former; but when the patient, the disease, and the physician (guru) are on one, and that the wrong, side, then nothing can save him from a descent on that downward path which it is the object of the sadhana to prevent. Verse 67 in Chapter I. of this Tantra is here in point.

Owing, however, to abuses, particularly as regards the tattva of madya and maithuna, this Tantra, according to the current version, prescribes in certain cases, limitations as regards their use. It prescribes that when the Kaliyuga is in full strength, and in the case of householders (grihastha) whose minds are engrossed with worldly affairs, the "three sweets" (madhuratraya) are to be substituted for wine. Those who are of virtuous temperament, and whose minds are turned towards the

*Brahman, are permitted to take five cups of wine. So
also as regards maithuna, this Tantra states that men
in this Kali age are by their nature weak and disturbed
by lust, and by reason of this do not recognize woman
(shakti) to be the image of the Deity. It accordingly
ordains that when the Kaliyuga is in full sway, the fifth
tattva shall only be accomplished with sviyashakti,
or the worshipper's own wife, and that union with a
woman who is not married to the sadhaka in either
Brahma or Shaiva form is forbidden. In the case of other
shakti (parakiya and sadharani) it prescribes, in lieu of
maithuna, meditation by the worshipper upon the lotus
feet of the Devi, together with japa of his ishtamantra.
This rule, however, the Commentator says, is not of universal application. Shiva has, in this Tantra, prohibited
sadhana with the last tattva, with parakiya, and sadharani shakti, in the case of men of ordinary weak intellect
ruled by lust; but for those who have by sadhana
conquered their passions and attained the state of a true
vira, or siddha, there is no prohibition as to the mode of
latasadhana. This Tantra appears to be, in fact, a protest
against the misuse of the tattwa, which had followed
upon a relaxation of the original rules and conditions
governing them. Without the panchatattva in one form
or another, the shaktipuja cannot be performed. The
Mother of the Universe must be worshipped with these
elements. By their use the universe (jagatbrahmanda)*

itself is used as the article of worship. Wine signifies the power (shakti) which produces all fiery elements; meat and fish all terrestrial and aquatic animals; mudra all vegetable life; and maithuna the will (ichchha) action (kriya) and knowledge (jnana) shakti of the Supreme Prakriti productive of that great pleasure which accompanies the process of creation. To the Mother is thus offered the restless life of Her universe.

The object of all sadhana is the stimulation of the sattvaguna. When by such sadhana this guna largely preponderates, the sattvika sadhana suitable for men of a high type of divyabhava is adopted. In this latter sadhana the names of the panchatattva are used symbolically for operations of a purely mental and spiritual character. Thus, the Kaivalya says that "wine" is that intoxicating knowledge acquired by yoga of the Parabrahman, which renders the worshipper senseless as regards the external world. Meat (mangsa) is not any fleshly thing, but the act whereby the sadhaka consigns all his acts to Me (Mam). Matsya (fish) is that sattvika knowledge by which through the sense of "mineness" the worshipper sympathizes with the pleasure and pain of all beings. Mudra is the act of relinquishing all association with evil which results in bondage, and maithuna is the union of the Shakti Kundalini with Shiva in the body of the worshipper. This, the Yogini Tantra says, is the best of all unions for those who have already con-trolled their passions (yati). According to the Agamasara, wine is the somadhara, or lunar ambrosia, which drops from the brahmarandhra; Mangsa (meat) is the tongue (ma), of which its part (angsha) is speech. The sadhaka, in "eating" it, controls his speech. Matsya (fish) are those two which are constantly moving in the two rivers Ida and Pingala. He who controls his breath by pranayama (q.v.), "eats" them by kumbhaka. Mudra is the awakening of knowledge in the pericarp of the great sahasrara Lotus, where the Atma, like mercury, resplendent as ten million suns, and deliciously cool as ten million moons, is united with the Devi Kundalini. The esoteric meaning of maithuna is thus stated by the Agama: The ruddy-hued letter Ra is in the Kunda, and the letter Ma, in the shape of vindu, is in the mahayoni. When Makara (m), seated on the Hangsa in the form of Akara (a), unites with rakara (r), then the Brahmajna-na, which is the source of supreme Bliss, is gained by the sadhaka, who is then called atmarama, for his enjoy-ment is in the Atma. in the sahasrara. This is the union on the purely sattvika plane, which corresponds on the rajasika plane to the union of Shiva and Shakti in the persons of their worshippers.

The union of Shiva and Shakti is described as a true yoga, from which, as the Yamala says, arises that joy which is known as the Supreme Bliss.

Chakrapuja

Worship with the panchatattva generally takes place in an assembly called a chakra, which is composed of men (sadhaka) and women (shakti), or Bhairava and Bhairavi. The worshippers sit in a circle (chakra), men and women alternately, the shakti sitting on the left of the sadhaka. The Lord of the chakra (chakrasvamin, or chakreshvara) sits with his Shakti in the centre, where the wine-jar and other articles used in the worship are kept. During the chakra all eat, drink, and worship together, there being no distinction of caste. No pashu should, however, be introduced. There are various kinds of chakra, such as the Vira, Raja, Deva, Maha – Chakras productive, it is said, of various fruits for the participators therein. Chapter VI. of the Mahanirvvana Tantra deals with the panchatattva, and Chapter VIII. gives an account of the Bhairavi and Tattva (or Divya) chakras. The latter is for worshippers of the Brahma-Mantra.

Yoga

This word, derived from the root Yuj ("to join"), is in grammar sandhi, in logic avayavashakti, or the power of the parts taken together, and in its most widely known and present sense the union of the jiva, or embodied spirit, with the Paramatma, or Supreme Spirit, and the

*practices by which this union may be attained. There
is a natural yoga, in which all beings are, for it is only
by virtue of this identity in fact that they exist. This
position is common ground, though in practice too
frequently overlooked. "Primus modus unionis est, quo
Deus, ratione suæ immensitatis est in omnibus rebus
per essentiam, præsentiam, et potentiam; per essentiam ut dans omnibus esse; per præsentiam ut omnia
prospiciens; per potentiam ut de omnibus disponens."
The mystical theologian cited, however, proceeds to say:
"Sed hæc unio animæ cum Deo est generalis, communis
omnibus et ordinis naturalis . . . illa namque de qua
loquimur est ordinis supernaturalis actualis et fructiva."
It is of this special yaga, though not in reality more "su-
pernatural" than the first, that we here deal. Yoga in its
technical sense is the realization of this identity, which
exists, though it is not known, by the destruction of the
false appearance of separation. "There is no bond equal
in strength to maya, and no force greater to destroy that
bond than yoga. There is no better friend than knowledge (jnana), nor worse enemy than egoism (ahangkara).
As to learn the Shastra one must learn the alphabet, so
yoga is necessary for the acquirement of tattvajnana
(truth)." The animal body is the result of action, and
from the body flows action, the process being compared
to the seesaw movement of a ghatiyantra, or water-lifter.
Through their actions beings continually go from birth*

*to death. The complete attainment of the fruit of yoga
is lasting and unchanging life in the noumenal world of
the Absolute.*

*Yoga is variously named according to the methods
employed, but the two main divisions are those of the
hathayoga (or ghatasthayoga) and samadhi yoga, of
which raja-yoga is one of the forms. Hathayoga is commonly misunderstood, both in its definition and aim
being frequently identified with exaggerated forms of
self-mortification.*

*The Gherandasanghita well defines it to be "the means
whereby the excellent rajayoga is attained." Actual
union is not the result of Hathayoga alone, which is
concerned with certain physical processes preparatory or
auxiliary to the control of the mind, by which alone union may be directly attained. It is, however, not meant
that all the processes of Hathayoga here or in the books
described are necessary for the attainment of rajayoga.
What is necessary must be determined according to the
circumstances of each particular case. What is suited
or necessary in one case may not be so for another. A
peculiar feature of Tan-trika virachara is the union of
the sadhaka and his shakti in latasadhana. This is a
process which is expressly forbidden to Pashus by the
same Tantras which prescribe it for the vira. The union*

*of Shiva and Shakti in the higher sadhana is different
in form, being the union of the Kundalini Shakti of the
Muladhara with the Vindu which is upon the Sahasrara. This process, called the piercing of the six chakra,
is described later on in a separate paragraph. Though,
however, all Hathayoga processes are not necessary,
some, at least, are generally considered to be so. Thus,
in the well-known ashtangayoga (eight-limbed yoga), of
which samadhi is the highest end, the physical conditions and processes known as asana and pranayama
(vide post) are prescribed.*

*This yoga prescribes five exterior (vahiranga) methods
for the subjugation of the body – namely (1) Yama,
forbearance or self-control, such as sexual continence, avoidance of harm to others (ahingsa), kindness,
forgiveness, the doing of good without desire for reward,
absence of covetousness, temperance, purity of mind and
body, etc. (2) Niyama, religious observances, charity,
austerities, reading of the Shastra and Ishvara Pranid-
hana, persevering devotion to the Lord. (3) Asana,
seated positions or postures (vide post). (4) Pranayama,
regulation of the breath. A yogi renders the vital airs
equable, and consciously produces the state of respiration which is favourable for mental concentration, as
others do it occasionally and unconsciously (vide post).
(5) Pratyahara, restraint of the senses, which follow in*

the path of the other four processes which deal with the subjugation of the body. There are then three interior (yogangga) methods for the subjugation of the mind – namely (6) Dharana, attention, steadying of the mind, the fixing of the internal organ (chitta) in the particular manner indicated in the works on yoga. (7) Dhyana or the uniform continuous contemplation of the object of thought; and (8) that samadhi which is called savikalpasamadhi. Savikalpasamadhi is a deeper and more intense contemplation on the Self to the exclusion of all other objects, and constituting trance or ecstasy. This ecstasy is perfected to the stage of the removal of the slightest trace of the distinction of subject and object in nirvikalpasamadhi, in which there is complete union with the Paramatma, or Divine Spirit. By vairagya (dispassion), and keeping the mind in its unmodified state, yoga is attained. This knowledge, Ahang Brahmasmi ("I am the Brahman"), does not produce liberation (moksha), but is liberation itself, Whether yoga is spoken of as the union of Kulakundalini with Paramashiva, or the union of the individual soul (jivatma) with the Supreme Soul (paramatma), or as the state of mind in which all outward thought is suppressed, or as the controlling or suppression of the thinking faculty (chittavritti), or as the union of the moon and the sun (Ida and Pingala), Prana and Apana, Nada and Vindu, the meaning and the end are in each case the same.

Yoga, in seeking mental control and concentration, makes use of certain preliminary physical processes (sadhana), such as the shatkarmma, asana, mudra, and pranayama. By these four processes and three mental acts, seven qualities, known as shodhana, dridhata, sthirata, dhairyya, laghava, pratyaksha, nirliptatva (vide post), are acquired.

Shodhana: Shatkarmma

The first, or cleansing, is effected by the six processes known as the shatkarmma. Of these, the first is Dhauti, or washing, which is fourfold, or inward washing (antar-dhauti), cleansing of the teeth, etc. (dantadhauti) of the "heart" (hriddhauti), and of the rectum (muladhauti). Antardhauti is also fourfold – namely, vatasara, by which air is drawn into the belly and then expelled; varisara, by which the body is filled with water, which is then evacuated by the anus; vahnisara, in which the nabhi-granthi is made to touch the spinal column (meru); and vahishkrita, in which the belly is by kakinimudra filled with air, which is retained half a yama, and then sent downward. Dantadhauti is fourfold, consisting in the cleansing of the root of the teeth and tongue, the ears, and the "hollow of the forehead" (kapalarandhra). By hriddhauti phlegm and bile are removed. This is done by a stick (dandadhauti) or cloth (vasodhauti) pushed into the throat, or swallowed, or by vomiting (vamanadhauti). Mudadhauti is done to cleanse the exit of the apanavayu either with the middle finger and water or the stalk of a turmeric plant.

Vasti, the second of the shatkarmma, is twofold, and is either of the dry (shuska) or watery (jala) kind. In the second form the yogi sits in the utkatasana posture in water up to the navel, and the anus is contracted and expanded by ashvini mudra; or the same is done in the pashchimottanasana, and the abdomen below the navel is gently moved. In neti the nostrils are cleansed with a piece of string. Lauliki is the whirling of the belly from side to side. In trataka the yogi, without winking, gazes at some minute object until the tears start from his eyes. By this the "celestial vision" (divya drishti) so often referred to in the Tantrika upasana is acquired. Kapalabhati is a process for the removal of phlegm, and is threefold – vatakrama by inhalation and exhalation; vyutkrama by water drawn through the nostrils and ejected through the mouth; and shitkrama the reverse process.

These are the various processes by which the body is cleansed and made pure for the yoga practice to follow.

Dridhata: Asana

Dridhata, or strength or firmness, the acquisition of which is the second of the above-mentioned processes, is attained by asana.

Asana are postures of the body. The term is generally described as modes of seating the body. But the posture is not necessarily a sitting one; for some asana are done on the belly, back, hands, etc. It is said that the asana are as numerous as living beings, and that there are 8,400,000 of these; 1,600 are declared to be excellent, and out of these thirty-two are auspicious for men, which are described in detail. Two of the commonest of these are muktapadmasana ("the loosened lotus seat"), the ordinary position for worship, and baddhapadmasana. Patanjali, on the subject of asana, merely points out what are good conditions, leaving each one to settle the details for himself according to his own requirements. There are certain other asana, which are peculiar to the Tantras, such as munddasana, chitasana, and shavasana, in which skulls, the funeral pyre, and a corpse respectively form the seat of the sadhaka. These, though they may have other ritual objects, form part of the discipline for the conquest of fear and the attainment of indifference, which is the quality of a yoga. And so the Tantras pre-scribe as the scene of such rites the solitary mountain-top, the lonely empty house and river-side, and the cremation-ground. The interior

*cremation-ground is there where the kamik body and its
passions are consumed in the fire of knowledge.*

Sthirata: Mudra

*Sthirata, or fortitude, is acquired by the practice of the
mudra. The mudra dealt with in works of hathayoga
are positions of the body. They are gymnastic, health-gi-
ving, and destructive of disease, and of death, such as
the jaladhara and other mudra. They also preserve
from injury by fire, water, or air. Bodily action and the
health resulting therefrom react upon the mind, and by
the union of a perfect mind and body siddhi is by their
means attained. The Gheranda Sanghita describes a
number of mudra, of which those of importance may
be selected. In the celebrated yonimudra the yogi in
siddhasana stops with his fingers the ears, eyes, nostrils,
and mouth. He inhales pranavayu by kakinimudra,
and unites it with apanavayu. Meditating in their order
upon the six chakra, he arouses the sleeping Kulakundalini by the mantra "Hung Hangsah," and raises Her
to the Sahasrara; then, deeming himself pervaded with
the Shakti, and in blissful union (sanggama) with Shiva,
he meditates upon himself, as by reason of that union
Bliss itself and the Brahman. Ashvinimudra consists of
the repeated contraction and expansion of the anus for
the purpose of shodhana or of contraction to restrain the*

*apana in Skatchakrabheda. Shaktichalana employs the
latter mudra, which is repeated until vayu manifests in
the sushumna. The process is accompanied by inhalation
and the union of prana and apana whilst in siddhasana.*

Dhairya: Pratyahara

*Dhairya, or steadiness, is produced by pratyahara. Pra-
tyahara is the restraint of the senses, the freeing of the
mind from all distractions, and the keeping of it under
the control of the Atma. The mind is withdrawn from
whatsoever direction it may tend by the dominant and
directing Self. Pratyahara destroys the six sins.*

Laghava: Pranayama

From pranayama (q.v.) arises laghava (lightness).

*All beings say the ajapa Gayatri, which is the expulsion
of the breath by Hangkara, and its inspiration by Sahka-
ra, 21,600 times a day. Ordinarily, the breath goes forth
a distance of 12 finger's breadth, but in singing, eating,
walking, sleeping, coition, the distances are 16, 20, 24,
30, and 36 breadths respectively. In violent exercise
these distances are exceeded, the greatest distance being
96 breadths. Where the breathing is under the normal
distance, life is prolonged. Where it is above that, it is*

shortened. Puraka is inspiration, and rechaka expi-ra-tion. Kumbhaka is the retention of breath between these two movements. Kumbhaka is, according to the Gheranda Sanghita of eight kinds: sahita, suryyabheda, ujjayi, shitali, bhastrika, bhramari, murchchha, and kevali. Pranayama similarly varies. Pranayama is the control of the breath and other vital airs. It awakens shakti, frees from disease, produces detachment from the world, and bliss. It is of varying values, being the best (uttama) where the measure is 20; middling (madhya-ma) when at 16 it produces spinal tremor; and inferior (adhama) when at 12 it induces perspiration. It is necessary that the nadi should be cleansed, for air does not enter those which are impure. The cleansing of the nadi (nadi-shuddhi) is either samau« or nirmanu – that is, with or without, the use of vija. According to the first form, the yogi in padmasana does gurunyasa according to the directions of the guru. Meditating on "yang," he does japa through Ida of the vija 16 times, kumbhaka with japa of vija 64 times, and then exhalation through the solar nadi and japa of vija 32 times. Fire is raised from manipura and united with prithivi. Then follows inhalation by the solar nadu with the vahni vija 16 times, kumbhaka with 64 japa of the vija, followed by exhalation through the lunar nadi and japa of the vija 32 times. He then meditates on the lunar brilliance, gazing at the tip of the nose. and inhales by Ida with

*japa of the vija "thang" 16 times. Kumbhaka is done
with the vija vang 64 times. He then thinks of himself as
flooded by nectar, and considers that the nadi have been
washed. He exhales by Pingala with 32 japa of the vija
lang, and considers himself thereby as strengthened. He
then takes his seat on a mat of kusha grass, a deerskin,
etc., and, facing east or north, does pranayama. For
its exercise there must be, in addition to nadi shuddhi,
consideration of proper place, time, and food. Thus, the
place should not be so distant as to induce anxiety, nor
in an unprotected place, such as a forest, nor in a city
or crowded locality, which induces distraction. The food
should be pure, and of a vegetarian character. It should
not be too hot or too cold, pungent, sour, salt, or bitter.
Fasting, the taking of one meal a day, and the like, are
prohibited. On the contrary, the Yogi should not remain
without food for more than one yama (three hours).
The food taken should be light and strengthening. Long
walks and other violent exercise should be avoided,
as also – cer-tainly in the case of beginners – sexual
intercourse. The stomach should only be half filled. Yoga
should be commenced, it is said, in spring or autumn.
As stated, the forms of pranayama vary. Thus, sahita,
which is either with (sagarbha) or without (nirgarbha)
vija, is, according to the former form, as follows: The
sadhaka meditates on Vidhi (Brahma), who is full of
rajoguna, red in colour, and the image of akara. He*

*inhales by Ida in six measures (matra). Before kum-
bhaka he does the uddiyanabandha mudra. Meditating
on Hari (Vishnu) as sattvamaya and the black vija
ukara, he does kumbhaka with 64 japa of the vija; then,
meditating on Shiva as tamomaya and his white vija
makara, he exhales through Pingala with 32 japa of the
vija; then, inhaling by Pingala, he does kumbhaka, and
exhales by Ida with the same vija. The process is repeated in the normal and reversed order.*

Pratyaksha: Dhyana

*Through dhyana is gained the third quality of realiza-
tion or pratyaksha. Dhyana, or meditation, is of three
kinds: (1) sthula, or gross; (2) jyotih; (3) sukshma, or
subtle. In the first the form of the Devata is brought
before the mind. One form of dhyana for this purpose
is as follows: Let the sadhana think of the great ocean
of nectar in his heart. In the middle of that ocean is the
island of gems, the shores of which are made of powdered gems. The island is clothed with a kadamba forest
in yellow blossom. This forest is surrounded by Malati,
Champaka, Parijata, and other fragrant trees. In the
midst of the Kadamba forest there rises the beautiful
Kalpa tree, laden with fresh blossom and fruit. Amidst
its leaves the black bees hum and the koel birds make
love. Its four branches are the four Vedas. Under the tree*

there is a great mandapa of precious stones, and within it a beautiful bed, on which let him picture to himself his Ishtadevata. The Guru will direct him as to the form, raiment, vahana, and the title of the Devata. Jyotirdhyana is the infusion of fire and life (tejas) into the form so imagined. In the muladhara lies the snake-like Kundalini. There the jivatma, as it were the tapering flame of a candle, dwells. The sadhaka then meditates upon the tejomaya Brahman, or, alternatively, between the eyebrows on pranavatmaka, the flame emitting its lustre.

Sukshmadhyana is meditation on Kundalini with sham-bhavi mudra after She has been roused. By this yoga (vide post) the atma is revealed (atmasakshatkara).

Nirliptatva: Samadhi

Lastly, through samadhi the quality of nirliptatva, or detachment, and thereafter mukti (liberation) is attained. Samadhi considered as a process is intense mental con-centration, with freedom from all sangkalpa, and attachment to the world, and all sense of "mineness," or self-interest (mamata). Considered as the result of such process it is the union of Jiva with the Paramatma.

Forms Of Samadhi Yoga

This samadhi yoga is, according to the Gheranda Sang-hita, of six kinds. (1) Dhyanayogasamadhi, attained by shambhavi mudra, in which, after meditation on the Vindu-Brahman and realization of the Atma (atmapra-tyaksha), the latter is resolved into the Mahakasha. (2) Nadayoga, attained by khechari mudra, in which the frenum of the tongue is cut, and the latter is lengthened until it reaches the space between the eyebrows, and is then introduced in a reversed position into the mouth. (3) Rasanandayoga, attained by kumbhaka, in which the sadhaka in a silent place closes both ears and does puraka and kumbhaka until he hears the word nada in sounds varying in strength from that of the cricket's chirp to that of the large kettledrum. By daily practice the anahata sound is heard, and the jyotih with the ma-nas therein is seen, which is ultimately dissolved in the supreme Vishnu. (4) Layasiddhiyoga, accomplished by the celebrated yonimudra already described. The sadha-ka, thinking of himself as Shakti and the Paramatma as Purusha, feels himself in union (sanggama) with Shiva, and enjoys with him the bliss which is shringararasa, and becomes Bliss itself, or the Brahman. (5) Bhakti Yoga, in which meditation is made on the Ishtadevata with devotion (bhakti) until, with tears flowing from the excess of bliss, the ecstatic condition is attained. (6) Rajayoga, accomplished by aid of the manomurchchha kumbhaka. Here the manas detached from all worldly

*objects is fixed between the eyebrows in the ajnachakra,
and Kumbhaka is done. By the union of the manas with
the atma, in which the jnani sees all things, rajayoga-
samadhi is attained.*

Shatchakra-bheda

*The piercing of the six chakra is one of the most impor-
tant subjects dealt with in the Tantras, and is part of
the practical yaga process of which they treat. Details of
practice can only be learnt from a Guru, but generally it
may be said that the particular is raised to the universal
life, which as chit is realizable only in the sahasrara in
the following manner: The jivatma in the subtle body,
the receptacle of the five vital airs (pancha prana), mind
in its three aspects of manas, ahangkara, and buddhi;
the five organs of action (panchakarmendriya) and the
five organs of perception (panchajnanendriya) is united
with the Kulakundalini. The Kandarpa or Kama Vayu
in the muladhara a form of the Apana Vayu is given a
leftward revolution and the fire which is round Kundalini is kindled. By the vija "Hung," and the heat of the fire
thus kindled, the coiled and sleeping Kundalini is wake-
ned. She who lay asleep around svayambhu-linga, with
her coils three circles and a half closing the entrance of
the brahma-dvara, will, on being roused, enter that door
and move upwards, united with the jivatma.*

*On this upward movement, Brahma, Savitri, Daki-
ni-Shakti, the Devas, vija, and vritti, are dissolved in
the body of Kundalini. The Mahimandala or prithivi
is converted into the vija "Lang," and is also merged in
Her body. When Kundalini leaves the muladhara, that
lotus which, on the awakening of Kundalini had opened
and turned its flower upwards, again closes and hangs
down-wards. As Kundalini reaches the svadhishtha-
na-chakra, that lotus opens out, and lifts its flower
upwards. Upon the entrance of Kundalini, Mahavishnu,
Mahalakshmi, Sarasvati, Rakini Shakti, Deva, Matrikas, and vritti, Vaikunthadhama, Golaka, and the
Deva and Devi residing therein are dissolved in the
body of Kundalini. The prithivi, or "earth" vija "Lang,"
is dissolved in apas, and apas converted into the vija
vang remains in the body of Kundalini. When the Devi
reaches the manipura chakra all that is in the chakra
merges in Her body. The Varuna vija "vang" is dissolved
in fire, which remains in the body of the Devi as the
Vija "rang." This chakra is called the Brahma-granthi
(or knot of Brahma). The piercing of this chakra may
involve considerable pain, physical disorder, and even
disease. On this account the directions of an experienced
Guru are necessary, and therefore also other modes of
yoga have been recommended for those to whom they
are applicable: for in such modes activity is provoked directly in the higher centre and it is not necessary that the*

*lower chakras should be pierced. Kundalini next reaches
the anahata chakra, where all which is therein is merged
in Her. The vija of Tejas, "rang," disappears in Vayu and
Vayu converted into its vija "Yang" merges into the body
of Kundalini. This chakra is known as Vishnu-granthi
(knot of Vishnu). Kundalini then ascends to the abode
of Bharati (or Sarasvati) or the vishuddha chakra. Upon
Her entrance, Arddha-narishvara Shiva, Shakini, the
sixteen vowels, mantra, etc., are dissolved in the body of
Kundalini. The vija of Vayu, "yang," is dissolved in akasha, which itself being transformed into the vija "hang,"
is merged in the body of Kundalini. Piercing the lalana
chakra, the Devi reaches the ajnachakra, where Parama
Shiva, Siddha-Kali, the Deva, guna, and all else therein,
are absorbed into Her body. The vija of akasha, "Hang,"
is merged in the manas chakra, and mind itself in the
body of Kundalini. The ajnachakra is known as Rud-
ra-granthi (or knot of Rudra or Shiva). After this chakra
has been pierced, Kundalini of Her own motion unites
with Parama Shiva. As She proceeds upwards from the
two-petalled lotus, the niralamba puri, pranava, nada,
etc., are merged in Her.*

*The Kundalini has then in her progress upwards absor-
bed in herself the twenty-four tattva commencing with
the gross elements, and then unites Herself and becomes
one. with Parama Shiva. This is the maithuna (coition)*

*of the sattvika-pancha-tattva. The nectar which flows
from such union floods the kshudrabrahmanda or human body. It is then that the sadhaka, forgetful of all in
this world, is immersed in ineffable bliss.*

*Thereafter the sadhaka, thinking of the vayu vija "yang"
as being in the left nostril, inhales through Ida, making
japa of the vija sixteen times. Then, closing both nostrils,
he makes japa of the vija sixty-four times. He then
thinks that the black "man of sin" (Papapurusha) in the
left cavity of the abdomen is being dried up (by air), and
so thinking he exhales through the right nostril Pingala,
making japa of the vija thirty-two times. The sadhaka
then meditating upon the red-coloured vija "rang" in
the manipura, inhales, making sixteen japa of the vija,
and then closes the nostrils, making sixteen japa. While
making the japa he thinks that the body of "the man
of sin" is being burnt and reduced to ashes (by fire). He
then exhales through the right nostril with thirty-two
japa. He then meditates upon the white chandravija
"thang." He next inhales through Ida, making japa of
the vija sixteen times, closes both nostrils with japa
done sixty-four times, and exhales through Pingala with
thirty-two japa. During inhalation, holding of breath,
and exhalation, he should consider that a new celestial
body is being formed by the nectar (composed of all the
letters of the alphabet, matrika-varna) dropping from*

the moon. In a similar way with the vija "vang," the
formation of the body is continued, and with the vija
"lang" it is completed and strengthened. Lastly, with the
mantra "So'hang," the sadhaka leads the jivatma into
the heart. Thus Kundalini, who has enjoyed Her union
with Paramashiva, sets out on her return journey the
way she came. As she passes through each of the chakra
all that she has absorbed therefrom come out from herself and take their several places in the chakra.

In this manner she again reaches the muladhara, when
all that is described to be in the chakras (see pp. lvii-lx-
iii) are in the positions which they occupied before her
awakening.

The Guru's instructions are to go above the ajna-chakra,
but no special directions are given; for after this chakra
has been pierced the sadhaka can reach the brahmast-
hana unaided. Below the "seventh month of Shiva" the
relationship of Guru and sishya ceases. The instructions
of the seventh amnaya is not expressed (aprakashita).

Sin and Virtue

According to Christian conceptions, sin is a violation of
the personal will of, and apostasy from, God. The flesh
is the source of lusts which oppose God's commands,

and in this lies its positive significance for the origin of a bias of life against God. According to St. Thomas, in the original state, no longer held as the normal, the lower powers were subordinate to reason, and reason subject to God. "Original sin" is formally a "defect of original righteousness," and materially "concupiscence." As St. Paul says (Rom. vii. 8, 14), the pneumatic law, which declares war on the lusts, meets with opposition from the "law in the members." These and similar notions involve a religious and moral conscious judgment which is assumed to exist in humanity alone. Hindu notions of papa (wrong) and punya (that which is pure, holy, and right) have a wider content. The latter is accordance and working with the will of Ishvara (of whom the jiva is itself the embodiment), as manifested at any particular time in the general direction taken by the cosmic process, as the former is the contrary. The two terms are relative to the state of evolution and the surrounding circumstances of the jiva to which they are applied. Thus, the impulse towards individuality which is necessary and just on the path of inclination or "going forth" (pra-vritti marga), is wrongful as a hindrance to the attainment of unity, which is the goal of the path of return (nivritti marga) where inclinations should cease. In short, what makes for progress on the one path is a hindrance on the other. The matter, when rightly undertsood, is not (except, perhaps, sometimes popularly) viewed from the juristic standpoint of an external Lawgiver, His commands, and those subject to it, but from that in which the exemplification of the moral law is regarded as the true and proper expression of the jiva's own evolution. Morality, it has been said, is the true nature of a being. For the same reason wrong is its destruction. What the jiva actually does is the result of his karmma. Further, the term jiva, though commonly applicable to the human embodiment of the atma, is not limited to it. Both papa and punya may therefore be manifested in beings of a lower rank than that of humanity in so far as what they (whether consciously or unconsciously) do is a hindrance to their true development. Thus, in the Yoga Vashishtha it is said that even a creeping plant acquired merit by association with the holy muni on whose dwelling it grew. Objectively considered, sin is concisely defined as duhkhajana-kam papam. It is that which has been, is, and will be the cause of pain, mental or physical, in past, present, and future births. The pain as the consequence of the action done need not be immediate. Though, however, the suffering may be experienced as a result later than the action of which it is the cause, the consequence of the action is not really something separate, but a part of the action itself – namely, that part of it which belongs to the future. The six chief sins are kama, krodha, lobha, moha, mada, matsaryya – lust, anger, covetousness, ignorance or delusion, pride and envy.

All wrong is at base self-seeking, in ignorance or disregard of the unity of the Self in all creatures. Virtue (punya), therefore, as the contrary of sin, is that which is the cause of happiness (sukhajanakam punyam). That happiness is produced either in this or future births, or leads to the enjoyment of heaven (Svarga). Virtue is that which leads towards the unity whose substance is Bliss (ananda). This good karmma produces pleasant fruit, which, like all the results of karmma, is transitory. As Shruti says: "It is not by acts or the pindas offered by one's children or by wealth, but by renunciation that men have attained liberation." It is only by escape from karmma through knowledge, that the jiva becoming one with the unchanging Absolute attains lasting rest. It is obvious that for those who obtain such release neither vice nor virtue, which are categories of phenomenal being, exist.

Karmma

Karmma is action, its cause, and effect. There is no uncaused action, nor action without effect. The past, the present, and the future are linked together as one whole. The ichchha, jnana, and kriya shakti manifest in the jivatma living on the worldly plane as desire, knowledge, and action. As the Brihadaranyaka Upanishad says: "Man is verily formed of desire. As is his desire, so is his thought. As is his thought, so is his action. As is his action, so is his attainment." These fashion the individual's Karmma. "He who desires goes by work to the object on which his mind is set." "As he thinks, so he becometh." Then, as to action, "whatsoever a man sows that shall he reap." The matter is not one of punishment and reward, but of consequence, and the consequence of action is but a part of it. If anything is caused, its result is caused, the result being part of the original action, whigh continues, and is transformed into the result. The jivatma experiences happiness for his good acts and misery for his evil ones.

Karmma is of three kinds – viz., sanchita karmma – that is, the whole vast accumulated mass of the unexhausted karmma of the past, whether good or bad, which has still to be worked out. This past karmma is the cause of the character of the succeeding births, and, as such, is called sangskara, or vasana. The second form of karmma is prarabdha, or that part of the first which is ripe, and which is worked out and bears fruit in the present birth. The third is the new karmma, which man is continually making by his present and future actions, and is called vartamana and agami. The embodied soul (jivatma), whilst in the sangsara or phenomenal world, is by its nature ever making present karmma and experiencing the past. Even the Devas themselves are subject to time and karmma. By his karmma a jiva may become an Indra.

Karmma is thus the invisible (adrishta), the product of ordained or prohibited actions capable of giving bodies. It is either good or bad, and together these are called the impurity of action (karmma mala). Even good action, when done with a view to its fruit, can never secure liberation. Those who think of the reward will receive benefit in the shape of that reward. Liberation is the work of Shiva-Shakti, and is gained only by brahmajnana, the destruction of the will to separate life, and realization of unity with the Supreme. All accompanying action must be without thought of self. With the cessation of desire the tie which binds man to the sangsara is broken.

According to the Tantra, the sadhana and achara (q.v.) appropriate to an individual depends upon his karmma. A man's tendencies, character, and temperament is moulded by his sanchita karmma. As regards prarabdha-karmma, it is unavoidable. Nothing can be done but to work it out. Some systems prescribe the same method for men of divers tendencies. But the Tantra recognizes the force of karmma, and moulds its method to the temperament produced by it. The needs of each vary, as also the methods which will be the best suited to each to lead them to the common goal. Thus, forms of worship which are permissible to the vira are forbidden to the pashu. The guru must determine that for which the sadhaka is qualified (adhikara).

Four Aims Of Being

There is but one thing which all seek – happiness – though it be of differing kinds and sought in different ways. All forms, whether sensual, intellectual, or spiritual, are from the Brahman, who is Itself the Source and Essence of all Bliss, and Bliss itself (rasovai sah). Though issuing from the same source – pleasure differs in its forms in being higher and lower, transitory or durable, or permanent. Those on the path of desire (pravritti marga) seek it through the enjoyments of this world (bhukti) or in the more durable, though still impermanent delights of heaven (svarga). He who is on the path of return (nivritti marga) seeks happiness, not in the created worlds, but in everlasting union with their primal source (mukti); and thus it is said that man can never be truly happy until he seeks shelter with Brahman, which is Itself the great Bliss (rasam hyevayam labdhva anandi bhavati).

The eternal rhythm of the Divine Breath is outwards from spirit to matter and inwards from matter to spirit. Devi as Maya evolves the world. As Mahamaya She recalls it to Herself. The path of outgoing is the way of pravritti; that of return nivritti. Each of these movements is Divine. Enjoyment (bhukti) and liberation (mukti) are each Her gifts. And in the third chapter of the work cited it is said that of Vishnu and Shiva mukti only can be had, but of Devi both bhukti and mukti; and this is so in so far as the Devi is, in a peculiar sense, the source whence those material things come from which enjoyment (bhoga) arises. All jiva on their way to humanity, and the bulk of humanity itself, is on the forward path, and rightly seeks the enjoyment which is appropriate to its stage of evolution.

The thirst for life will continue to manifest itself until the point of return is reached and the outgoing energy is exhausted. Man must, until such time, remain on the path of desire. In the hands of Devi is the noose of desire. Devi herself is both desire and that light of knowledge which in the wise who have known enjoyment lays bare its futilities. But one cannot renounce until one has enjoyed, and so of the world-process itself it is said: that the unborn ones, the Purushas, are both subservient to Her (prakriti), and leave Her by reason of viveka.

Provision is made for the worldly life which is the "outgoing" of the Supreme. And so it is said that the Tantrika has both enjoyment (bhukti) and liberation (mukti). But enjoyment itself is not without its law. Desire is not to be let loose without bridle. The mental self is, as is commonly said, the charioteer of the body, of which the senses are the horses. Contrary to mistaken notions on the subject, the Tantras take no exception to the ordinary rule that it is necessary not to let them run away. If one would not be swept away and lost in the mighty force which is the descent into matter, thought and action must be controlled by Dharmma. Hence the first three of the aims of life (trivarga) on the path of pravritti are dharmma, artha, and kama.

Dharmma

Dharmma means that which is to be held fast or kept – law, usage, custom, religion, piety, right, equity, duty, good works, and morality. It is, in short, the eternal and immutable (sanatana) principles which hold together the universe in its parts and in its whole, whether organic or inorganic matter. "That which supports and holds together the peoples (of the universe) is dharmma." "It was declared for well-being and bringeth well-being. It upholds and preserves. Because it supports and holds together, it is called Dharmma. By Dharmma are the people upheld." It is, in short, not an artificial rule, but the principle of right living. The mark of dharmma and of the good is achara (good conduct), from which dharm-

ma is born and fair fame is acquired here and hereafter. The sages embraced achara as the root of all tapas. Dharmma is not only the principle of right living, but also its application. That course of meritorious action by which man fits himself for this world, heaven, and liberation. Dharmma is also the result of good action – that is, the merit acquired thereby. The basis of the sanatana dharmma is revelation (shruti) as presented in the various Shastra.– Smriti, Purana, and Tantra. In the Devi Bhagavata it is said that in the Kaliyuga Vishnu in the form of Vyasa divides the one Veda into many parts, with the desire to benefit men, and with the knowledge that they are short-lived and of small intelligence, and hence unable to master the whole. This dharmma is the first of the four leading arms (chaturvarga) of all being.

Kama

Kama is desire, such as that for wealth, success, family, position, or other forms of happiness for self or others. It also involves the notion of the necessity for the posses-sion of great and noble aims, desires, and ambitions, for such possession is the characteristic of greatness of soul. Desire, whether of the higher or lower kinds, must, however, be lawful, for man is subject to dharmma, which regulates it.

Artha

Artha (wealth) stands for the means by which this life may be maintained – in the lower sense, food, drink, money, house, land, and other property; and in the higher sense the means by which effect may be given to the higher desires, such as that of worship, for which artha may be necessary, aid given to others, and so forth. In short, it is all the necessary means by which all right desire, whether of the lower or higher kinds, may be fulfilled. As the desire must be a right desire – for man is subject to dharmma, which regulates them – so also must be the means sought, which are equally so governed.

This first group is known as the trivarga, which must be cultivated whilst man is upon the pravritti marga. Unless and until there is renunciation on entrance upon the path of return, where inclination ceases (nivritti marga), man must work for the ultimate goal by me-ritorious acts (dharmma), desires (kama), and by the lawful means (artha) whereby the lawful desires which give birth to righteous acts are realized. Whilst on the pravritti marga "the trivarga should be equally culti-vated, for he who is addicted to one only is despicable" (dharmmartha-kamah samameva sevyah yo hyekasak-tah sa jano-jagha-nyah).

Moksha

Of the four aims, moksha or mukti is the truly ultimate end, for the other three are ever haunted by the fear of Death the Ender.

Mukti means "loosening" or liberation. It is advisable to avoid the term "salvation," as also other Christian terms, which connote different, though in a loose sense, analogous ideas. According to the Christian doctrine (soteriology), faith in Christ's Gospel and in His Church effects salvation, which is the forgiveness of sins mediated by Christ's redeeming activity, saving from judgment, and admitting to the Kingdom of God. On the other hand, mukti means a loosening from the bonds of the sangsara (phenomenal existence), resulting in a union (of various degrees of completeness) of the embodied spirit (jivatma) or individual life with the Supreme Spirit (paramatma). Liberation can be attained by spiritual knowledge (atmajnana) alone, though it is obvious that such knowledge must be preceded by, and accompanied with, and, indeed, can only be attained in the sense of actual realization, by freedom from sin and right action through adherence to dharmma. The idealistic system of Hinduism, which posits the ultimate reality as being in the nature of mind, rightly, in such cases, insists on what, for default of a better term, may be described as the intellectual, as opposed to the ethical, nature. Not that it fails to recognize the importance of the latter, but regards it as subsidiary and powerless of itself to achieve that extinction of the modifications of the energy of consciousness which constitute the supreme mukti known as Kaivalya. Such extinction cannot be effected by conduct alone, for such conduct, whether good or evil, pro-duces karmma, which is the source of the modifications which it is man's final aim to suppress. Moksha belongs to the nitvritti marga, as the trivarga appertain to the pravritti marga.

There are various degrees of mukti, some more perfect than the others, and it is not, as is generally supposed, one state.

There are four future states of Bliss, or pada, being in the nature of abodes – viz., salokya, samipya, sarupya, and sayujya – that is, living in the same loka, or region, with the Deva worshipped; being near the Deva,; receiving the same form or possessing the same aishvaryya (Divine qualities) as the Deva, and becoming one with the Deva worshipped. The abode to which the jiva attains depends upon the worshipper and the nature of his worship, which may be with, or without, images, or of the Deva regarded as distinct from the worshipper, and with attributes, and so forth. The four abodes are the

*result of action, transitory and conditioned. Mahanir-
vvana, or Kaivalya, the real moksha, is the result of
spiritual knowledge (jnana), and is unconditioned and
permanent. Those who know the Brahman, recognizing
that the worlds resulting from action are imperfect,
reject them, and attain to that unconditioned Bliss
which transcends them all. Kaivalya is the supreme state
of oneness without attributes, the state in which, as the
Yogasutra says, modification of the energy of consciousness is extinct, and when it is established in its own real
nature.*

*Liberation is attainable while the body is yet living, in
which case there exists the state of jivanmukti celebrated
in the Jivanmuktigita of Dattatreya. The soul, it is true,
is not really fettered, and any appearance to the contrary is illusory. There is, in fact, freedom, but though
moksha is already in possession still, because of the
illusion that it is not yet attained, means must be taken
to remove the illusion, and the jiva who succeeds in this
is jivanmukta, though in the body, and is freed from
future embodi-ments. The enlightened Kaula, according to the Nitya-nita, sees no difference between mud
and sandal, friend and foe, a dwelling-house and the
cremation-ground. He knows that the Brahman is all,
that the Supreme soul (paramatma) and the individual
soul (jivatma) are one, and freed from all attachment he*

is jivanmukta, or liberated, whilst yet living. The means whereby mukti is attained is the yoga process (vide ante).

Siddhi

Siddhi is produced by sadhana. The former term, which literally means "success," includes accomplishment, achievement, success, and fruition of all kinds. A person may thus gain siddhi in speech, siddhi in mantra, etc. A person is siddha also who has perfected his spiritual development. The various powers attainable – namely, anima, mahima, laghima, garima, prapti, prakamya, ishitva, vashitva, the powers of becoming small, great, light, heavy, attaining what one wills, and the like – are known as the eight siddhi. The thirty-ninth chapter of the Brahmavaivarta Purana mentions eighteen kinds, but there are many others, including such minor accomplishments as nakhadarpana siddhi or "nail-gazing." The great siddhi is spiritual perfection. Even the mighty powers of the "eight siddhi" are known as the "lesser siddhi," since the greatest of all siddhi is full liberation (mahanirvana) from the bonds of phenomenal life and union with the Paramatma, which is the supreme object (paramartha) to be attained through human birth.

A. A.

CHAPTER 1

Questions relating to the Liberation of Beings

*THE enchanting summit of the Lord of Mountains,
resplendent with all its various jewels, clad with many
a tree and many a creeper, melodious with the song
of many a bird, scented with the fragrance of all the
season's flowers, most beautiful, fanned by soft, cool, and
perfumed breezes, shadowed by the still shade of stately
trees; where cool groves resound with the sweet-voiced
songs of troops of Apsara, and in the forest depths flocks
of kokila maddened with passion sing; where (Spring)
Lord of the Seasons with his followers ever abide (the
Lord of Mountains, Kailasa); peopled by (troops of)
Siddha, Charana, Gandharva, and Ganapatya (1-5).
It was there that Parvati, finding Shiva, Her gracious
Lord, in mood serene, with obeisance bent low and for
the benefit of all the worlds questioned Him, the Silent
Deva, Lord of all things movable and immovable, the
ever Beneficent and ever Blissful One, the nectar of
Whose mercy abounds as a great ocean, Whose very
essence is the Pure Sattva Guna, He Who is white as
camphor and the Jasmine flower, the Omnipresent One,
Whose raiment is space itself, Lord of the poor and the
beloved Master of all yogi, Whose coiled and matted*

hair is wet with the spray of Ganga and (of Whose naked body) ashes are the adornment only; the passionless
One, Whose neck is garlanded with snakes and skulls of
men, the three-eyed One, Lord of the three worlds, with
one hand wielding the trident and with the other be-
stowing blessings; easily appeased, Whose very substance is unconditioned Knowledge; the Bestower of eternal
emancipation, the Ever-existent, Fearless, Changeless,
Stainless, One without defect, the Benefactor of all, and
the Deva of all Devas (5-10).

Shri Parvati said:

*O Deva of the Devas, Lord of the world, Jewel of Mercy,
my Husband, Thou art my Lord, on Whom I am ever
dependent and to Whom I am ever obedient. Nor can I
say ought without Thy word. If Thou hast affection for
me, I crave to lay before Thee that which passeth in my
mind. Who else but Thee, O Great Lord, in the three
worlds is able to solve these doubts of mine, Thou Who
knowest all and all the Scriptures (11-13).*

Shri Sadashiva said:

*What is that Thou sayest, O Thou Great Wise One and
Beloved of My heart, I will tell Thee anything, be it
ever so bound in mystery, even that which should not*

be spoken of before Ganesha and Skanda Commander of the Hosts of Heaven. What is there in all the three worlds which should be concealed from Thee? For Thou, O Devi, art My very Self. There is no difference between Me and Thee. Thou too art omnipresent. What is it then that Thou knowest not that Thou questionest like unto one who knoweth nothing (14-16).

The pure Parvati, gladdened at hearing the words of the Deva, bending low made obeisance and thus questioned Shangkara.

Shri Adya said:

O Bhagavan! Lord of all, Greatest among those who are versed in Dharmma, Thou in former ages in Thy mercy didst through Brahma reveal the four Vedas which are the propagators of all dharmma and which ordain the rules of life for all the varying castes of men and for the different stages of their lives (18-19). In the First Age, men by the practice of yaga and yajna prescribed by Thee were virtuous and pleasing to Devas and Pitris (20). By the study of the Vedas, dhyana and tapas, and the conquest of the senses, by acts of mercy and charity men were of exceeding power and courage, strength and vigour, adherents of the true Dharmma, wise and truthful and of firm resolve, and, mortals though they

*were, they were yet like Devas and went to the abode
of the Devas (21, 22). Kings then were faithful to their
engagements and were ever concerned with the protection of their people, upon whose wives they were wont
to look as if upon their mothers, and whose children
they regarded as their very own (23). The people, too,
did then look upon a neighbour's property as if it were
mere lumps of clay, and, with devotion to their Dharmma, kept to the path of righteousness (24). There were
then no liars, none who were selfish, thievish, malicious,
foolish, none who were evil-minded, envious, wrathful,
gluttonous, or lustful, but all were good of heart and
of ever blissful mind. Land then yielded in plenty all
kinds of grain, clouds showered seasonable rains, cows
gave abundant milk, and trees were weighted with
fruits (25-27). No untimely death there was, nor famine
nor sickness. Men were ever cheerful, prosperous, and
healthy, and endowed with all qualities of beauty and
brilliance. Women were chaste and devoted to their husbands. Brahmanas, Kshatriyas, Vaishyas, and Shudras
kept to and followed the customs, Dharmma, yajna, of
their respective castes, and attained the final liberation
(28-29).*

*After the Krita Age had passed away Thou didst in the
Treta Age perceive Dharmma to be in disorder, and
that men were no longer able by Vedic rites to accom-*

plish their desires. For men, through their anxiety and perplexity, were unable to perform these rites in which much trouble had to be overcome, and for which much preparation had to be made. In constant distress of mind they were neither able to perform nor yet were willing to abandon the rites.

Having observed this, Thou didst make known on earth the Scripture in the form of Smriti, which explains the meaning of the Vedas, and thus delivered from sin, which is cause of all pain, sorrow, and sickness, men too feeble for the practice of tapas and the study of the Vedas. For men in this terrible ocean of the world, who is there but Thee to be their Cherisher, Protector, Saviour, their fatherly Benefactor, and Lord? (30-33).

Then, in the Dvapara Age when men abandoned the good works prescribed in the Smritis, and were deprived of one half of Dharmma and were afflicted by ills of mind and body, they were yet again saved by Thee, through the instructions of the Sanghita and other religious lore (34-36).

Now the sinful Kali Age is upon them, when Dharmma is destroyed, an Age full of evil customs and deceit. Men pursue evil ways. The Vedas have lost their power, the Smritis are forgotten, and many of the Puranas, which *contain stories of the past, and show the many ways (which lead to liberation), will, O Lord! be destroyed. Men will become averse from religious rites, without restraint, maddened with pride, ever given over to sinful acts, lustful, gluttonous, cruel. heartless, harsh of speech, deceitful, short-lived, poverty-stricken, harassed by sickness and sorrow, ugly, feeble, low, stupid, mean, and addicted to mean habits, companions of the base, thievish, calumnious, malicious, quarrelsome, depraved, cowards, and ever-ailing, devoid of all sense of shame and sin and of fear to seduce the wives of others. Vipras will live like the Shudras, and whilst neglecting their own Sandhya will yet officiate at the sacrifices of the low. They will be greedy, given over to wicked and sinful acts, liars, insolent, ignorant, deceitful, mere hangers-on of others, the sellers of their daughters, degraded, averse to all tapas and vrata. They will be heretics, impostors, and think themselves wise. They will be without faith or devotion, and will do japa and puja with no other end than to dupe the people. They will eat unclean food and follow evil customs, they will serve and eat the food of the Shudras and lust after low women, and will be wicked and ready to barter for money even their own wives to the low. In short, the only sign that they are Brahmanas will be the thread they wear. Observing no rule in eating or drinking or in other matters, scoffing at the Dharmma Scriptures, no thought of pious speech ever so much as entering their minds, they will be but bent upon the injury of the good (37-50).*

By Thee also have been composed for the good and liberation of men the Tantras, a mass of Agamas and Nigamas, which bestow both enjoyment and liberation, containing Mantras and Yantras and rules as to the sadhana of both Devis and Devas. By Thee, too, have been described many forms of Nyasa, such as those called srishti, sthiti (and sanghara). By Thee, again, have been described the various seated positions (of yoga), such as that of the "tied" and "loosened" lotus, the Pashu, Vira, and Divya classes of men, as also the Devata, who gives success in the use of each of the mantras (50-52). And yet again it is Thou Who hast made known in a thousand ways rites relating to the worship with woman, and the rites which are done with the use of skulls, a corpse, or when seated on a funeral pyre (53). By Thee, too, have been forbidden both pashu-bhava and divya-bhava. If in this Age the pashu-bhava cannot exist, how can there be divya-bhava? (54). For the pashu must with his own hand collect leaves, flowers, fruits, and water, and should not look at a Shudra or even think of a woman (55). On the other hand, the Divya is all but a Deva, ever pure of heart, and to whom all opposites are alike, free from attachment to worldly things, the same to all creatures and forgiving (56). How can men with the taint of this Age upon them, who are ever of restless mind, prone to sleep and sloth, attain to purity of disposition? (57). By Thee, too, have been spoken the rites of Vira-sadhana, relating to the Pancha-tattva – namely, wine, meat, fish, parched grain, and sexual union of man and woman (58-59). But since the men of the Kali Age are full of greed, lust, gluttony, they will on that account neglect sidhana and will fall into sin, and having drunk much wine for the sake of the pleasure of the senses, will become mad with intoxication, and bereft of all notion of right and wrong (61). Some will violate the wives of others, others will become rogues, and some, in the indiscriminating rage of lust, will go (whoever she be) with any woman (62). Over eating and drinking will disease many and deprive them of strength and sense. Disordered by madness, they will meet death, falling into lakes, pits, or in impenetrable forests, or from hills or house-tops (63-64). While some will be as mute as corpses, others will be for ever on the chatter, and yet others will quarrel with their kinsmen and elders. They will be evil-doers, cruel, and the destroyers of Dharmma (65-66). I fear, O Lord! that even that which Thou hast ordained for the good of men will through them turn out for evil (67). O Lord of the World! who will practise Yoga or Nyasa, who will sing the hymns and draw the Yantra and make Purashcharana? (68). Under the influences of the Kali Age man will of his nature become indeed wicked and bound to all manner of sin (69). Say, O Lord of all the distressed! in Thy mercy how without great pains men may obtain longevity, health, and energy, increase of strength and courage, learning, intelligence, and happiness; and how they may become great in strength and valour, pure of heart, obedient to parents, not seeking the love of others' wives, but devoted to their own, mindful of the good of their neighbour, reverent to the Devas and to their gurus, cherishers of their children and kinsmen (70-72), possessing the knowledge of the Brahman, learned in the lore of, and ever meditating on, the Brahman. Say, O Lord! for the good of the world, what men should or should not do according to their different castes and stages of life. For who but Thee is their Protector in all the three worlds? (73-74).

End of the First Joyful Message, entitled "Questions relating to the Liberation of Beings."

CHAPTER 2

Introduction to the Worship of

Brahman

HAVING heard the words of the Devi, Shangkara, Bestower of happiness on the world, great Ocean of mercy, thus of the truth of things spoke.

Sadashiva said:

O Exalted and Holy One! Benefactress of the universe, well has it been asked by Thee. By none has such an auspicious question been asked aforetime (2). Worthy of all thanks art Thou, Who knoweth all good, Benefactress of all born in this age, O Gentle One! Thou art Omniscient. Thou knowest the past, present, and future, and Dharmma. What Thou hast said about the past, present, and future, and, indeed, all things, is in accordance with Dharmma, and is the truth, and is without a doubt accepted by Me. O Sureshvari! I say unto you most truly and without all doubt that men, whether they be of the twice born or other castes, afflicted as they are by this sinful Age, and unable to distinguish the pure from the impure, will not obtain purity or the success of their desired ends by the Vedic ritual, or that prescribed by the Sanghitas and Smritis (3-6). Verily, verily, and yet again

*verily, I say unto you that in this Age there is no way to
liberation but that proclaimed by the Agama (7). I, O
Blissful One, have already foretold in the Vedas, Smritis,
and Puranas,' that in this Age the wise shall worship
after the doctrine of the Agama (8). Verily, verily, and
beyond all doubt, I say to you that there is no liberation for him who in this Age, heedless of such doctrine,
follows another (9). There is no Lord but I in this world,
and I alone am He Who is spoken of in the Vedas, Puranas, and Smritis and Sanghitas (10). The Vedas and the
Puranas proclaim Me to be the cause of the purity of the
three worlds, and they who are averse to My doctrine
are unbelievers and sinners, as great as those who slay a
Brahmana (11). Therefore, O Devi! the worship of him
who heeds not My precepts is fruitless, and, moreover,
such an one goes to hell (12). The fool who would follow
other doctrine heedless of Mine is as great a sinner as
the slayer of a Brahmana or of a woman, or a parricide;
have no doubt of that (13).*

*In this Age the Mantras of the Tantras are efficacious,
yield immediate fruit, and are auspicious for Japa,
Yajna, and all such practices and ceremonies (14).
The Vedic rites and Mantras which were efficacious
in the First Age have ceased to be so in this. They are
now as powerless as snakes, the poison-fangs of which
are drawn and are like to that which is dead (15). The*

whole heap of other Mantras have no more power than the organs of sense of some pictured image on a wall. To worship with the aid of other Mantras is as fruitless as it is to cohabit with a barren woman. The labour is lost (16-17). He who in this Age seeks salvation by ways prescribed by others is like a thirsty fool who digs a well on the bank of the Jahnavi (18), and he who, knowing My Dharmma, craves for any other is as one who with nectar in his house yet longs for the poisonous juice of the akanda plant (19). No other path is there to salvation and happiness in this life or in that to come like unto that shown by the Tantras (20). From my mouth have issued the several Tantras with their sacred legends and practices both for Siddhas and Sadhakas (21). At times, O My Beloved! by reason of the great number of men of the pashu disposition, as also of the diversity of the qualifications of men, it has been said that the Dharmma spoken of in the Kulachara Scriptures should be kept secret (22). But some portions of this Dharmma, O Beloved! have been revealed by Me with the object of inclining the minds of men thereto. Various kinds of Devata and worshippers are mentioned therein, such as Bhairava, Vetala, Vatuka, Nayika, Shaktas, Shaivas, Vaishnavas, Sauras, Ganapatyas, and others. In them, too, are described various Mantra and Yantra which aid men in the attainment of siddhi, and which, though they demand great and constant effort, yet yield the desired

*fruit (23-25). Hitherto My answer has been given accor-
ding to the nature of the case and the questioner, and for
his individual benefit only (26).*

*None before has ever questioned Me as Thou hast done
for the advantage of all mankind – nay, for the benefit
of all that breathes, and that, too, in such detail and
with reference to the Dharmma of each of the different
Ages. Therefore, out of My affection for Thee, O Parvati!
I will speak to Thee of the essence of essences and of the
Supreme (27-28). O Deveshi! I will state before Thee the
very essence distilled from the Vedas and Agamas, and
in particular from the Tantras (29). As men versed in
the Tantras are to other men, as the Jahnavi is to other
rivers, as I am to all other Devas, so is the Mahanirvana
Tantra to all other Agamas (30).*

*O Auspicious One! of what avail are the Vedas, the
Puranas, or the Shastras, since he who has the knowledge of this great Tantra is Lord of all Siddhi? (31). Since
Thou hast questioned Me for the good of the world, I
will speak to Thee of that which will lead to the benefit
of the universe (32).*

*O Parameshvari! should good be done to the univer-
se, the Lord of it is pleased, since He is its soul, and it
depends on Him (33). He is One. He is the Ever-exis-*

tent. He is the Truth. He is the Supreme Unity without a second. He is Ever-full and Self-manifest. He is Eternal Intelligence and Bliss (33-34). He is without change, Self-existent, and ever the Same, Serene, above all attributes. He beholds and is the Witness of all that passes, Omni-present, the Soul of everything that is. He, the Eternal and Omnipresent, is hidden and pervades all things. Though Himself devoid of sense, He is the Illuminator of all the senses and their powers (35-36). The Cause of all the three worlds, He is yet beyond them and the mind of men. Ineffable and Omniscient, He knows the universe, yet none know Him (37). He sways this incompre-hensible universe, and all that has movement and is motionless in the three worlds depends on Him; and lighted by His truth, the world shines as does Truth itself. We too have come from Him as our Cause (38-39). He, the one Supreme Lord, is the Cause of all beings, the Manifestation of Whose creative Energy in the three worlds is called Brahma (40). By His will Vishnu protects and I destroy, Indra and all other Guardian Devas of the world depend on Him and hold rule in their respective regions under His command. Thou His supreme Prakriti art adored in all the three worlds (41-42). Each one does his work by the power of Him who exists in his heart. None are ever independent of Him (43). Through fear of Him the Wind blows, the Sun gives heat, the Clouds shower seasonable rain, and the Trees in the forest flower (44).

It is He who destroys Time at the Great Dissolution, of Whom even Fear and Death itself are afraid. He is Bhagavan, Who is known as Yat Tat in the Vedanta (45).O Adored of the Devas! all the Devas and Devis – nay, the whole universe, from Brahma to a blade of grass – are His forms (46). If He be pleased, the Universe is pleased. If aught be done to gratify Him, then the gratification of All is caused (47). As the pouring of water at the root of a tree satisfies the wants of the leaves and branches, so by worshipping Him all the Deathless Ones are satisfied (48). Just as, O Virtuous One! all the beautiful Ones are pleased when Thou art worshipped and when men meditate on and make Japa and pray to Thee (49). As all rivers must go to the ocean, so, O Parvati! all acts of worship must reach Him as the ultimate goal (50). Whoever be the worshipper, and whoever be the Devata, he reverentially worships for some desired end, all that is given to him through the Deva he so worships comes from Him as the Supreme (51). Oh, what use is it to say more before Thee, O My Beloved?

There is none other but Him to meditate upon, to pray to, to worship for the attainment of liberation (52). Need there is none to trouble, to fast, to torture one's body, to follow rules and customs, to make large offerings; need there is none to be heedful as to time nor as to Nyasa or Mudra, wherefore, O Kuleshani! who will strive to seek shelter elsewhere than with Him? (53-54).

End of the Second Joyful Message, entitled "Introduction

to the Worship of Brahman."

CHAPTER 3

Description of the Worship of
the Supreme Brahman

SHRI DEVI said:

O Deva of the Devas, great Deva, Guru of Brihaspati himself, Thou Who discourseth of all Scriptures, Mantra, Sadhana, and hast spoken of the Supreme Brahman by the adoration of Whom mortals attain happiness and liberation, do Thou, O Lord! deign to instruct us in the way of service of the Supreme Soul and of the observances, Mantra, and meditation in His worship. It is my desire, O Lord! to hear the essential substance of all these from Thee (1-4).

Shri Sadashiva said:

Listen, then, O Beloved of My life! to the most secret and supreme Truth, the mystery whereof has nowhere yet been revealed (5).

Because of My affection for Thee I shall speak to Thee of that Supreme Brahman, Who is ever Existent, Intelligent, and Who is dearer to Me than life itself. O Mahes-

hvari! the eternal, intelligent, infinite Brahman may be known in Its real Self or by Its external signs (5-6). That Which is changeless, existent only, and beyond both mind and speech, Which shines as the Truth amidst the illusion of the three worlds, is the Brahman according to Its real nature (7). That Brahman is known in samadhi-yoga by those who look upon all things alike, who are above all contraries, devoid of doubt, free of all illusion regarding body and soul (8). That same Brahman is known from His external signs, from Whom the whole universe has sprung, in Whom when so sprung It exists, and into Whom all things return (9). That which is known by intuition may also be perceived from these external signs. For those who would know Him through these external signs, for them sadhana is enjoined (10).

Attend to me, Thou, O dearest One! while I speak to Thee of such sadhana. And firstly, O Adye! I tell Thee of the Mantroddhara of the Supreme Brahman (11). Utter first the Pranava, then the words "existence" and "intelligence," and after the word "One" say "Brahman."

MANTRA

Ong Sachchidekam Brahma (12).

This is the Mantra. These words, when combined ac-

cording to the rules of Sandhi, form a Mantra of seven letters. If the Pranava be omitted, it becomes a Mantra of six letters only (13). This is the most excellent of all the Mantras, and the one which immediately bestows Dharmma, Artha, Kama, and Moksha. In the use of this Mantra there is no need to consider whether it be efficacious or not, or friendly or inimical, for no such considerations affect it (14). Nor at initiation into this Mantra is it necessary to make calculations as to the phases of the Moon, the propitious junction of the stars, or as to the Signs of the Zodiac. Nor are there any rules as to whether the Mantra is suitable or not. Nor is there need of the ten Sangskara. This Mantra is in every way efficacious in initiation. There is no necessity for considering anything else (15). Should one have obtained, through merit acquired in previous births, an excellent Guru, from whose lips this Mantra is received, then life indeed becomes fruitful (16), and the worshipper receiving in his hands Dharmma, Artha, Kama, and Moksha, rejoices both in this world and the next (17).

He whose ears this great jewel of Mantra reaches is indeed blest, for he has attained the desired end, being virtuous and pious, and is as one who has bathed in a the sacred places, been initiated in all Yajnas, versed in all Scriptures, and honoured in all the worlds (18-19). Happy is the father and happy the mother of such a one

*– yea, and yet more than this, his family is hallowed and
the gladdened spirits of the Pitris rejoice with th Devas,
and in the excess of their joy sing (20): "In our family
is born the most excellent of our race, one initiate in
the Brahma-mantra. What need have we now of pinda
offered at Gaya, or of shraddha, tarpana, pilgrimage
at holy places (21); of what use are alms, japa, homa,
or sadhana, since now we have obtained imperishable
satisfaction?" (22)*

*Listen, O Devi! Adored of the world, whilst I tell You
the very truth that for the worshippers of the Supreme
Brahman there is no need for other religious observances (23). At the very moment of initiation into this
Mantra the disciple is filled with Brahman, and for such
an one, O Devi! what is there which is unattainable in
all the three worlds? (24). Against him what can adverse
planets or Vetala, Chetaka, Pishacha, Guhyaka, Bhuta,
the Matrika, Dakini, and other spirits avail?*

*The very sight of him will drive them to flight with av-
erted faces (25). Guarded by the Brahma-mantra, clad
with the splendour of Brahman, he is as it were another
Sun. What should he fear, then, from any planet? (26).
They flee, frightened like elephants at the sight of a lion,
and perish like moths in a flame (27). No sin can touch,
and none but one as wicked as a suicide can harm, him,*

who is purified by truth, without blemish, a benefactor of all beings, a faithful believer in Brahman (28). The wicked and sinful who seek to harm him who is initiate in the knowledge of the Supreme Brahman do but harm themselves, for are they not indeed in essence inseparate from the ever-existent One? (29). For he is the holy sage and well-wisher, working for the happiness of all, and, O Devi! should it be possible to harm such an one who can go in peace? (31). For him, however, who has no knowledge of the meaning of nor of the awakening of the Mantra, it is fruitless, even though it were inwardly uttered ten million times (31).

Listen, then, O My Beloved! while I tell Thee of the meaning and awakening of Mantra. By the letter A is meant the Protector of the world; the letter U denotes its Destroyer; and M stands for its Creator (32). The meaning of Sat is Ever-existent; of Chit, Intelligence; and of Ekam, One without a second. Brahman is so called because He exists everywhere. Now, O Devi! I have given You the meaning of the Mantra, which grants the fulfilment of desires. The awakening of the Mantra is the knowledge of Him, Who is the pervading Devata of the Mantra, and such knowledge, O Supreme Devi! yields the fruit of worship to the worshipper (35). O Devi! the presiding Devata of the Mantra is the omnipresent, eternal, inscrutable, formless, passionless, and ineffable

Brahman (36). When introduced by the Vija of Saras-vati, Maya, or Kamala, instead of the Mantra Om, it bestows various kinds of learning, siddhi, and prosperity in every quarter (37). The Mantra may be varied either by the prefixing or omitting of Om, or by the placing of it before each word or every two words of the Mantra (38). Sadashiva is the Rishi of this Mantra. The verse is called Anushtup, and its presiding Devata is the Supre-me Brahman, Who is without attributeand Who abides in all things. It avails for the attainment of Dharmma, Artha, Kama, and Moksha.

Now listen, dear One, whilst I speak to You of Anga-ny-asa and Kara-nyasa (39-40). O great and adorable Devi! the syllable Om, the words Sat, Chit, Ekam, Brahma, should be pronounced over the thumb, the th-reatening finger, the middle, nameless, and little fingers respectively, followed in each case by the words Namah, Svaha, Vashat, Hung, and Vaushat; and Ong Sachchide-kam Brahma should be said over the palm and back of the hand, followed by the Mantra Phat (41, 42).

The worshipper disciple should in the like manner, with his mind well under control, perform Anga-nyasa in accordance with the rules thereof, commencing with the heart and ending with the hands (43).

After this, whilst reciting the Mantra Om or the Mula-mantra, Pranayama should be performed thus: He should close the left nostril with the middle of the fourth finger, and then inhale through the right nostril, meanwhile making japa of the Pranava or the Mula-mantra eight times. Then, closing the right nostril with the thumb and shutting also the mouth, make japa of the Mantra thirty-two times. After that gently exhale the breath through the right nostril, doing japa of the Mantra the while sixteen times.

In the same way perform these three acts with the left nostril, and then repeat the same process with the right nostril. O adored of the Devas! I have now told Thee of the method of Pranayama to be observed in the use of the Brahma-Mantra (44-48). The Sadhaka should then make meditation which accomplishes his desire (49).

DHYANA

In the lotus of my heart I contemplate the Divine Intelligence, the Brahman without distinctions and difference, Knowable by Hari, Hara, and Vidhi, whom Yogis approach in meditation, He Who destroys the fear of birth and death, Who is Existence, Intelligence, the Root of all the three worlds (50)

*Having thus contemplated the Supreme Brahman,
the worshipper should, in order to attain union with
Brahman, worship with offerings of his mind (51). For
perfume let him offer to the Supreme Soul the essence of
the Earth, for flowers the ether, for incense the essence of
the air, for light the Lustre of the universe, and for food
the essence of the Waters of the world (52). After mentally repeating the great mantra and offering the fruit of
it to the Supreme Brahman, the excellent disciple should
commence external worship*

*Meditating with closed eyes on the Eternal Brahman,
the worshipper should with reverence offer to the Supreme whatever be at hand, such as perfumes, flowers,
clothes, jewels, food, and drink, after having purified
them with the following (54-55):*

MANTRA

*The vessel in which these offerings are placed is Brah-
man, and so, too, is the gheeoffered therein. Brahman is
both the sacrificial Fire and he who makes the sacrifice,
and to Brahman he will attain whose mind is fixed
on the Brahman by the performance of the rites which
lead to Brahman (56). Then, opening the eyes, and
inwardly and with all his power making japa with the
Mula-mantra, the worshipper should offer the japa to*

Brahman and then recite the hymn that follows and the Kavacha-mantra (57). Hear, O Maheshvari! the hymn to Brahman, the Supreme Spirit, by the hearing whereof the disciple becomes one with the Brahman (58).

Stotra

Ong! I bow to Thee, the eternal Refuge of all:

I bow to Thee, the pure Intelligence manifested in the universe.

I bow to Thee Who in His essence is One and Who grants liberation.

I bow to Thee, the great, all-pervading attributeless One (59).

Thou art the only Refuge and Object of adoration.

The whole universe is the appearance of Thee Who art its Cause.

Thou alone art Creator, Preserver, Destroyer of the world.

Thou art the sole immutable Supreme, Who art neither this nor that (60);

Dread of the dreadful, Terror of the terrible.

Refuge of all beings, Purificator of all purificators.

Thou alone rulest the high-placed ones,

Supreme over the supreme, Protector of the Protectors (61).

O Supreme Lord in Whom all things are, yet Unmanifest in all,

Imperceptible by the senses, yet the very truth.

Incomprehensible, Imperishable, All-pervading hidden Essence.

Lord and Light of the Universe! save us from harm (62).

On that One alone we meditate, that One alone we in mind worship,

To that One alone the Witness of the Universe we bow.

Refuge we seek with the One Who is our sole Eternal Support,

The Self-existent Lord, the Vessel of safety in the ocean of being (63).

This is the five-jewelled hymn to the Supreme Soul.

He who pure in mind and body recites this hymn is united with the Brahman (64). It should be said daily in the evening, and particularly on the day of the Moon. The wise man should read and explain it to such of his kinsmen as believe in Brahman (65). I have spoken to You, O Devi! of the five-jewelled hymn, O Graceful One! listen now to the jagan-mangala Mantra of the amulet, by the wearing and reading whereof one becomes a knower of the Brahman (66).

MANTRA

May the Supreme Soul protect the head,

May the Supreme Lord protect the heart,

May the Protector of the world protect the throat,

May the All-pervading, All-seeing Lord protect the face (67),

May the Soul of the Universe protect my hands,

May He Who is Intelligence itself protect the feet,

May the Eternal and Supreme Brahman protect my body in all its parts always (68).

The Rishi of this world-beneficent amulet is Sada-shiva; the verse is anushtup, its presiding Devata is the Supreme Brahman, and the object of its use is the attainment of Dharmma, Artha, Kama, and Moksha (69). He who recites this protective Mantra after offering it to its Rishi attains knowledge of Brahman, and is one immediately with the Brahman (70). If written on birch-bark and encased in a golden ball, it be worn round the neck or on the right arm, its wearer attains all kinds of powers (71). I have now revealed to Thee the amulet Mantra of the Supreme Brahman. It should be given to the favourite disciple who is both devoted to the Guru and possessed of understanding (72). The excellent Sadhaka shall, after reciting the Mantra and the hymn with reverence, salute the Supreme (73).

Salutation

Ong

I bow to the Supreme Brahman.

I bow to the Supreme Soul.

I bow to Him Who is above all qualities.

I bow to the Ever-existent again and again (74).

*The worship of the Supreme Lord may be by body or
mind or by word; but the one thing needful is purity
of disposition (75). After worshipping in the manner
of which I have spoken, the wise man should with his
friends and kinsmen partake of the holy food consecrated to the Supreme Spirit. (76) In the worship of the
Supreme there is no need to invoke Him to be present or
to desire Him to depart.*

*It may be done always and in all places (77). It is of no
account whether the worshipper has or has not bathed,
or whether he be fasting or have taken food. But the
Supreme Spirit should ever be worshipped with a pure
heart (78). After purification by the Brahma-Mantra,
whatever food or drink is offered to the Supreme Lord
becomes itself purifying (79). The touch of inferior castes
may pollute the water of Ganga and the Shaligrama,
but nothing which has been consecrated to the Brahman
(80) can be so polluted. If dedicated to Brahman with
this Mantra, the worshipper with his people may eat
of anything, whether cooked or uncooked (81). In the
partaking of this food no rule as to caste or time need
be observed. No one should hesitate to take the leavings*

from the plate of another, whether such another be pure or impure. (82).

Whenever and whatsoever the place may be, howsoever it may have been attained, eat without scruple or inquiry the food dedicated to the Brahman (83). Such food, O Devi! even the Devas do not easily get, and it purifies even if brought by a Chamdala, or if it be taken from the mouth of a dog (84). As to that which the partaking of such food affects in men, what, O Adored of the Devas! shall We say of it? It is deemed excellent even by the Devas. Without a doubt the partaking of this holy food, be it but once only, frees the greatest of sinners and all sinners of their sins (85-86). The mortal who eats of it acquires such merit as can only otherwise be earned by bathing and alms at thirty-five millions of holy places (87). By the eating of it ten million times greater merit is gained than by the Horse-sacrifice, or indeed by any other sacrifice whatever (88). Its excellence cannot be described by ten million tongues and a thousand million mouths (89). Wherever the Sadhaka may be, and though he be a Chandala, he attains to union with the Brahman the very moment he partakes of the nectar dedicated to Him (90). Even Brahmans versed in the Vedanta should take food prepared by low-caste men if it be dedicated to the Brahman (91). No distinction of caste should be observed in eating food dedicated to

*the Supreme Spirit. He who thinks it impure becomes
a great sinner (92). It would be better, O Beloved! to
commit a hundred sins or to kill a Brahmana than to
despise food dedicated to the Supreme Brahman (93).
Those fools who reject food and drink made holy by the
great Mantra. cause the fall of their ancestors into the
lower regions, and they themselves go headlong into
the Hell of blind darkness, where they remain until the
Dissolution of things. No liberation is there for such
as despise food dedicated to Brahman (94-95). In the
sadhana of this great Mantra, even acts without merit
become meritorious; in slumber merit is acquired; and
acts are accepted as rightful which are done according to
the worshipper's desires (96). For such what need is there
of Vedic practices, or for the matter of that what need is
there even of those of the Tantra? Whatever he does according to his desire, that is recognized as lawful in the
case of the wise believer in the Brahman (97). For them
there is neither merit nor demerit in the performance or
non-performance of the customary rites. In the sadhana
of this Mantra his faults or omissions are no obstacle
(98). By the sadhana of this Mantra, O Great Devi! man
becomes truthful, conqueror of the passions devoted to
the good of his fellow-men, one to whom all things are
indifferent, pure of purpose, free of envy and arrogance, merciful and pure of mind, devoted to the service
and seeking the of his parents, a listener ever to things*

devine, a meditator ever on the Brahman. His mind is ever turned to the search for Brahman. With strength of determination holding his mind in close control, he is ever conscious of the nearness of Brahman (99-101). He who is initiated in the Brahma-Mantra will not lie or think to harm, and will shun to go with the wives of others (102). At the commencement of all rites, let him say, "Tat Sat"; and before eating or drinking aught let him say, "I dedicate this to Brahman" (103). For the knower of Brahman, duty consists in action for the well-being of fellow-men. This is the eternal Dharmma.

I will now, O Shambhavi! speak to Thee of the duties relating to Sandhya in the practice of the Brahma Mantra, whereby men acquire that real wealth which comes to them in the form of Brahman (105). Wheresoever he may be, and in whatsoever posture, the excellent and well-intentioned sadhaka shall, at morning, noon and eventide, meditate upon the Brahman in the manner prescribed. Then, O Devi! let him make japa of th Gayatri one hundred and eight times. Offering the japa to the Devata, let him make obeisance in the way of which I have spoken (106-108). I have now told thee of the sandhya to be used by him in the sadhana of the Brahma-Mantra, and by which the worshipper shall become pure of heart (106-108). Listen to Me now, Thou Who art figured with grace, to the Gayatri, which destroys all sin.

Say "Parameshvara" in the dative singular, then "vidma-he," and, Dear One, after the word "Paratattvaya" say "dhimahi," adding, O Devi! the words, "tanno Brahma prachodayat."

MANTRA

"May we know the Supreme Lord; let us contemplate the Supreme Essence, and may that Brahman direct us."

This is the auspicious Brahma-Gayatri which confers Dharmma, Artha, Kama, and Moksha (109-111).

Let everything which is done, be it worship or sacrifice, bathing, drinking, or eating, be accompanied by the recitation of the Brahma-Mantra (112). When arising at the middle of the fourth quarter of the night, and after bowing to the Preceptor who gave initiation in the Brah-ma-Mantra, let it be recited with all recollection. Then obeisance should be made to the Brahman as aforesaid, after meditating upon Him. This is the enjoined mor-ning rites (113). For Purashcharana, O Beautiful One! japa of the Mantra should be done thirty-two thousand times, for oblations three thousand two hundred times; for the presenting of or offering water to the Devata, three hundred and twenty times; for purification before worship thirty-two times; and Rrahmanas should be

*feasted four times(114-115). In Purashcharana no rule
need be observed touching food or as regards what
should be accepted or rejected. Nor need an auspicious time nor place for performance be selected (116).
Whether he be fasting or have taken food, whether with
or without bathing, let the Sadhaka, as he be so inclined, make sadhana with this supreme Mantra (117).
Without trouble or pain, without hymn, amulet, nyasa,
mudra, or setu, without the worship of Ganesha as the
Thief, yet surely and shortly the most Supreme Brahman
is met face to face (118-119).*

*In the sadhana of this great Mantra no other Sangkalpa
is necessary than the inclination of the mind thereto and
purity of disposition. The worshipper of Brahman sees
Brahman in everything (120). The worshipper does not
sin, nor does he suffer harm should he perchance in such
sadhana omit anything. On the contrary, if there be any
omission, the use of this great Mantra is the remedy
therefor (121). In this terrible and sinful Age devoid
of tapas which is so difficult to traverse, the very seed
of liberation is the use of the Brahma-Mantra (122).
Various Tantras and Agamas have prescribed various
modes of sadhana, but these, O Great Devi! are beyond
the powers of the feeble men of this Age (123). For these,
O Beloved! are short-lived, without enterprise, their life
dependent on food, covetous, eager to gain wealth, so*

unsettled in their intellect that it is without rest, even in its attempts at yoga. Incapable, too, are they of suffering and impatient of the austerities of yoga. For the happiness and liberation of such have been ordained the Way of Brahman (124-125). O Devi! verily and verily I say to You that in this Age there is no other way to happiness and liberation than that by initiation in Brahma-Mantra; I again say to You there is no other way (126). The rule in all the Tantras is that that which is prescribed for the morning should be done in the morning, Sandhya thrice daily and worship at midday, but, O Auspicious One! in the worship of Brahman there is no other rule but the desire of the worshipper (127). Since in Brahma-worship rules are but servants and the prohibitions of other worships do not prevail, who will seek shelter in any other? (128). Let the disciple obtain a Guru who is a knower of Brahman, peaceful and of placid mind, and then, clasping his lotus-like feet, let him supplicate him as follows:

Supplication to the Guru

O merciful one! Lord of the distressed! to thee I have come for protection: cast then the shadows of thy lotus-like feet over my head, oh thou whose wealth is fame (130).

Having thus with all his powers prayed to and worshipped his Guru, let the disciple remain before him in silence with folded hands (131). The Guru will the carefully examine the signs on and qualities of the disciple, kindly call the latter to him, and give to the good disciple the great Mantra (132). Let the wise one sitting on a seat, with his face to the East or to the North place his disciple on his left, and gaze with tenderness upon him (133). The Guru, after performing Rishi-nyasa, will then place his hand on his disciple's head, and for the siddhi of the latter make japa of the Mantra one hundred and eight times (134).

Let the excellent Guru, ocean of kindness, next whisper the Mantra seven times into the right ear of the disciple if he be a Brahmana, or into the left ear if he be of another caste (135). O Kalika! I have now described the manner in which instructions in Brahma-Mantra should be given. For this there is no need of puja, and his Sangkalpa should be mental only (136). The Guru should then raise the disciple, now become his son, who is lying prostrate at his lotus-feet, and say with affection the following (137).

Reply of the Guru

Rise, my son, thou art liberated: Be ever devoted to the

*knowledge of Brahman: Conquer thy passions: May
thou be truthful, and have strength and health (138).*

*Let the excellent disciple on rising make an offering of
his own self, money or a fruit, as he may afford. Remaining obedient to his preceptor's commands, he may then
roam the world like a Deva (139). Immediately upon
his initiation into this Mantra his soul is suffused with
the Divine Being. What need, then, O Deveshi! for such
an one to practise various kinds of sadhana? O Dearest One! I have now briefly told You of the initiation
into the Brahma-Mantra (140). For such initiation the
merciful mood of the Guru is alone necessary (141). The
worshipper of the Divine Power, of Shiva, of the Sun, of
Vishnu, Ganesha, Brahmanas versed in the Vedas and
all other castes may be initiated (142).*

*It is by the grace of this Mantra, O Devi! that I have
become the Deva of Devas, have conquered Death, and
have become the Guru of the whole world. By it I have
done whatever I will, casting from Me ignorance and
doubt (143). Brahma was the First to receive the Mantra
from Me, and He taught it to the Brahmarshis, who
taught it to the Devas. From these the Devarshis learnt
it. The Sages learnt it of these last, and royal Rishis
learnt it of Sages, and all have thus, through the grace
of the Supreme Spirit and this Mantra, become one with*

Brahman (144-145).

*In the use of this Brahma-Mantra, O Great Devi there
are no restrictions. The Guru may without hesitation
give his disciple his own Mantra, a father may initiate
his sons, a brother his brothers, a husband his, wife, a
maternal uncle his nephews, a maternal grand father
his grandsons (146-147). Such fault as elsewhere there is
in other worships, in the giving of one's own Mantra, in
initiation by a father or other near relative does not exist
in the case of this great and successfu Mantra (148). He
who has heard it, however it may be from the lips of one
initiate in the knowledge of Brahman, is purified, and
attains the state of Brahman, and is affected neither by
virtue nor sin (149). The householder of the Brahmanas
and other castes who pray with the Brahma Mantra
should be respected and worshipped as being the greatest
of their respective classes (150).*

*Brahmanas at once become like those who have conqu-
ered their passions, and lower castes become equal to
Brihmanas: therefore let all worship those initiate in the
Brahma-Mantra, and thus possessed of Divine knowledge (151). They who slight them are as wicked as the
slayers of Brahmanas, and go to a terrible Hell,where
they remain as long as the Sun and Stars endure (152).
To revile and calumniate a worshipper of the Supreme*

Brahman is a sin ten million times worse than that of killing a woman or bringing about an abortion (153). As men by initiation in the Brahma-Mantra become freed of all sins, so, O Devi! also may they be freed by the worship of Thee (154).

End of Third Joyful Message, entitled "Description of the Worship of the Supreme Brahman."

CHAPTER 4

Introduction of the Worship of the Supreme Prakriti

*HAVING listened with attention to that which has been
said concerning the worship of the Supreme Brahman,
the Supreme Devi greatly pleased again thus questioned
Shankara (1).*

Shri Devi said:

*O Lord of the Universe and Husband! I bathe with
contentment in the nectar of Thy words concerning the
excellent worship of the Supreme, which lead to the
well-being of the world and to the path of Brahman, and
gives light, intelligence, strength, and prosperity (2-3).
Thou hast said, O Ocean of Mercy! that as union with
the Brahman is attainable through worship of Him, so,
it may be attained by worship of Me (4). I wish to know,
O Lord! of this excellent worship of Myself, which as
Thou sayest is the cause of union of the worshipper with
the Brahman (5). What are its rites, and by what means
may it be accomplished? What is its Mantra, and what
the form of its meditation and mode of worship? (6). O
Shambhu! who but Thee, great Physician of earthly ills,
is fit to speak of it, from its beginning to its end, and in*

all its detail agreeable as it is to Me and beneficent to all humanity? (7).

Hearing the words of the Devi, the Deva of Devas, Husband of Parvati, was delighted, and spoke to Her thus: (8)

Shri Sadashiva said:

Listen, O Thou of high fortune and destiny, to the reasons why Thou shouldst be worshipped, and how thereby the individual becomes united with the Brahman (9). Thou art the only Para Prakriti of the Supreme Soul Brahman, and from Thee has sprung the whole Universe – O Shiva – its Mother (10). O gracious One ! whatever there is in this world, of things which have and are without motion, from Mahat to an atom, owes its origin to and is dependent on Thee (11). Thou art the Original of all the manifestations; Thou art the birthplace of even Us; Thou knowest the whole world, yet none know Thee (12).

Thou art Kali, Tarini, Durga, Shodashi, Bhuvaneshvari, Dhumavati. Thou art Bagala, Bhairavi, and Chhinna-mastaka. Thou art Anna-purna, Vagdevi, Kama-lalaya. Thou art the Image or Embodiment of all the Shaktis and of all the Devas (13-14). Thou art both

Subtle and Gross, Manifested and Veiled, Formless, yet with form. Who can understand Thee? (15). For the accomplishment of the desire of the worshipper, the good of the world, and the destruction of the Danavas, Thou dost assume various forms (16). Thou art four-armed, two-armed, six-armed, and eight-armed, and holdest various missiles and weapons for the protection of the Universe (17). In other Tantras I have spoken of the different Mantras and Yantras, with the use of which Thou shouldst be worshipped according to Thy different forms, and there, too, have I spoken of the different dispositions of men (18). In this Kali Age there is no Pashu-bhava: Divya-bhava is difficult of attainment, but the practices relating to Vira-sadhana yield visible fruit (19).

In this Kali Age, O Devi! success is achieved by Kaulika worship alone, and therefore should it be performed with every care (20). By it, O Devi! is acquired the knowledge of Brahman, and the mortal endowed therewith is of a surety whilst living freed from future births and exonerated from the performance of all religious rites (21). According to human knowledge the world appears to be both pure and impure, but when Brahma-jnana has been acquired there is no distinction between pure and impure (22). For to him who knows that the Brahman is in all things and eternal, what is there that can be impure? (23). Thou art the Image of all, and above all Thou art the Mother of all. If Thou art pleased, O Queen of the Devas! then all are pleased (24).

Before the Beginning of things Thou didst exist in the form of a Darkness which is beyond both speech and mind, and of Thee by the creative desire of the Supreme Brahman was the entire Universe born (25). This Universe, from the great principle of Mahat down to the gross elements, has been created by Thee, since Brahman Cause of all causes is but the instrumental Cause (26). It is the Ever-existent, Changeless, Omnipresent, Pure Intelligence unattached to, yet existing in and enveloping all things (27). It acts not, neither does It enjoy. It moves not, neither is It motionless. It is the Truth and Knowledge, without beginning or end, Ineffable and Incomprehensible (28).

Thou the Supreme Yogini dost, moved by his mere desire, create, protect, and destroy this world with all that moves and is motionless therein (29). Mahakala, the Destroyer of the Universe, is Thy Image. At the Dissolution of things, it is Kala Who will devour all (30), and by reason of this He is called Mahakala, and since Thou devourest Mahakala Himself, it is Thou who art the Supreme Primordial Kalika (31).

Because Thou devourest Kala, Thou art Kali, the original form of all things, and because Thou art the Origin of and devourest all things Thou art called the Adya Kali (32). Resuming after Dissolution Thine own form, dark and formless, Thou alone remainest as One ineffable and inconceivable (33). Though having a form, yet art Thou formless; though Thyself without beginning, multiform by the power of Maya, Thou art the Beginning of all, Creatrix, Protectress, and Destructress that Thou art (34). Hence it is, 0 Gentle One! that whatsoever fruit is attained by initiation in the Brahma-Mantra, the same may be had by the worship of Thee (35).

According to the differences in place, time, and capacity of the worshippers I have, O Devi! in some of the Tantras spoken of secret worship suited to their respective customs and dispositions (36). Where men perform that worship which they are privileged to perform, there they participate in the fruits of worship, and being freed from sin will with safety cross the Ocean of Being (37). By merit acquired in many previous births the mind inclines to Kaulika doctrine, and he whose soul is purified by such worship himself becomes Shiva (38). Where there is abundance of enjoyment, of what use is it to speak of Yoga, and where there is Yoga there is no enjoyment, but the Kaula enjoys both (39).

*If one honours but one man versed in the knowledge
of the essence of Kula doctrine, then all the Devas and
Devis are worshipped – there is no doubt of that (40).*

*The merit gained by honouring a Kaulika is ten million
times that which is acquired by giving away the world
with all its gold (41). A Chandala versed in the knowledge of Kaulika doctrine excels a Brahmana, and a
Brahmana who is wanting in such knowledge is beneath
even a Chandala. (42).*

*I know of no Dharmma superior to that of the Kaulas,
by adherence to which man becomes possessed of Divine
knowledge (43). I am telling Thee the truth, O Devi! Lay
it to the heart and ponder over it. There is no doctrine
superior to the Kaulika doctrine, the most excellent of
all (44). This is the most excellent path kept hidden by
reason of the crowd of Pashus, but when the Kali Age
advances this pathway will be revealed (45).*

*Verily and verily I say unto you that when the Kali
Age reaches the fullness of its strength there will be no
Pashus, and all men on earth will be followers of the
Kaulika doctrine (46). O Vararohe! know that when
Vedic and Puranic initiations cease then the Kali Age
has become strong (47). O Shive! 0 Peaceful One! when
virtue and vice are no longer judged by the Vedic rules,*

then know that the Kali Age has become strong (48).

*O Sovereign Mistress of Kaula doctrine! when the
Heavenly Stream is at some places broken, and at others
diverted from its course, then know that the Kali Age
has become strong (49). O Wise One! when kings of the
Mlechchha race become excessively covetous, then know
that the Kali Age has become strong (50).*

*When women become difficult of control, heartless
and quarrelsome, and calumniators of their husbands,
then know that the Kali Age has become strong (51).
When men become subject to women and slaves of lust,
oppressors of their friends and Gurus, then know that
the Kali Age has become strong (52). When the fertility
of the earth has gone and yields a poor harvest, when
the clouds yield scanty rain, and trees give meagre fruit,
then know that the Kali Age has become strong (53).
When brothers, kinsmen, and companions, prompted
by the desire for some trifle, will strike one another, then
know that the Kali Age has become strong (54). When
the open partaking of flesh and liquor will pass without
condemnation and punishment, when secret drinking
will prevail, then know that the Kali Age has become
strong (55).*

As in the Satya, Treta, and Dvapara Ages wine and the

like could be taken, so they may be taken in the Kali Age in accordance with the Kaulika Dharmma (56). The Kali Age cannot harm those who are purified by truth, who have conquered their passions and senses, who are open in their ways, without deceit, are compassionate and follow the Kaula doctrine (57). The Kali Age cannot harm those who are devoted to the services of their Guru, to the lotus of their mothers' feet, and to their own wives (58). The Kali Age cannot harm those who are vowed to and grounded in truth, adherents of the true Dharmma, and faithful to the performance of Kaulika rites and duties (59). The Kali Age cannot harm those who give to the truthful Kaulika Yogi the elements of worship, which have been previously purified by Kaulika rites (60).

The Kali Age cannot harm those who are free of malice, envy, arrogance, and hatred, and who are firm in the faith of Kaulika dharmma (61). The Kali Age cannot harm those who keep the company of Kaulikas, or live with Kaulika Sages, or serve the Kaulikas (62). The Kali Age cannot harm those Kaulikas who, whatever they may appear outwardly to be, yet remain firm in their Kaulika Dharmma, worshipping Thee according to its doctrine (63). The Kali Age cannot harm those who perform their ablutions, charities, penances, pilgrimages, devotions, and offerings of water according to the Kaulika ritual (64).

The Kali Age cannot harm those who perform the ten
purificatory ceremonies, such as the blessing of the
womb, obsequial ceremonies of their fathers, and other
rites according to Kaulika ritual (65). The Kali Age
cannot harm those who respect the Kaula-tattva, Kau-
la-dravya, and Kaula-yogi (66).

The Kali Age is but the slave of those who are free of all
crookedness and falsehood, men of candour, devoted
to the good of others, who follow Kaulika ways (67). In
spite of its many blemishes, the Kali Age possesses one
great merit, that from the mere intention of a Kaulika
of firm resolution desired result ensues (68). In the other
Ages, O Devi! effort of will produced both religious
merit and demerit, but in the Kali Age men by intention
merely acquire merit only, and not demerit (68). The
slaves of the Kali Age, on the other hand, are those who
know not Kulachara, and who are ever untruthful and
the persecutors of others (70). They too are the slaves of
the Kali Age who have no faith in Kulacharas, who lust
after others' wives, and hate them who are faithful to
Kaulika doctrine (71).

In speaking of the customs of the different Ages, I have,
O Gentle One! and out of love, O Parvati! truly re-
counted to Thee the signs of the dominance of the Kali
Age (72). When the Kali Age is made manifest, piety is

enfeebled and Truth alone remains; therefore should one be truthful (73). O Thou Virtuous One! know this for certain, that whatsoever man does with Truth that bears fruit (74). There is no Dharmma higher than Truth, there is no sin greater than falsehood; therefore should man seek protection under Truth with all his soul (75). Worship without Truth is useless, and so too without Truth is the Japa of Mantras and the performance of Tapas. It is in such cases just as if one sowed seed in salt earth (76).

Truth is the appearance of the Supreme Brahman; Truth is the most excellent of all Tapas; every act is rooted in Truth. Than Truth there is nothing more excellent (77). Therefore has it been said by Me that when the sinful Kali Age is dominant, Kaula ways should be practised truthfully and without concealment (78). Truth is divorced from concealment. There is no concealment without untruth. Therefore is it that the Kaulika-sadhaka, should perform his Kaulika-sadhana openly (79). What I have said in other Kaulika Tantras about the concealment of Kaulika-dharmma not being blameworthy is not applicable when the Kali Age becomes strong (80).

In the (First or) Satya. Age, O Devi! Virtue possessed the four quarters of its whole; in the Treta Age it lost one-quarter of its Virtue; in the Dvapara Age there was *of Virtue but two quarters, and in the Kali Age it has but one (81). In spite of that Truth will remain strong, though Tapas and Charity become weakened. If Truth goes Virtue goes also, therefore of all acts Truth should be the abiding support (82). O Sovereign Mistress of the Kaula-Dharmma! since men can in this Age have recourse to Kaulika Dharmma only, if that doctrine be itself infected with untruth, how can there be liberation? (83). With his soul purified in every way by Truth, man should, according to his caste and stage of life, perform the following acts in the manner shown by Me (84): initiation, worship, recitation of Mantras, the worship of Fire with ghee, repetition of Mantras, private devotions, marriage, the conception ceremony, and that performed in the fourth, sixth, or eighth months of pregnancy, the natal rite, the naming and tonsure ceremonies, and obsequial rites upon cremation and after death. All such ceremonies should be performed in the manner appro-ved by the Agamas (85-86).*

The ritual which I have ordained should be followed, too, as regards Shraddha at holy places, dedication of a bull, the autumnal festival, on setting out on a jour-ney, on the first entry into a house, the wearing of new clothes or jewels, dedication of tanks, wells, or lakes, in the ceremonies performed at the phases of the Moon, the building and consecration of houses, the installation of

Devas, and in all observances to be performed during the day or at night, in each month, season, or year, and in observances both daily or occasional, and also in deciding generally what ought and what ought not to be done, and in determining what ought to be rejected and what ought to be adopted (87-90). Should one not follow the ritual ordained, whether from ignorance, wickedness, or irreverence, then one is disqualified for all observances, and becomes a worm in dung (91). O Maheshi! if when the Kali Age has become very powerful any act be done in violation of My precepts, then that which happens is the very contrary of that which is desired (92). Initiation of which I have not approved destroys the life of the disciple, and his act of worship is as fruitless as oblations poured on ashes, and the Deva whom he worships becomes angry or hostile, and at every step he encounters danger (93). Ambika! he who during the dominance of the Kali Age, knowing My ordinances, yet performs his religious observances in other ways, is a great sinner (94). The man who performs any Vrata, or marries according to other ways, will remain in a terrible Hell so long as the Sun and Moon endure (95). By his performance of Vrata he incurs the sin of killing a Brahmana, and similarly by being invested with the sacred thread he is degraded. He merely wears the thread, and is lower than a Chandala (96), and so too the woman who is married according to other ways than Mine is to be despised, and, 0 Sovereign Mistress of the Kaulas! the man who so marries is her associate in wrong, and is day after day guilty of the sin of going with a prostitute (97). From him the Devata will not accept food, water, and other offerings, nor will the Pitris eat his offerings, considering them to be as it were mere dung and pus (98). Their children are bastards, and disqualified for all religious, ancestral, and Kaulika observances and rites (99). To an image dedicated by rites other than those prescribed by Shambhu the Deva never comes. Benefit there is none either in this or the next world. There is but mere waste of labour and money (100).

A Shraddha performed according to other rites than those prescribed by the Agamas is fruitless, and he who performs it will go to Hell together with his Pitris (101). The water offered by him is like blood, and the funeral cake like dung. Let the mortal then follow with great care the precepts of Shankara (102). What is the need of saying more? Verily and verily I say to You, O Devi! that all that is done in disregard of the precepts of Shambhu is fruitless (103). For him who follows not His precepts there is no future merit. That which has been already acquired is destroyed, and for him there is no escape from Hell (104). O Great Ruler! the performance of daily and occasional duties in the manner spoken of by Me is the same as worshipping Thee (105). Listen, O Devi! to the particulars of the worship with its Mantras and Yantras, which is the medicine for the ills of the Kali Age (106).

End of the Fourth Chapter, entitled "Introduction of the Worship of the Supreme Prakriti."

CHAPTER 5

The Formation of the Mantras, Placing of the Jar, and Purification of the Elements of Worship

Thou art the Adya Parama Shakti, Thou art all Power. It is by Thy power that We (the Trinity) are powerful in the acts of creation, preservation, and destruction. Endless and of varied colour and form are Thy appearances, and various are the strenuous efforts whereby the worshippers may realize them. Who can describe them? (1-2). In the Kula Tantras and Agamas I have, by the aid of but a small part of Thy mercies and with all My powers, described the Sadhana and Archana of Thy appearances; yet nowhere else is this very secret Sadhana revealed. It is by the grace of this (Sadhana), O Blessed One! that Thy mercy in Me is so great (3-4). Questioned by Thee I am no longer able to conceal it. For Thy pleasure, O Beloved! I shall speak of that which is dearer to Me than even life itself (5). To all sufferings it brings relief. It wards off all dangers. It gives Thee pleasure, and is the way by which Thou art most swiftly obtained (6). For men rendered wretched by the taint of the Kali Age, short-lived and unfit for strenuous effort, this is the greatest wealth (7). In this (sadhana) there is no need for a multiplicity of Nyasa, for fasting or other practices of self-restraint. It is simple and pleasurable, yet yields great fruit to the worshipper (8). Then first listen, O Devi! to the Mantroddhara of the Mantra, the mere hearing of which liberates man from future births while yet living (9).

By placing "Pranesha" on "Taijasa," and adding to it "Bherunda" and the Vindu, the first Vija is formed. After this, proceed to the second (to). By placing "Sandhya" on "Rakta," and adding to it "Vama-netra" and Vindu, the second Mantra is formed. Now listen, O Blessed One! to the formation of the third Mantra.

Prajapati is placed on Dipa, and to them is added Govinda and Vindu. It yields happiness to the worshippers: After making these three Mantras add the word Parameshvari in the vocative, and then the word for Vahni-kanta. Thus, O Blessed One! is the Mantra of ten letters formed. This Vidya of the Supreme Devi contains in itself all Mantras (11-13).

The most excellent worshipper should for the attainment of wealth and all his desires make Japa of each or all of the first three Vijas (14). By omitting the first three Devi the Vidya of ten letters become one of seven. By prefixing the Vija of Kama, or the Vagbhava, or the Tara, three Mantras of eight letters each are formed (15).

*At the end of the Mantra of ten letters the word Kalika
in the vocative should be uttered, and then the first three
Vija, followed by the name of the Wife of Vahni (16).
This Vidya is called Shodashi, and is concealed in all
the Tantras. If it be prefixed by the Vija of Vadhu or by
the Pranava, two Mantras of seventeen letters each are
formed (17).*

*O Beloved! there are tens of millions upon tens of mil-
lions, nay an hundred millions, nay countless Mantras
for Thy worship. I have here but shortly stated twelve
of them (18). Whatsoever Mantras are set forth in the
various Tantras, they are all Thine, since Thou art the
Adya Prakriti (19). There is but one sadhana in the case
of all these Mantras, and of that I shall speak for Thy
pleasure and the benefit of humanity (20).*

*Without Kulachara, O Devi! the Shakti-Mantra is
powerless to give success, and therefore the worshipper
should worship the Shakti with Kulachara rites*

*O Adya! the five essential Elements in the worship of
Shakti have been prescribed to be Wine, Meat, Fish,
parched Grain, and the Union of man with woman
(22). The worship of Shakti without these five elements
is but the practice of evil magic. That Siddhi which is
the object of sadhana is never attained thereby, and ob-*

stacles are encountered at every step (23). As seed sown on barren rocks does not germinate, so worship without these five elements is fruitless (24).

Without the prior performance of the morning rites a man is not qualified to perform the others. And therefore, O Devi! I shall first speak of those which are to be performed in the morning (25). In the second half of the last quarter of the night the disciple should rise from sleep. Having seated himself and shaken off drowsiness, let him meditate upon the image of his Guru:

Dhyana

As two-eyed and two-armed, situate in the white lotus of the head (26); clad in white raiment, engarlanded with white flowers, smeared with sandal paste. With one hand he makes the sign which dispels fear, and with the other that which bestows blessings. He is calm, and is the image of mercy. On his left his Shakti, holding in her hand a lotus, embraces him. He is smiling and gracious, the bestower of the fulfilment of the desires of his disciples (27-28).

O Kuleshvari! the disciple should, after having thus meditated upon his Teacher and worshipped him with the articles of mental worship, make Japa with the excellent Mantra, the Vagbhava-Vija. (29).

After doing Japa of the Mantra as best lies in his power, the wise disciple should, after placing the Japa in the right palm of his excellent Guru, bow before him, saying meanwhile the following (30):

Mantra

I bow to thee, O Sad-guru,

Thou who destroyeth the bonds which hold us to this world,

Thou who bestoweth the vision of Wisdom,

Together with worldly enjoyment and final liberation,

Dispeller of ignorance,

Revealer of the Kula-dharmma,

Image in human form of the Supreme Brahman (31-32).

The disciple, having thus made obeisance to his Guru, should meditate upon his Ishta-devata, and worship Her as aforesaid, inwardly reciting the Mula-mantra meanwhile (33). Having done this to the best of his powers, he should place the Japa in the left palm of the

Devi, and then make obeisance to his Ishta-devata with
the following (34):

Mantra

To thee I bow Who art one with, and the Supporter of,
the Universe,

I bow to Thee again and yet again, the Adya Kalika,
both Creatrix and Destructress (35).

Having thus made obeisance to the Devi, he should
leave his house, placing his left foot first, and then make
water, discharge his bowels, and cleanse his teeth (36).
He then should go towards some water, and make his
ablutions in the manner prescribed (37). First of all
let him rinse his mouth, and then enter the water, and
stand therein up to his navel. He should then cleanse his
body by a single immersal only, and then, standing up
and rubbing himself, rinse his mouth, saying the Mantra
the while (38). That best of worshippers, the Kula-Sad-
haka, should then sip a little water and say:

Mantra

Atma-tattvaya Svaha

After that he should again sip water twice, followed in each case by the

Mantras

Vidya-tattvaya Svaha.

Shiva-tattvaya Svaha, respectively. Lastly, he should rinse the upper lip twice (39).

Then, O Beloved! the wise disciple should draw on the water the Kula-yantra with the Mantra in its centre, and do Japa over it with the Mula-mantra twelve times (40). Then meditating on the Water as the Image of Fire, let him offer it thrice to the Sun in his joined palms. Sprinkling it thrice over his head, let him close the seven openings therein (41). Then for the pleasure of the Devi he should immerse himself thrice, leave the water, dry his body, and put on two pieces of clean cloth.

Tying up his hair whilst reciting the Gayatri, he should mark on his forehead with pure earth or ashes the tilaka and tri-pundra, with a Vindu over it (42). Let the worshipper then perform both the Vaidika and Tantrika forms of Sandhya in their respective order. Listen while I now describe to you the Tantrika Sandhya (4g).

After rinsing his mouth in the manner described, he should, O Blessed One! invoke into the water the Waters of the holy Rivers thus (45):

Mantra

O Ganga, Yamuna, Godavari, Sarasvati, Narmmada,

Sindhu, Kaveri, come into this water (46).

The intelligent worshipper having invoked the sacred Rivers with this Mantra, and made the angkusha-mudra, should do Japa with the Mula-mantra twelve times (47). Let him then again utter the Mula-mantra, and with the middle and nameless fingers joined together throw drops of that water thrice upon the ground (48).

He should then sprinkle his head seven times with the water, and taking some in the palm of his left hand cover it up with his right (49). Then inwardly reciting the Vija of Ishana, Vayu, Varuna, Vahni, and Indra four times, the water should be transferred to the right palm (50). Seeing (in his mind's eye) and meditating upon the water as Fire, the worshipper should draw it through the nose by Ida, expel it through Pingala (into his palm), and so wash away all inward impurity (51).

The worshipper should then three times dash the water (so expelled into his palm) against an (imaginary) adamant. Uttering the Astra-Mantra, let him then wash his hands (52). Then rinsing his mouth, oblation of water should be offered to the Sun with the following (53):

Mantra

Ong Hring Hangsa

To Thee, O Sun, full of heat, shining, effulgent, I offer this oblation; Svaha (54).

Then let him meditate morning, midday, and evening upon the great Devi Gayatri, the Supreme Devi, as manifested in her three different forms and according to the three qualities (55).

Dhyana

In the morning meditate upon Her in Her Brahmi form, as a Maiden of ruddy hue, with a pure smile, with two hands, holding a gourd full of holy water, garlanded with crystal beads, clad in the skin of a black antelope, seated on a Swan (56). At midday meditate upon Her in Her Vaishnavi form, of the colour of pure gold, youthful, with full and rising breasts, situated in the Solar disc, with four hands holding the conch-shell, discus, mace, and lotus, seated on Garuda, garlanded with wild-flowers (57-58). In the evening the Yati should meditate upon Her as of a white colour, clad in white raiment, old and long past her youth, with three eyes, beneficent, propitious, seated on a Bull, holding in Her lotus-like hands a noose, a trident, a lance, and a skull (59-60).

Having thus meditated on the great Devi Gayatri, and offered water three times in the hollow of his joined hands, the worshipper should make Japa with the Gayatri either ten or a hundred times (61). Listen now, O Devi of the Devas! while I out of my love for Thee recite the Gayatri (62).

After the word "Adyayai" say "vidmahe," and then "Parameshvaryyai dhimahi: tannah Kali prachodayat." This is Thy Gayatri which destroys all great sins (63). The inward recitation of this Vidya thrice daily obtains the fruit of the performance of Sandhya. Water should then be offered to the Devas, Rishis, and the Pitris (64). First say the Pranava, and then the name of the Deva (the Rishi or the Pitri) in the accusative case, and after that the words "tarpayami namah." When, however, oblation is offered to Shakti, the Maya Vija should be said in place of the Pranava, and in lieu of Namah the Mantra Svaha (65).

After uttering the Mula-mantra, say "Sarvva-bhuta-ni-vasinyai," and then "Sarvva-svarupa" and "Sayudha" in the dative singular, as also "Savarana" and "Paratpara," and then "Adyayai, Kalikayai, te, idam arghyam: Svaha" (66-67). (When the Mantra will be.)

Mantra

Hring, Shring, Kring, to the Supreme Devi. O Supreme Devi, Thou Who dwelleth in all things and Whose image all things are, Who art surrounded by attendant deities, and Who bearest arms, Who art above even the most high to Thee, Who art the Adya Kalika, I offer this oblation: Svaha.

Having offered this arghya to the Mahadevi, the wise one should make Japa with the Mula-mantra with all his powers, and then place the Japa in the left hand of the Devi (68). Then let the Sadhaka bow to the Devi, take such water as is needed for his worship, bowing to the water whence he has drawn it, and proceed to the place of worship, earnestly meditating on and reciting hymns of praise to the Devi meanwhile. On his arrival there let him wash his hands and feet, and then make in front of the door the Samanyarghya (69-70). The wise one should draw a triangle, and outside it a circle, and outside the circle a square, and after worshipping the

243

Adhara-shakti place the vessel on the figure (71).

Let him wash the vessel with the Weapon-Mantra, and while filling it with water let him say the Heart-Mantra. Then, throwing flowers and perfume into the water, let him invoke the holy Rivers into it (72). Worshipping Fire, Sun, and Moon in the water of the vessel, let him say the Maya Vija over it (73). The Dhenu and Yoni Mudras should then be shown. This is known as Samanyarghya. With the water and flowers of this oblation the Devata of the entrance to the place of worship should be worshipped (74), such as Ganesha, Kshetrapala, Vatuka, Yogini, Ganga, Yamuna, Lakshmi, and Vani (75). The wise one, lightly touching that part of the door-frame which is on his left, should then enter the place of worship with his left foot forward, meditating the while on the lotus-feet of the Devi (76). Then, after worship of the presiding Deva of the site, and of Brahma in the south-west corner, the place of worship should be cleansed with water taken from the common offering (77). Let the best of worshippers then with a steady gaze remove all celestial obstacles, and by the repetition of the Weapon-Mantra remove all obstacles in the Anta-riksha (78).

Striking the ground three times with his heel, let him drive away all earthly obstacles, and then fill the place of worship with the incense of burning sandal, fragrant aloe, musk, and camphor. He should then mark off a rectangular space as his seat, draw a triangle within it, and therein worship Kama-rupa with the

Mantra

To Kama-rupa, Namah: (79-80).

Then for his seat spreading a mat over it, let him worship the Adhara-Shakti with the

Mantra

Kling, Obeisance to the Adhara-Shakti of the lotus-seat (81).

The learned worshipper should then seat himself according to the "tied heroic" mode, with his face towards the East or the North, and should consecrate the Vijaya (81). (With the following)

Mantra

Ong Hring. Ambrosia, that springeth from ambrosia, Thou that showereth ambrosia, draw ambrosia for me again and again. Bring Kalika within my control. Give siddhi; Svaha.

This is the Mantra for the consecration of Vijaya (83-84). Then inwardly reciting the Mula-mantra seven times over the Vijaya, show the Dhenu, the Yoni, the Avahani, and other Mudras (85).

Then satisfy the Guru who resides in the Lotus of a thousand petals by thrice offering the Vijaya with the Sangketa-Mudra, and the Devi in the heart by thrice offering the Vijaya with the same Mudra, and reciting the Mula-mantra (86). Then offer oblations to the mouth of the Kundali, with the Vijaya reciting the following

Mantra

Aing (0 Devi Sarasvati), Thou Who art the Ruler of all the essences, do Thou inspire me, do Thou inspire me, and remain ever on the tip of my tongue; Svaha (87).

After drinking the Vijaya he should bow to the Guru, placing his folded palms over the left ear, then to Ganesha, placing his folded palms over his right ear, and lastly to the Eternal Adya Devi, by placing his folded palms in the middle of his forehead, and should the meanwhile meditate on the Devi. (88).

The wise worshipper should place the articles necessary for worship on his right, and scented water and other

Kula articles on his left (89). Saying the Mula-mantra terminated by the Weapon-Mantra, let him take water from the common offering and sprinkle the articles of worship with it, and then enclose himself and the articles in a circle of water. After that, O Devi! let him by the Vahni Vija surround them with a wall of fire (90). Then for the purification of the palms of his hands he should take up a flower which has been dipped in sandal paste, rub it between the palms, reciting meanwhile the Mantra Phat, and throw it away (91).

Then in the following manner let him fence all the quarters so that no obstructions proceed from them. Join the first and second fingers of the right hand, and tap the palm of the left hand three times, each time after the first with greater force, thus making a loud sound, and then snap the fingers while uttering the weapon-Mantra (92). He should then proceed to perform the purification of the elements of his body. The excellent disciple should place his hands in his lap with the palms upwards, and fixing his mind on the Muladhara Chakra let him rouse Kundalini by uttering the Vija "Hung." Having so roused Her, let him lead Her with Prithivi by means of the Hangsa Mantra to the Svadhishthana Chakra, and let him there dissolve each one of the elements of the body by means of another of such elements (93-94). Then let him dissolve Prithivi together with odour, as also the organ of smell, into water. Dissolve water and taste, as also the sense of taste itself, into Fire (95). Dissolve Fire and vision and form, and the sense of sight itself, into air (96).

Let air and touch, as also the sense of touch itself, be dissolved into ether. Dissolve ether and sound into the conscious Self and the Self into Mahat, Mahat itself into Prakriti, and Prakriti Herself into Brahman (97). Let the wise one, having thus dissolved (the twenty-four) tatt-vas, then think of an angry black man in the left side of the cavity of his abdomen of the size of his thumb with red beard and eyes, holding a sword and shield, with his head ever held low, the very image of all sins (98-99).

Then the foremost of disciples should, thinking of the purple Vayu Vija as on his left nostril, inhale through that nostril sixteen times. By this let him dry the sinful body (100). Next, meditating on the red Vija of Agni as being situate in the navel, the body with all its sinful inclinations should be burnt up by the fire born of the Vija, as also by sixty-four Kumbhakas (101). Then, thinking of the white Varuna Vija in his forehead, let him bathe (the body which has been so burnt) with the nectar-like water dropping from the Varuna Vija by thirty-two exhalations (102).

Having thus bathed the whole body from feet to head, let him consider that a Deva body has come into being (103). Then, thinking of the yellow Vija of the Earth as situate in the Muladhara circle, let him strengthen his body by that Vija and by a steadfast and winkless gaze (104). Placing his hand on his heart and uttering the

Mantra

Ang, Hring, Krong, Hangsah, So'hang.

let him infuse into his body the life of the Devi (105).

O Ambika! having thus purified the elements (the disciple) with a mind well under control, and intent upon the nature of the Devi, should do Matrika-nyasa. The Rishi of Matrika is Brahma, and the verse is Gayatri, and Matrika is presiding Devi thereof; the consonants are its Seed, and the vowels its Shaktis, and Visarga is the End. In Lipi-nyasa, O Mahadevi! each letter should be separately pronounced as it is placed in the different parts of the body. Having similarly performed Rishi-ny-asa, Kara-nyasa and Ang-ga-nyasa should be perfor-med (106-108).

O Beauteous Face! the Mantras enjoined for Shad-ang-ga-nyasa are Ka-varga between Ang and Āng, Cha-var-

ga between Ĭng and Īng, Ta-varga between Ŭng and Ūng, Ta-varga between Eng and Aing, and Pa-varga between Ong and Aung, and the letters from Ya to Ksha between Vindu and Visarga respectively (109-110), and having placed the letters according to the rules of Nyasa, the Sadhaka should then meditate upon Sarasvati:

Dhyana

I seek refuge in the Devi of Speech, three-eyed, encircled with a white halo, whose face, hands, feet, middle body, and breast are composed of the fifty letters of the alphabet, on whose radiant forehead is the crescent moon, whose breasts are high and rounded, and who with one of her lotus hands makes Jnana-mudra, and with the other holds the rosary of Rudraksha beads, the jar of nectar, and learning (112).

Having thus meditated upon the Devi Matrika, place the letters in the six Chakras as follows: Ha and Kska in the Ajna Lotus, the sixteen vowels in the Vishuddha Lotus, the letters from Ka to Tha in the Anahata Lotus, the letters from Da to Pha in Manipura Lotus, the letters from Ba to La in the Svadhishthana Lotus, and in the Muladhara Lotus the letters Va to Sa. And having thus in his mind placed these letters of the alphabet, let the worshipper place them outwardly (113-115). Having placed them on the forehead, the face, eyes, ears, nose, cheeks, upper lip, teeth, head, hollow of the mouth, back, the hump of the back, navel, belly, heart, shoulders, (four) joints in the arms, end of the arms, heart, (four) joints of the legs, ends of legs, and on all parts from the heart to the two arms, from the heart to the two legs, from the heart to the mouth, and from the heart to the different parts as above indicated, Pranayama should be performed (116-118). Draw in the air by the left nostril whilst muttering the Maya Vija sixteen times, then fill up the body by Kumbhaka by stopping the passage of both the nostrils with the little, third finger, and thumb whilst making japa of the Vija sixty-four times, and, lastly, exhale the air through the right nostril whilst making japa of the Vija thirty-two times (119-120). The doing of this thrice through the right and left nostrils alternately is Pranayama.

After this has been done, Rishi-nyasa should be perfor-med (121). The Revealers of the Mantra are Brahma and the Brahmarshis, the metre is of the Gayatri and other forms, and its presiding Devata is the Adya Kali (122). The Vija is the Vija of the Adya, its Shakti is the Maya Vija, and that which comes at the end is the Kamala Vija (123). Then the Mantra should be assigned to the head, mouth, heart, anus, the two feet, and all the parts of the body (123). The passing of the two hands

*three or seven times over the whole body from the feet
to the head, and from the head to the feet, making japa
meanwhile of the Mula-mantra, is called Vyapaka-nyasa, which yields the declared result (124).*

*O Beloved! by adding in succession the six long vowels to
the first Vija of the Mula-mantra, six Vidya are formed.
The wise worshipper should in Angga-kalpana utter in
succession these or the Mula-mantra alone (125), and
then say "to the two thumbs," "to the two index fingers,"
"to the two middle fingers," "to the two ring fingers," "to
the two little fingers," "to the front and back of the two
palms," concluding with Namah, Svaha, Vashat, Hung,
Vaushat, and Phat in their order respectively (126).*

*When touching the heart say "Namah," when touching
the head "Svaha," and when touching the crown lock
thereon "Vashat." Similarly, when touching the two
upper portions of the arms, the three eyes and the two
palms, utter the Mantras Hung and Vaushat and Phat
respectively. In this manner nyasa of the six parts of
the body should be practised, and then the Vira should
proceed to Pithanyasa (127-128). Then let the Vira
place in the lotus of the heart, the Adhara-shakti, the
tortoise, Shesha serpent, Prithivi, the ocean of ambrosia, the Gem Island, the Parijata tree, the chamber of
gems which fulfil all desires, the jewelled altar, and the*

lotus seat (129-130). Then he should place on the right shoulder, the left shoulder, the right hip, the left hip, respectively and in their order, Dharmma, Jnana, Aishvaryya, and Vairagya (131), and the excellent worshipper should place the negatives of these qualities on the mouth, the left side, the navel, and the right side respectively (132). Next let him place in the heart Ananda Kanda, Sun, Moon, Fire, the three qualities, adding to the first of their letters the sign Vindu, and the filaments and pericarp of the Lotus, and let him place in the petals of the lotus the eight Pitha Nayikas – Mangala, Vijaya, Bhadra, Jayanti, Aparajita, Nandini, Narasinghi, Vaishnavi, and in the tips of the petals of the lotus the eight Bhairavas – Asitanga, Chanda, Kapali, Krodha, Bhishana, Unmatta, Ruru, Sanghari (133-135).

Then the worshipper should, after forming his hands into the Kachchhapa Mudra, take two fragrant flowers, and, placing his hands on his heart, let him meditate upon the ever-existent Devi (136). The nature of meditation upon Thee, O Devi! is of two kinds, according as Thou art imagined formless or with a form. As formless Thou art ineffable and incomprehensible, imperceptible. Of Thee it cannot be said that Thou art either this or that, Thou art omnipresent, unobtainable, attainable only by Yogis through penances and acts of self-restraint (137-138). I will now speak of meditation upon Thee in

*corporeal form in order that the mind may learn con-
centration, that desires be speedily achieved, and that
the power to meditate according to the subtle form may
be aroused (139).*

*The form of the greatly lustrous Kalika, Mother of Kala
Who devours all things, is imagined according to Her
qualities and actions (140).*

Dhyana

*I adore the Adya Kalika Whose body is of the hue of
the (dark) rain-cloud, upon Whose forehead the Moon
gleams, the three-eyed One, clad in crimson raiment,
Whose two hands are raised – the one to dispel fear, and
the other to bestow blessing – Who is seated on a red
lotus in full bloom, Her beautiful face radiant, watching
Maha-Kala, Who, drunk with the delicious wine of the
Madhuka flower, is dancing before Her (141).*

*After having meditated upon the Devi in this form, and
placed a flower on his head, let the devotee with all devotion worship Her with the articles of mental worship
(142). Let him offer the lotus of the heart for Her seat,
the ambrosia trickling from the lotus of a thousand petals for the washing of Her feet, and his mind as arghya
(143). Then let him offer the same ambrosia as water for*

*rinsing of Her mouth and bathing of Her body, let him
offer the essence of the ether to be raiment of the Devi,
the essence of scent to be the perfumes, his own heart
and vital air the essence of fire, and the ocean of nectar
to be respectively the flowers, incense, light, and food
offerings (of worship).*

*Let him offer the sound in the Anahata Chakra for
the ringing of the bell, the essence of the air for the fan
and fly-whisk, and the functions of the senses and the
restlessness of the mind for the dance before the Devi
(144-146). Let various kinds of flowers be offered for the
attainment of the object of one's desire: amaya, ana-
hangkara, araga, amada, amoha, adambha, advesha,
akshobha, amatsaryya, alobha, and thereafter the five
flowers – namely, the most excellent flowers, ahingsa,
indriya-nigraha, daya, kshama, and jnana. With these
fifteen flowers, fifteen qualities of disposition, he should
worship the Devi (147-149).*

*Then let him offer (to the Devi) the ocean of ambrosia, a
mountain of meat and fried fish, a heap of parched food,
grain cooked in milk with sugar and ghee, the Kula
nectar, the Kula flower, and the water which has been
used for the washing of the Shakti. Then, having sacrificed all lust and anger, the cause of all impediments, let
him do japa (150-151).*

The mala (rosary) prescribed consists of the letters of the alphabet, strung on Kundalini as the thread (152). After reciting the letters of the alphabet from A to La, with the Vindu superposed upon each, the Mula-mantra should be recited. This is known as Anuloma. Again, beginning with La and ending with A, let the sadhaka make japa of the Mantra. This is known as Viloma and Ksha-kara is called the Meru (153-154).

The last letters of the eight groups should be added to the Mula-mantra, and having made japa of this Mantra of one hundred and eight letters the japa should be offered (to the Devi) with the following (155):

Mantra

O Adya Kali, Who abidest in the innermost soul of all, Who art the innermost light, O Mother! accept this japa of my heart. I bow to Thee (156).

Having finished the japa, he should mentally prostrate himself, touching the ground with the eight parts of his body. Having concluded the mental worship, let him commence the outer worship (157).

I am now speaking of the consecration of the Vishesh-arghya, by the mere placing whereof the Devata is exceedingly pleased. Do Thou listen (158). At the mere sight of the cup of this offering the Yoginis, Bhairavas, Brahma, and other Devatas dance for joy and grant siddhi (159). The disciple should on the ground in front of him and on his left draw with water taken from the Samanyarghya a triangle, with the Maya Vija in its centre, outside the triangle a circle, and outside the circle a square, and let him there worship the Shakti of the Adhara with the Mantra

Hring!

Obeisance to the Shakti of the Adhara (160-161).

He should then wash the Adhara, and place it on the Mandala, and worship the region of Fire with the

Mantra

Mang!

Obeisance to the circle of Fire possessed of ten sections.

And having washed the arghya vessel with the Mantra Phat, the worshipper should place it on the Adhara with the Mantra Namah (162-163). He should then worship the cup with the

Mantra

Ang!

Obeisance to the circle of Sun who has twelve divisions;

*and fill the vessel (in which the offering is made) whilst
repeating the Mula-mantra three parts with wine and
one part with water, and having placed scent and flower
in it, he should there worship, O Mother! with the Mantra following (164-165):*

Mantra

Ung!

Obeisance to the Moon with its sixteen digits (166).

*He should then place in front of the special offering,
on bael leaves dipped in red sandal paste, durva grass,
flowers, and sun-dried rice (167).*

*Having invoked the holy waters (of the sacred Ri-
vers into the arghya) by the Mula-mantra and Angkusha-mudra, the Sadhaka should meditate upon
the Devi, and worship Her with incense and flowers,
making japa of the Mula-mantra twelve times (168).*

*After this let him display over the arghya the Dhenu
Mudra and the Yoni Mudra, incense sticks and a light.
The worshipper should then pour a little water from the
arghya into the vessel kept for that purpose, and sprinkle
himself and the offering therewith. The vessel containing the offering must not, however, be moved until the
worship is concluded (169-170). O Thou of pure Smiles!
I have now spoken of the consecration of the special
offering. I will now pass to the principal Yantra which
grants the aims of all human existence (171).*

*Draw a triangle with the Maya Vija within it, and
around it two concentric circles (the one outside the
other). In the space between the two circumferences
of the circles draw in pairs the sixteen filaments, and
outside these the eight petals of the lotus, and outside
them the Bhu-pura, which should be made of straight
lines with four entrances, and be of pleasing appearance
(172-173). In order to cause pleasure to the Devata the
disciple should (reciting the Mula-mantra the meanwhile) draw the Yantra either with a gold needle, or with
the thorn of a bael tree on a piece of gold, silver, or
copper, which has been smeared with either the Svayambhu, Kunda, or Gola flowers, or with sandal, fragrant
aloe, kungkuma, or with red sandal paste. A clever
carver may also carve the Yantra on crystal, coral, or
lapis lazuli (174-176).*

After it has been consecrated by auspicious rites, it should be kept inside the house; and on this being done all wicked ghosts, all apprehensions from (adverse) planets, and diseases are destroyed; and by the grace of this Yantra the worshipper's house becomes of pleasing aspect. With his children and grandchildren, and with happiness and dominion, he becomes a bestower of gifts and charities, a protector of his dependents, and his fame goes abroad (177-178). After having drawn the Yantra and placed it on a jewelled altar in front of the worshipper, and having worshipped the Devata of the Pitha according to the rules of Pitha-nyasa, the principal Devi should be adored in the pericarp of the Lotus (179).

I will now speak of the placing of the jar and the formation of the circle of worship by the mere institution of which the Devata is well pleased, the Mantra becomes fruitful, and the wishes of the worshipper are accomplished (180). The jar is called kalasa, because Vishva-karma made it from the different parts of each of the Devatas (181).

It should be thirty-six fingers breadth (in circumference) in its widest part, and sixteen in height. The neck should be four fingers breadth, the mouth six fingers, and the bottom five fingers breadth. This is the rule for the design of the kalasha (182). It should be made either of gold, silver, copper, bell-metal, mud, stone, or glass, and without hole or crack. In its making all miserliness should be avoided, since it is fashioned for the pleasure of the Devas (183). A kalasha of gold, one of silver, one of copper, and one of bell-metal give enjoyment, emancipation, pleasure of mind, and nourishment respectively to the worshipper. One of crystal is good for the attainment of Vashikarana, and one of stone for the attainment of Stambhana. A kalasha made of mud is good for all purposes. Whatever it is made of it should be clean and of pleasing design (184).

On his left side the worshipper should draw a hexagon with a point in its centre, around it a circle, and outside the circle a square (185). These figures should be drawn either with vermilion or Rajas (Kula-pushpa), or red sandal paste; the Devata of the support should then be worshipped thereon (186). The Mantra for the worship of the Shakti or Devi of the support is –

Mantra

Hring,

salutation to the Shakti of the support (187).

The support for the jar should be washed with the Mantra namah, and placed on the Mandala, and the jar itself with the Mantra Phat, and then placed on the support (188).

Let the disciple then fill the kalasha with wine, uttering meanwhile the Mula-mantra and the Matrika Varnas, with Vindu in Viloma order (189). The wise one who is then himself possessed of the disposition of the Devi should worship the region of Fire, Sun, and Moon in the support in the jar and in the wine in the manner already described (190). After decorating the jar with vermilion, red sandal paste, and a garland of crimson flowers, the worshipper should perform Panchikarana (191).

Strike the wine-jar with a wisp of kusha grass, saying Phat; then, whilst uttering the Vija Hung, veil it by the Avagunthana Mudra, next utter the Vaja Hring, and look with unwinking eye upon the jar, then sprinkle the jar with the Mantra Namah. Lastly, whilst reciting the Mula-mantra, smell the jar three times. this is the Panchikarama ceremony (192).

Making obeisance to the jar, purify the wine therein by throwing red flowers into it, and say the following (193):

Mantra

*Ong, O Devi Sudhe! by the Supreme Brahman, Who is
One without a second: and who is always both gross and
subtle, destroy the sin of slaying a Brahmana which attached to thee (the wine) by the death of Kacha (194). O
Thou Who hast Thy abode in the region of the Sun, and
Thy origin in the dwelling-place of the Lord of Ocean (in
the churning of which thou, O Nectar! wast produced),
thou who art one with the Ama Vija, mayest Thou be
freed from the curse of Shukra (195). O Devi! as the
Pranava of the Vedas is one with the bliss of Brahman,
may by that truth be destroyed Thy sin of slaying a
Brahmana.*

Mantra

*Hring: the Supreme Hangsa dwells in the brilliant
Heaven, as Vasu It moves throughout the space between
Heaven and Earth. It dwells on earth in the form of the
Vedic Fire, and in the Sacrificer, and is honoured in
the Guest. It is in the household Fire and in the consciousness of man, and dwells in the honoured region. It
resides in Truth and in the Ether.*

*It is born in water, in the rays of light in Truth and in
the Eastern Hill where the Sun rises. Such is the great*

Aditya, the Truth, Which cannot be bound or concealed, the Great Consciousness Who dwelleth everywhere –Brahman (196-197).

Exchange the vowel of the Varuna Vija for each of the long vowels, then say "Salutation to the Devi of Ambrosia, who is relieved of the curse of Brahma." By the repetition of the entire Mantra seven times, the curse of Brahma is removed (198). Substituting in their order the six long vowels in place of the letter o in Angkusha, and adding thereto the Shri and Maya Vijas, say the following:

Mantra

"Remove the curse of Krishna in the wine: pour nectar again and again: Svaha" (199).

Having thus removed the curse of Shukra, of Brahma and of Krishna, the worshipper should with mind controlled worship Ananda-Bhairava and Ananda-Bhairavi (200). The Mantra of the former is:

Mantra

"Ha-Sa-Ksha-Ma-La-Va-Ra-Yung:

Salutation to Ananda-Bhairava: Vashat" (201);

and in the worship of the Ananda-Bhairavi the Mantra is the same, except that its face is reversed, and in place of its Ear the left Eye should be placed, and then should be said:

Mantra

"Sa-Ha-Ksha-Ma-La-Va-Ra-Ying:

Salutation to the Wine Devi: Vaushat" (202).

Then, meditating upon the union of the Deva and Devi in the wine, and thinking that the same is filled with the ambrosia of such union, japa should be made over it of the Mula-mantra twelve times (203). *Then, considering the wine to be the Devata, handfuls of flowers should be offered with japa of the Mula-Mantra. Lights and incense-sticks should be waved before it to the accompaniment of the ringing of a bell* (204). *Wine should be always thus purified in all ceremonies, whether puja of the Devata, Vrata, Homa, marriage, or other festivals* (205).

The disciple, after placing the meat on the triangular Mandala in front of him, should sprinkle it with the

Mantra Phat, and then charge it thrice with the Vijas of Air and Fire (206). Let him then cover it up with the Gesture of the Veil, uttering the Kavacha-Mantra, and protect it with the Weapon-Mantra Phat. Then, uttering the Vija of Varuna, and displaying the Dhenu-Mudra, make the meat like unto nectar with the following (207):

Mantra

May that Devi whose abode is in the breast of Vishnu and in the breast of Shankara purify this my meat, and give me a resting-place at the excellent foot of Vishnu (208).

In a similar manner, placing the fish and sanctifying it with the Mantras already prescribed, let the wise one say the following Mantra over it (208):

Mantra

"We worship the Father of the Three; He Who causes nourishment, He Who is sweet-scented. As the fruit of the Urvaruka is detached of itself from the stalk on which it grows, so may He free us whilst living from the bond of Karmma, until we are finally liberated, and made one with the Supreme" (210).

Then, O Beloved! the disciple should take and purify the parched grain with the following:

Mantras

Ong! As the Eye of Heaven is plainly visible to those of the common man, so do the Wise have constant vision of the Excellent Foot of Vishnu (211). The Intelligent and Prayerful, whose mind is awake and controlled, see the most excellent Foot of Vishnu (212).

Or all the Tattvas may be consecrated by the Mula-Mantra itself. To him who has belief in the root, of what use are the branches and leaves? (213).

I say that anything which is sanctified by the Mula-Mantra alone is acceptable for the pleasure of the Devata (214). If the time be short, or if the disciple be pressed for time, everything should be sanctified with the Mula-Mantra, and offered to the Devi (215). Truly, truly, and again truly, the ordinance of Shankara is that if the Tattvas be so offered, there is no sin or shortcoming (216).

End of Fifth Joyful Message, entitled "The Formation of the Mantras, Placing of the Jar, and Purification of the Elements of Worship."

CHAPTER 6

Placing of the Shri-patra, Homa, Formation of the Chakra, and other Rites

SHRI DEVI said:

*As Thou hast kindness for Me, pray tell Me, O Lord!
more particularly about the Pancha-tattvas and the
other observances of which Thou hast spoken (1).*

Shri Sadashiva said:

*There are three kinds of wine which are excellent –
namely, that which is made from molasses, rice, or the
Madhuka flower. There are also various other kinds
made from the juice of the palmyra and date tree, and
known by various names according to their substance
and place of production. They are all declared to be equally appropriate in the worship of the Devata (2).*

*Howsoever it may have been produced, and by
whomsoever it is brought, the wine, when purified, gives
to the worshipper all siddhi. There are no distinctions
of caste in the taking of wine so sanctified (3). Meat,
again, is of three kinds, that of animals of the waters, of
the earth, and of the sky. From wheresoever it may be*

brought, and by whomsoever it may have been killed, it gives, without doubt, pleasure to the Devas (4). Let the desire of the disciple determine what should be offered to the Devas. Whatsoever he himself likes, the offering of that conduces to his well-being (5). Only male animals should be decapitated in sacrifice. It is the command of Shambhu that female animals should not be slain (6). There are three superior kinds of Fish – namely, Shala, Pathina and Rohita. Those which are without bones are of middle quality, whilst those which are full of bones are of inferior quality. The latter may, however, if well fried, be offered to the Devi (7-8).

There are also three kinds of parched food, superior, middle, and inferior. The excellent and pleasing kind is that made from Shali rice, white as a moonbeam, or from barley or wheat, and which has been fried in clarified butter. The middling variety is made of fried paddy. Other kinds of fried grain are inferior (9-10). Meat, fish, and parched food, fruits and roots, or anything else offered to the Devata along with wine, are called Shuddhi (11). O Devi! the offering of wine without Shuddhi, as also puja and tarpana (without Shuddhi), become fruitless, and the Devata is not propitiated (12). The drinking of wine without Shuddhi is like the swallowing of poison. The disciple is ever ailing, and lives for a short time and dies (13). O Great Devi! when the weakness *of the Kali Age becomes great, one's own Shakti or wife should alone be known as the fifth Tattva. This is devoid of all defects (14). O Beloved of My Life! in this (the last Tattva) I have spoken of Svayambhu and other kinds of flower. As substitutes for them, however, I enjoin red sandal paste (15). Neither the Tattvas nor flowers, leaves, and fruits should be offered to the Mahadevi unless purified. The man who offers them without purification goes to hell (16).*

The Shri-patra should be placed in the company of one's own virtuous Shakti; she should be sprinkled with the purified wine or water from the common offering (17). The Mantra for the sprinkling of the Shakti is –

Mantra

Aing, Kling, Sauh. Salutation to Tripura; purify this Shakti, make her my Shakti; Svaha (18-19).

If she who is to be Shakti is not already initiated, then the Maya Vija should be whispered into her ear, and other Shaktis who are present should be worshipped and not enjoyed (20).

The worshipper should then, in the space between himself and the Yantra, draw a triangle with the Maya Vija in its centre, and outside the triangle and in the order here stated a circle, a hexagon, and a square (21). The excellent disciple should then worship in the four corners of the square the Pithas, Purna-shaila, Uddiyana, Jalandhara, and Kama-rupa, with the Mantras formed of their respective names, preceded by Vijas formed by the first letter of their respective names, and followed by Namah (22).

Then the six parts of the body should be worshipped in the six corners of the hexagon. Then worship the triangle, with the Mula-Mantra, and then the Shakti of the receptacle with the Maya Vija and Namah (23). Wash the receptacle with the Mantra Namah, and then place it (as in the case of the jar) on the Mandala, and worship in it the ten parts of Vahni with the first letters of their respective names as Vijas (24). These parts, which are ten in number – viz., Dhumra, Archih, Jvalini, Sukshma, Jvalini, Vishphulingini, Sushri, Surupa, Kapila,Havya-kavya-vaha – should be uttered in the Dative singular, and followed by the Mantra Namah (25-26).

Then worship the region of Vahni (in the adhara or receptacle) with the following:

Mantra

Mang: Salutation to the region of Vahni with his ten qualities (27).

Then, taking the vessel of offering and purifying it with the Mantra Phat, place it on the receptacle, and, having so placed it, worship therein the twelve parts of the Sun with the Vijas, commencing with Ka-Bha to Tha-Da (28). These twelve parts are – Tapini, Tapini, Dhumra, Marichi, Jvalini, Ruchi, Sudhumra, Bhoga-da, Vishva, Bodhini, Dharini, Kshama (29). After this, worship the region of Sun in the vessel of offering with the following:

Mantra

Ang: Salutation to the circle of Sun, with His twelve parts (30).

Then the worshipper should fill the cup of offering th-ree-quarters full with wine taken from the jar, uttering the Matrika Vijas in the reverse order (31). Filling the rest of the cup with water taken from the special offering, let him worship with a well-controlled mind the sixteen digits of the Moon, saying as Vijas each of the sixteen vowels before each of the sixteen digits spoken in the dative singular, followed by the Mantra Namah (32).

The sixteen desire-granting digits of Moon are – Amrita,

Pranada, Pusha, Tushti, Pushti, Rati, Dhriti, Shashini, Chandrika, Kanti, Jyotsna, Skri, Priti, Angada, Purna, and Purnamrita (33). As in the case of the other Devas mentioned, the disciple should then worship the region of the Moon with the following:

Mantra

Ung: Salutation to the region of Moon with its sixteen digits (34).

Durva grass, sun-dried rice, red flowers, Varvara, leaf, and the Aparajita flower should be thrown into the vessel with the Mantra Hring, and the sacred waters should be invoked into it (35). Then, covering the wine and the vessel of offering with the Avagunthana Mudra, and uttering the Armour Vija, protect it with the Weapon-Vija, and converting it into ambrosia with the Dhenu-Mudra, cover it with the Matsya-Mudra (36). Making japa of the Mula-Mantra ten times, the Ishta-devata should be invoked and worshipped with flowers offered in the joined palms.

Then charge the wine with the following five Mantras, beginning with akhanda: (37)

Mantras

O Kula-rupini! infuse into the essence of this excellent wine which produces full and unbroken bliss its thrill of joy (38).

Thou who art like the nectar which is in Ananga, and art the embodiment of Pure Knowledge, place into this liquid the ambrosia of Brahmananda (39).

O Thou, who art the very image of That! do Thou unite this arghya with the image or self of That, and having become the kulamrita, blossom in me (40).

Bring into this sacred vessel, which is full of wine, essence of ambrosia produced from the essence of all that is in this world, and containing all kinds of taste (41).

May this cup of self, which is filled with the nectar of self, Lord, be sacrificed in the Fire of the Supreme Self (42).

Having thus consecrated the wine with the Mantra, think of the union in it of Sadashiva and Bhagavati and wave lights and burning incense-sticks before it (43).

This is the consecration of the Shri-patra in Kaulika worship. Without such purification the disciple is guilty of sin, and the worship is fruitless (44). The wise one should then, according to the rules prescribed for the placing of the common offering, place between the jar and the Shri-patra the cups of the Guru, the cup of Enjoyment, the cup of the Shakti, the cups of the Yoginis of the Vira and of Sacrifice, and those for the washing of the feet and the rinsing of the mouth respectively, making nine cups in all (45-46).

Then, filling the cups three-quarters full of wine from the jar, a morsel of Shuddhi of the size of a pea should be placed in each of them (47). Then, holding the cup between the thumb and the fourth finger of the left hand, taking the morsel of Shuddhi in the right hand, making the Tattva-mudra, Tarpana should be done. This is the practice which has been enjoined (48). Taking an excellent drop of wine from the Shripatra and a piece of Shuddhi, Tarpana should be made to the Deva Ananda-Bhairava and the Devi Ananda-Bhairavi (49).

Then, with the wine in the cup of the Guru, offer oblations to the line of Gurus. in the first place to the worshipper's own Guru seated together with his wife on the lotus of a thousand petals, and then to the Parama Guru, the Parapara Guru, the Parameshti Guru successively. In offering oblations to the four Gurus, the Vagbhava Vija should first be pronounced, followed in each case by the names of each of the four Gurus (50). Then, *with wine from the cup of enjoyment, the worshipper should, in the lotus of his heart, offer oblations to the Adya-Kali. In this oblation Her own Vija should precede, and Svaha should follow Her name. This should be done thrice (51).*

Next, with wine taken from the cup of the Shakti, oblation should be similarly offered to the Devata of the parts of Her body and their Avarana-Devatas (52). Then, with the wine in the cup of the Yogini, oblation should be offered to the Adya-Kalika, carrying all Her weapons and with all Her followers.

Then should follow the sacrifice to the Vatukas (53). The wise worshipper should draw on his left an ordinary rectangular figure, and after worshipping it, place therein food with wine, meat, and other things (54). With the Vijas of Vak, Maya, Kamala, and with the Mantra:

"Vang, Salutation to Vatuka," he should be worshipped in the East of the rectangle, and then sacrifice should be offered to him (55).

Then, with the

Mantra

"Yang to the Yogin is Svaha,"

sacrifice should be made to the Yoginis on the South (56), and then to Kshetra-pala on the West of the rectangle, with the

Mantra

"To Kshetra-pala namah,"

preceded by the letter Ksha, to which in succession the six long vowels are added with the Vindu (57). Following this, sacrifice should be made to Gana-pati on the North, adding to Ga the six long vowels in succession with the Vindu thereon, followed by the name of Ganesha in the dative singular, and ending with Svaha. Lastly, sacrifice should be made inside the rectangle to all Bhutas, according to proper form (58-59).

Uttering "Hring, Shring, Sarvva-vighna-kridbhyah," add "Sarvva-bhutebhyah," and then "Hung Phat Svaha;" this is how the Mantra is formed (60). Then a sacrifice to Shiva should be made with the following:

Mantra

Ong, O Dev! O Shiva, O Exalted One, Thou art the ima-

*ge of the final conflagration at the dissolution of things,
deign to accept this sacrifice, and to reveal clearly to me
the good and evil which is my destiny. To Shiva I bow.*

This is the Mula-Mantra in the worship of Shiva.

*Having said this, perform the sacrifice, saying, "This is
Thy Vali. To Shiva, Namah. O Holy One! I have now
described to Thee the mode of formation of the circle
of worship (and the placing of the cup and other rites)
(61-62). Then, making with the two hands the Kach-
chhapa-Mudra, let the worshipper take up with his
hands a beautiful flower scented with sandal, fragrant
aloes, and musk, and, carrying it to the lotus of his
heart, let him meditate therein (in the lotus) upon the
most supreme Adya (63-64).*

*Then let him lead the Devi along the Sushumna Nadi,
which is the highway of Brahman to the great Lotus of
a thousand petals, and there make Her joyful. Then,
bringing Her through his nostrils, let him place Her
on the flower (her presence being communicated) as it
were, by one light to another, and place the flower on the
Yantra and with folded hands pray with all devotion to
his Ishta-devata thus (65-66):*

Mantra

O Queen of the Devas! Thou who art easily attained by devotion. Remain here, I pray Thee, with all Thy following, the while I worship Thee (67).

Then, uttering the Vija Kring, say the following:

Mantra

O Adya Devi Kalika! come here with all Thy following, come here (and then say), stay here, stay here (68); (and then say) place Thyself here, (and then say) be Thou detained here. Accept my worship (69).

Having thus invoked (the Devi) into the Yantra, the Vital Airs of the Devi should be infused therein by the following pratishtha Mantra (70):

Mantra

Ang, Hring, Krong, Shring, Svaha; may the five Vital Airs of this Devata be here: Ang, Hring, Krong, Shring, Svaha (71). Her Jiva is here placed – Ang, Hring, Krong, Shring, Svaha – all senses – Ang, Hring, Krong, Shring, Svaha. Speech, mind, sight, smell, hearing, touch, and the Vital Airs of the Adya-Kali Devata, may they come here and stay happily here for ever. Svaha (72-74).

Having recited the above three times, and having in due form placed the Vital Airs (of the Devi) in the Yantra with the Lelihina-Mudra, with folded palms, he (the worshipper) should say (75):

Mantra

O Adya Kali! hast Thou had a good journey, hast Thou had a good journey? O Parameshvari! mayest Thou be seated on this seat (76)?

Then, whilst repeating the primary Mantra, sprinkle thrice the water of the special oblation over the Devi, and then make Nyasa of the Devi with the six parts of Her body. This ceremony is called Sakalikarama or Sakalikriti. Then worship the Devi with all the sixteen offerings (77). These are: water for washing the feet, the water for the offering, water for rinsing the mouth and for Her bath, garments, jewels, perfume, flowers, incense-sticks, lights, food, water for washing the mouth, nectar, pan, water of oblation, and obeisance. In worship these sixteen offerings are needed (78-79).

Uttering the Adya Vija, and then saying "this water is for washing the feet of the (Adya). To the Devata Namah," offer the water at the feet of the Devi. Similarly with the word Svaha, in place of Namah, the offering

should be placed at the head of the Devi (80). Then the
wise worshipper with Svadha should offer the water for
rinsing the mouth to the mouth of the Devi, and then
the worshipper should offer to the lotus-mouth of the
Devi Madhu-parka with the Mantra Svadha. He should
then offer water to rinse the mouth (a second time) with
the Mantra "Vang Svadha" (81). Then the worshipper,
saying:

Mantra

Hring, Shring, Kring, Parameshvari, Svaha: I offer
this water for bathing, this apparel, these jewels, to the
Supreme Devi, the Primordial Kalika. Svaha,

make an offer of them to all parts of the body of the
Devi (82).

Then the worshipper should, with the same Mantra, but
ending with Namah, offer scent with his middle and
third finger to the heart-lotus (of the Devi), and with
the same Mantra, but ending with Vaushat, he should
similarly offer to Her flowers (83). Having placed the
burning incense and lighted lamp in front of Devi, and
sprinkling them with water, they should be given away
with the

Mantra

*Hring, Shring, Kring, Parameshvari, Svaha: This incen-
se-stick and light I humbly offer to Adya-Kalika. Svaha.*

After worship of the Bell with the

Mantra

*O Mother, Who produces the sound which proclaims
triumph to Thee. Svaha,*

*he should ring it with his left hand, and, taking up the
incense-stick with his right hand, he should wave it
up to the nostrils of the Devi. Then, placing the incense-stick on Her left, he should raise and wave the light
ten times up to and before the eyes of the Devi (84-86).
Then, taking the Cup and the Shuddhi in his two hands,
the worshipper should, whilst uttering the Mula-Mantra, offer them to the centre of the Yantra (87).*

Mantra

*O Thou who hast brought to an end a crore of kalpas,
take this excellent wine, as also the Shuddhi, and grant
to me endless liberation (88).*

Then, drawing a figure (in front of the Yantra), according to the rules of ordinary worship, place the plate with food thereon (89). Sprinkle the food (with the Mantra Phat) and veil it with the Avagunthana-Mudra (and the Mantra Hung), and then again protect it (by the Mantra Phat) (Saying Vang), and, exhibiting the Dhenu-Mudra over it, make it into the food of immortality. Then, after recitation of the Mula-Mantra seven times, it should be oftered to the Devi with the water taken from the vessel of offering (90).

The worshipper, after reciting the Mula-Mantra, should say: "This cooked food, with all other necessaries, I offer to the Adya-Kali, my Ishta-devi." He should then say: "O Shiva! partake of this offering" (91). Then he should make the Devi eat the offering by means of the five Mudras called Prana, Apana, Samana, Vyana, and Udana (90).

Next, form with the left hand the Naivedya-Mudra, which is like a full-blown lotus. Then, whilst reciting the Mula-Mantra, give away the jar with wine to the Devi for Her to drink. After that offer again water for rinsing the mouth, and following that a threefold oblation should be made to the Devi with wine from the cup of the Shri-patra (93-94). Then, reciting the Mula-Mantra, let the worshipper offer five handfuls of flowers to the

*head, heart, Muladhara Lotus, the feet, and all parts
of the body of the Devi (95), and thereafter with folded
palms he should pray to his Ishta-devata thus:*

Mantra

*O Ishta-devata! I am now worshipping the Devatas who
surround thee, namah (96).*

*The six parts of the body of the Devi should then be
worshipped at the four corners of the Yantra, and in
front and behind it in their order; and then the line of
Gurus should be worshipped (97). Then, with scent and
flowers, worship the four Kula-gurus – namely, Guru,
Parama-guru, Parapara-guru, Parameshti-guru (98).*

*Then, with the wine in the cup of the Guru, make
three Tarpanas to each, and on the lotus of eight petals
worship the eight Mother Nayikas – namely, Mangala,
Vijaya, Bhadra, Jayanti, Aparajita, Nandini, Narasinghi, and Kaumari (99-100), and on the tips of the petals
worship the eight Bhairavas – Asitanga, Ruru, Chanda,
Krodhonmatta, Bhayangkara, Kapali, Bhishana, and
Sanghara (101-102). Indra and the other Dik-palas
should be worshipped in the Bhu-pura, and their weapons outside the Bhu-pura, and then Tarpana should be
made to them (103).*

*After worshipping (the Devi) with all the offerings,
sacrifice should be carefully made to Her (104). The
ten approved beasts which may be sacrificed are – deer,
goat, sheep, buffalo, hog, porcupine, hare, iguana, and
rhinoceros (105); but other beasts may also be sacrificed
if the worshipper so desires (106). The worshipper versed
in the rules of sacrifice should select a beast with good
signs, and, placing it before the Devi, should sprinkle
it with the water from the Vishesharghya, and by the
Dhenu-Mudra should make it into nectar.*

*Let him then worship the goat (sheep, or whatever other
animal is being sacrificed) with (the Mantra) "Namah to the goat," which is a beast, and with perfumes,
flowers, vermilion, food, and water. Then he should
whisper into the ears of the beast the Gayatri Mantra,
which severs the bond of its life as a beast (107-108).
The Pashu-Gayatri, which liberates a beast from its life
of a beast, is as follows: After the word "Pashu-pashaya"
say " Vidmahe," then, after the word "Vishva-karmane,"
say "Dhimahi," and then "Tanno jivah prachodayat."*

Mantra

*Let us bring to mind the bonds of the life of a beast. Let
us meditate upon the Creator of the Universe. May He
liberate us from out of this life (of a beast) (109-110).*

Then, taking the sacrificial knife, the excellent worshipper should worship it with the Vija "Hung," and worship Sarasvati and Brahma at its end, Lakshmi and Narayana at its middle, and Uma and Maheshvara at the handle (111-112). Then the sacrificial knife should be worshipped with the

Mantra

Namah to the sacrificial knife infused with the presence of Brahma, Vishnu, Shiva, and their Shaktis (113).

Then, dedicating it with the Great Word, he should, with folded hands, say: "May this dedication to Thee be according to the ordained rites" (114).

Having thus offered the beast to the Devi, it should be placed on the ground (115). The worshipper then, with mind intent upon the Devi, should sever the head of the beast with one sharp stroke. This may be done either by the worshipper himself or by his brother, brother's son, a friend, or a kinsman, but never by one who is an enemy (116). The blood, when yet warm, should be offered to the Vatukas. Then the head with a light on it should be offered to the Devi with the following:

Mantra

"This head with the light upon it I offer to the Devi with obeisance " (117).

This is the sacrificial rite of the Kaulikas in Kaula worship. If it be not observed, the Devata is never pleased (118). After this Homa should be performed. Listen, O Beloved One! to the rules which relate to it (119). The worshipper should, with sand, make on his right a square, each side of which is one cubit. Let him, then, while reciting the Mula-Mantra, gaze at it, stroke it with a wisp of kusha grass, uttering the Weapon-Vija, and then sprinkle it with water to the accompaniment of the same Vija (120).

Then, veiling it with the Kurchcha-Vija, he should say: "Obeisance to the sthandila of the Devi," and with this Mantra worship the square (121). Then, inside the square three lines should be drawn from East to West, and three lines from South to North, of the length of a pradesha. When this has been done, the (following Devatas, whose names are hereinafter given) should be worshipped over these lines (122). Over the lines from West to East worship Mukunda, Isha, and Purandara: over the lines from South to North, Brahma, Vaivasvata, and Indu (123).

Then a triangle should be drawn within the square, and

within the triangle the Vija Hsauh should be written. Outside the triangle draw a hexagon, outside this a circle, and outside the circle a lotus with eight petals, and outside this a (square) Bhu-pura, with four entrances; so should the wise one draw the excellent Yantra (124). Having worshipped with the Mula-Mantra and with offerings of handfuls of flowers, the space thus marked off and washed, the articles for the Homa sacrifice with the Pranava, the intelligent one, should, after first uttering the Maya Vija, worship in the pericarp of the lotus the Adhara-shakti and others, either individually or collectively (125). Piety, Knowledge, Dispassion, and Dominion should be worshipped in the Agni, Ishana, Vayu, and Nairrita corners of the Yantra respectively, and the negation of the qualities in the East, North, West, and South respectively, and in the centre Ananta and Padma (126-127). Then let him worship Sun with his twelve parts, and Moon with her sixteen digits, and, on the filament commencing from the East, worship Pita, and then Shveta, Aruna, Krishna, Dhumra, Tibra, Sphulingini, Ruchira, in their order, and in the centre Jvalini (128-129). In all worship Pranava should commence the Mantra, and Namah should end it. The seat of Fire should be worshipped with the

Mantra

Rang, Salutation to the seat of Fire.

Then the Mantrin should meditate upon the Devi Sarasvati after She has bathed, with eyes like the blue lotus on the seat of Fire in the embrace of Vagishvara, and worship in the seat of Fire with the Maya-Vija (130).

Then let him bring Fire in the manner prescribed, and gaze intently on it, and, whilst repeating the Mula-Mantra, invoke Vahni into it with the Mantra Phat (131-132). Then the seat of Fire should be worshipped in the Yantra with the

Mantra

Ong Salutation to the Yoga-pitha of Fire,

and on the four sides, beginning on the East and ending on the South, Vama, Jyeshtha, Raudri, Ambika, should be worshipped in the order given (133).

Then the marked-off space should be worshipped with the

Mantra

Salutation to the sthandila of the revered Devata, the

Primeval Kalika:

*and then within this place the worshipper should med-
itate upon the Devi Vagishvari under the form of the
Mula-Devata. After lighting the Fire with the Vija Rang,
and reciting the Mula-Mantra, and then the*

Mantra

Hung Phat: to the eaters of raw flesh: Svaha,

*the share of the raw meat eaters (Rakshasas) should be
put aside. Gaze at the Fire, saying the Weapon-Mantra,
and surround it with the Veil Mudra, uttering the Vija
Hung (134-136). Make the Fire into nectar with the
Dhenu-Mudra. Take some Fire in both palms, and wave
it thrice in a circle over the sthandila from right to left.
Then with both knees on the ground, and meditating on
Fire as the male seed of Shiva, the worshipper should
place it into that portion of the Yoni Yantra which is
nearest him (137-138). Then, first, worship the Image of
Fire with the*

Mantra

*Hring, Salutation to the Image of Fire, and after that the
Spirit of Fire with the Mantra*

Rang: to the Spirit of Fire namah (139).

The Mantrin will then think in his mind of the awakened form of Vahni, and kindle the fire with the following (140)

Mantra

Ong, yellow Spirit of Fire, which knows all, destroy, destroy, burn, burn, ripen, ripen command: Svaha.

This is the Mantra for kindling Fire. After this, with folded hands, Fire should again be adored (141-142).

Mantra

I adore the kindled Fire of the colour of gold, free from impurity, burning, author of the Veda the devourer of oblations, which faces every quarter (143).

After adoration of Fire in this manner, cover the marked-off space with kusha grass, and then the worshipper, giving Fire the name of his own, Ishta-devata, should worship him (144).

Mantra

*Ong,O Red-eyed One! Vaishvanara, origin of the Veda,
come here, come, come here, (help me to) accomplish all
(my) works: Svaha.*

*Then the seven Tongues of Fire, Hiranya and others,
should be worshipped (145-146). The worshipper should
next adore the six Limbs of Vahni uttering the word "of
a thousand rays" in the dative singular, and at the end
"obeisance to the heart" (147).*

*Then the wise one should worship the forms of Vahni
(147), the eight forms Jata-veda and others (148), and
then the eight Shaktis – namely, Brahmi and others, the
eight Nidhis – namely, Padma and others, and the ten
Dik-palas – namely, Indra and others (149).*

*After worshipping the thunderbolt and other weapons,
the sacrificer should take two blades of kusha grass of
the length of the space between his stretched-out thumb
and forefinger, and place them lengthwise in the ghee
(150). He should meditate on the Nadi Ida in the left
part of the ghee, and on the Nadi Pingala in the right
portion, and on the Nadi Sushumna in the centre, and
with a well-controlled mind take ghee from the right
side, and offer it to the right eye of Vahni with the
following:*

Mantra

Ong to Agni Svaha.

*Then, taking ghee from the left side, offer it to the left
eye of Vahni with the*

Mantra

Ong to Soma Svaha (151-153).

*Then, taking ghee from the middle portion, offer it to the
forehead of Vahni with the*

Mantra

Ong to Agni and Soma Svaha (154).

*Then, saying namah, take the ghee again from the right
side, say first the Pranava, and then*

Mantra

To Agni the Svishti-krit Svaha.

*With this Mantra he should offer oblation to the mouth
of Vahni. Then, uttering the Vyahriti with the Pranava*

*at the commencement, and Svaha at the end, the Homa
sacrifice should be performed (155-156). Then he should
offer oblations thrice with the*

Mantra

*Om,O Vaishvanara, origin of the Veda, come hither,
come hither, O Red-eyed One! and fulfil all my works
(157)*

*Then, invoking the Ishta-Devata with the proper Mantra
into the Fire, let him worship Her and the Pitha-Devata.
Twenty-five oblations should then be offered (uttering
the Mula-Mantra with Svaha at the end), and, contemplating on the union (or identity) of his own soul
with Vahni and the Devi, eleven oblations should also
be offered with the Mula-Mantra to the Anga-Devatas,
concluding with Svaha (158-159).*

*Then, with a mixture of ghee, tila-seed, honey, or with
flowers and bael-leaves, or with (other prescribed)
articles, oblation should be made for the attainment of
one's desire. This oblation should be made not less than
eight times, and with every attention and care (160-
161). Then, reciting the primary Mantra ending with
Svaha, complete oblation should be made (with a full
ladle) with fruits and leaves. The worshipper, with the*

*Sanghara-Mudra, transferring the Devi from the Fire
to the lotus of his heart (162), should then say "Pardon
me," and dismiss Him who feeds on oblations. Then,
distributing presents, the Mantrin should consider that
the Homa has been duly performed (163).*

*Then the excellent worshipper should place between the
eyebrows what is left over of the oblations (164). This is
the ordinance relating to Homa in all forms of Agama
worship. After performance of Homa the worshipper
should proceed to do japa (165). Now, listen,O Devi! to
the instructions which relate to japa by which the Vidya
is pleased. During japa, the Devata, the Guru, and the
Mantra should be considered as one (166). The letters
of the Mantra are the Devata, and the Devata is in the
form of the Guru. To him who worships them as one
and the same, his is the greatest success (167).*

*The worshipper should then meditate upon his Guru as
being in his head, the Devi in his heart, the Mula-Mantra in the form of tejas on his tongue, and himself as
united with the glory of all three (168). Then, adding the
Tara to the beginning and the end of the Mula-Mantra, it should be made japa of seven times, and then
it should be recapitulated with the Matrika Vija at its
beginning and end (169). The wise worshipper should
make japa of the Maya-Vija over his head ten times,*

*and of the Pranava ten times over his mouth, and of the
Maya-Vija again seven times in the lotus of his heart,
and then perform Pranayama (170).*

*Then, taking a rosary of coral, etc, let him worship it
thus:*

Mantra

*O rosary, O rosary, O great rosary, thou art the image of
all Shaktis. Thou art the repository of the fourfold blessings. Do thou therefore be the giver to me of all success.*

*Having thus worshipped the Mala, and also made
Tarpana to it thrice with wine taken from the Shri-patra, accompanied by recitation of the Mula-Mantra, the
worshipper should, with well-controlled mind, make
japa one thousand and eight, or at least one hundred
and eight times (171-173). Then, doing Pranayama, he
should offer on the left lotus-hand of the Devi the fruit
of his japa, whose form is Tejas, together with water and
flowers from the Shri-patra, and, bowing down his head
to the ground, say the following:*

Mantra

O Great Queen! Thou Who protectest that which is most

secret, deign to accept this my recitation. May by Thy grace success attend my effort.

After this, let him with folded hands recite the hymn and the protective Mantra (174-176). Then the Sadhaka should, with the special oblation in his hand, going round the Devi, keeping Her to his right, say the following, and dedicate his own self by offering Vilomarghya (177).

Mantra

Om, whatsoever ere this I in the possession of life, intelligence, body, or in action, awake, in dream or dreamless sleep have done, whether by word or deed, by my hands, feet, belly, or organ of generation, whatsoever I have remembered or spoken – of all that I make an offering to Brahman. I and all that is mine I lay at the lotus-feet of the Adya Kali. I make the sacrifice of myself Ong tat sat (178-179).

Then, with folded hands, let him supplicate his Ishta-Devata, and reciting the Maya-Mantra, say:

Mantra

"O Primordial Kalika! I have worshipped Thee with all

my powers and devotion,"

and then saying, "Forgive me," let him bid the Devi go. Let him with his hands formed into Sanghara-Mudra take up a flower, smell it, and place it on his heart (182-183). A triangular figure well and clearly made should next be drawn in the North-East corner, and there he should worship the Devi Nirmalya-vasini with the

Mantra

Hring salutation to the Devi Nirmalya-vasini (184).

Then, distributing Naivedya to Brahma, Vishnu, and Shiva, and all the other Devas, the worshipper should partake of it (185). Then, placing his Shakti on a separate seat to his left, or on the same seat with himself, he should make a pleasing drink in the cup (186), The cup should be so formed as to hold not more than five and not less than three tolas of wine, and may be of either gold or silver (187), or crystal, or made of the shell of a cocoa-nut. It should be kept on a support on the right side of the plate containing the prepared food (188).

Then the wise one should serve the sacred food and wine either himself or by his brother's sons among the worshippers according to the order of their seniority

(189). The purified wine should be served in the drinking-cups, and the purified food in plates kept for that purpose, and then should food and drink be taken with such as are present at the time (190). First of all, some purified food should be eaten to make a bed as it were (for the wine which is to be drunk). Let the assembled worshippers then joyously take up each his own cup filled with excellent nectar.

Then let him take up each his own cup and meditate upon the Kula-Kundalini, who is the Chit, and who is spread from the Muladhara lotus to the tip of the tongue, and, uttering the Mula-Mantra, let each, after taking the others' permission, offer it as oblation to the mouth of the Kundali (191-193). When the Shakti is of the household, the smelling of the wine is the equivalent of drinking it. Worshippers who are householders may drink five cups only (194). Excessive drinking prevents the attainment of success by Kula worshippers (195).

They may drink until the sight or the mind is not affected. To drink beyond that is bestial (196). How is it possible for a sinner who becomes a fool through drink and who shows contempt for the Sadhaka of Shakti to say "I worship the Adya Kalika"? (197). As touch cannot affect food, etc, offered to Brahman, so there is no distinction of caste in food offered to Thee (198).

*As I have directed, so should eating and drinking be
done. After partaking of food offeredto Thee, the hands
should not be washed, but with a piece of cloth or a
little water remove that which has adhered to the hands
(199). Lastly, after placing a flower from the nirmalya
on his head, and wearing a tilaka mark made from
the remnants of the oblation on the Yantra between his
eyebrows, the intelligent worshipper may roam the earth
like a Deva (200).*

*End of the Sixth Joyful Message, entitled "Placing of the
Shri-patra, Homa, Formation of the Chakra, and other
Rites."*

CHAPTER 7

Hymn of Praise (Stotra), Amulet (Ka-vacha), and the description of the Kula-tattva

PARVATI was pleased at hearing the revelation of the
auspicious Mantra of the Adya Kalika, which yields
abundant blessings, is the only means of attaining to a
knowledge of the Divine essence, and leads to liberation;
as also at hearing of the morning rites, the rules relating
to bathing, Sandhya, the purification of Bhang, the
methods of external and internal Nyasa and worship,
the sacrifice of animals, Homa, the formation of the
circle of worship, and the partaking of the holy food.
Bowing low with modesty, the Devi questioned Shankara (1-3).

Shri Devi said:

O Sadashiva! Lord, and Benefactor of the Universe,
Thou hast in Thy mercy spoken of the mode of worship
of the supreme Prakriti (4), which benefits all being, is
the sole path both for enjoyment and final liberation,
and which gives, in this Age, in particular, immediate
success (5). My mind, immersed in the ocean of the

nectar of Thy word, has no desire to rise therefrom, but craves for more and more (6). O Deva, in the directions Thou hast given relating to the worship of the great Devi, Thou hast but given a glimpse of the hymn of praise, and of the protective Mantra. Do Thou reveal them now (7).

Shri Sadashiva said:

Listen, then, O Devi, Who art the adored of the worlds-,to this unsurpassed hymn, by the reciting of or listening to which one becomes the Lord of all the Siddhis (8), (a hymn) which allays evil fortune, increases happiness and prosperity, destroys untimely death, and removes all calamities (9), and is the cause of the happy approach to the gracious Adya Kalika. It is by the grace of this hymn,O Happy One, that I am Tripurari (10).

O Devi! the Rishi of this hymn is Sadashiva, its metre is Anushtup, its Devata is the Adya Kalika, and the object of its use is the attainment of Dharmma, Artha, Kama, and Moksha (11).

Hymn Entitled Adya-Kali-Svarupa.

Hring, O Destroyer of Time,
Shring, O Terrific One,

Kring, Thou Who art beneficent,

Possessor of all the Arts,

Thou art Kamala,

Destroyer of the pride of the Kali Age,

Who art kind to Him of the matted hair, (12)

Devourer of Him Who devours,

Mother of Time,

Thou Who art brilliant as the Fires of the final Dissolu-

tion,

Wife of Him of the matted hair,

O Thou of formidable countenance,

Ocean of the nectar of compassion, (13)

Merciful,

Vessel of Mercy,

Whose Mercy is without limit,

Who art attainable alone by Thy mercy,

Who art Fire,

Tawny,

Black of hue,

Thou Who increasest the joy of the Lord of Creation,

(14)

Night of Darkness,

Image of Desire,

Yet Liberator from the bonds of desire,

Thou Who art (dark) as a bank of Clouds,

And bearest the crescent-moon,

Destructress of sin in the Kali Age, (15)

Thou Who art pleased by the worship of virgins,

Thou Who art the Refuge of the worshippers of virgins,

Who art pleased by the feasting of the virgins,

Who art the Image of the virgin, (16)

Thou Who wanderest in the kadamba forest,

Who art pleased with the flowers of the kadamba forest,

Who hast Thy abode in the kadamba forest,

Who wearest a garland of kadamba flowers, (17)

Thou Who art youthful,

Who hast a soft low voice,

Whose voice is sweet as the cry of a Chakravaka bird,

Who drinkest and art pleased with the kadambari wine,

(18)

And Whose cup is a skull,

Who wearest a garland of bones,

Who art pleased with,

And Who art seated on the Lotus, (19)

Who abidest in the centre of the Lotus,

Whom the fragrance of the Lotus pleases,

Who movest with the swaying gait of a Hangsa,

Destroyer of fear,

Who assumest all forms at will,

Whose abode is at Kama-rupa, (20)

Who ever plays at the Kama-pitha,

O beautiful One,

O Creeper Which givest every desire,

Who art the Possessor of beautiful ornaments, (21)

Adorable as the Image of all tenderness,

Thou with a tender body,

And Who art slender of waist,

Who art pleased with the nectar of purified wine,

Giver of success to them whom purified wine rejoices,

(22)

The own Deity of those who worship Thee when joyed

with wine,

Who art gladdened by the worship of Thyself with

purified wine,

Who art immersed in the ocean of purified wine,

Who art the Protectress of those who accomplish vrata

with wine, (23)

Whom the fragrance of musk gladdens,

And Who art luminous with a tilaka-mark of musk,

Who art attached to those who worship Thee with musk,

Who lovest those who worship Thee with musk, (24)

Who art a Mother to those who burn musk as incense,

Who art fond of the musk-deer and art pleased to eat its

musk,

Whom the scent of camphor gladdens,

Who art adorned with garlands of camphor,

And Whose body is smeared with camphor and sandal

paste, (25)

Who art pleased with purified wine flavoured with

Camphor,

Who drinkest purified wine flavoured with camphor,

Who art bathed in the ocean of camphor,

Whose abode is in the ocean of camphor, (26)

Who art pleased when worshipped with the Vija Hung,

Thou Who threatenest with the Vija Hung,

Embodiment of Kulachara,

Adored by Kaulikas,

Benefactress of the Kaulikas, (27)

Observant of Kulachara,

Joyous One, Revealer of the path of the Kaulikas,

Queen of Kashi,

Allayer of sufferings,

Giver of blessings to the Lord of Kashi,(28)

Giver of pleasure to the Lord of Kashi,

Beloved of the Lord of Kashi, (29)

Thou Whose toe-ring bells make sweet melody as Thou movest,

Whose girdle bells sweetly tinkle,

Who abidest in the mountain of gold,

Who art like a Moon-beam on the mountain of gold, (30)

Who art gladdened by the recitation of the Mantra Kling,

Who art the Kama Vija,

Destructress of all evil inclinations,

And of the afflictions of the Kaulikas,

Lady of the Kaulas, (31)

O Thou Who by the three Vijas, Kring, Hring, Shring,

art the Destructress of the fear of Death.

(To Thee I make obeisance.)

These are proclaimed as the Hundred Names of Kalika (32), beginning with the letter Ka. They are all identical with the image of Kali (33). He who in worship recites these names with his mind fixed on Kalika, for him Mantra-siddhi is quickly obtained, and with him Kali is pleased (34). By the mere bidding of his Guru he acquires intelligence, knowledge, and becomes wealthy, famous, munificent, and compassionate (35). Such an one enjoys life happily in this world with his children and grandchildren with wealth and dominion (36). He who, on a new moon night, when it falls on Tuesday, worships the great Adya Kali, Mistress of the three worlds, with the five Ma-karas, and repeats Her hundred names, becomes suffused with the presence of the Devi, and for him there remains nothing in the three worlds which is beyond his powers (37-38).

He becomes in learning like Brihaspati himself, in wealth like Kuvera. His profundity is that of the ocean, and his strength that of the wind (39). He shines with the blinding brilliance of the Sun, yet pleases with the soft glamour of the Moon. In beauty he becomes like the God of Love, and reaches the hearts of women (40). He comes forth as conqueror everywhere by the grace of this hymn of praise. Singing this hymn, he attains all his

*desires (41). All these desires he shall attain by the grace
of the gracious Adya, whether in battle, in seeking the
favour of Kings, in wagers, or in disputes, and when his
life be in danger (42), at the hands of robbers, amidst
burning villages, lions, or tigers (43), in forests and
lonely deserts, when imprisoned, threatened by Kings or
adverse planets, in burning fever, in long sickness, when
attacked by fearful disease (44), in the sickness of children caused by the influence of adverse planets, or when
tormented by evil dreams, when fallen in boundless
waters, and when he be in some storm-tossed ship (45).*

*O Devi! he who with firm devotion meditates upon
the Parama Maya–image of the most excellent Kali–is
without a doubt relieved of all dangers. For him there is
never any fear, whether arising from sin or disease (46-
47). For him there is ever victory, and defeat never. At
the mere sight of him all dangers flee (48). He expounds
all Scriptures, enjoys all good fortune, and becomes
the leader in all matters of caste and duty, and the lord
among his kinsmen (49). In his mouth Vani ever abides,
and in his home Kamala. Men bow with respect at the
mere mention of his name (50). The eight Siddhis, such
as Anima and others, he looks upon as but mere bits of
grass.*

I have now recited the hymn of a hundred names, which

is called "The Very Form of the Adya Kali" (51).

Purashcharana of this hymn, which is its repetition one hundred and eight times, yields all desired fruit (52). This hymn of praise of a hundred names, which is the Primeval Kali Herself, if read, or caused to be read, if heard, or caused to be heard, frees from all sins and leads to union with Brahman (53-54).

Shri Sadashiva said.

I have spoken of the great hymn of the Prakriti of the Supreme Brahman, hear now the protective Mantra of the sacred Adya Kalika (55). The name of the Mantra is "Conqueror of the three Worlds," its Rishi is Shiva, the verse is Anushtup, and its Devata the Adya Kali (56).

Its Vija is the Maya Vija, its Shakti is Kama Vija, and its Kilaka is Kring. It should be used for the attainment of all desired objects (57).

The Protective Mantra

(Known As Trailokya-Vijaya)

*Hring, may the Adya protect my head;
Shring, may Kali protect my face;*

Kring, may the Supreme Shakti protect my heart;

May She Who is the Supreme of the Supreme protect my throat (58);

May Jagaddhatri protect my two eyes;

May Shankari protect my two ears;

May Mahamaya protect my power of smell;

May Sarvva-mangala protect my taste (58);

May Kaumari protect my teeth;

May Kamalalaya protect my cheeks;

May Kshama protect my upper and lower lips;

May Charu-hasini protect my chin (60);

May Kuleshani protect my neck;

May Kripa-mayi protect the nape of my neck;

May Bahu-da protect my two arms;

May Kaivalya-dayini protect my two hands; (61)

May Kapardini protect my shoulders;

May Trailokya-tarini protect my back;

May Aparna protect my two sides;

May Kamathasana protect my hips (62);

May Vishalakshi protect my navel;

May Prabha-vati protect my organ of generation;

May Kalyani protect my thighs;

May Parvati protect my feet;

May Jaya-durga protect my vital breaths,

And Sarvva-siddhi-da protect all parts of my body (63).

As to those parts as have not been mentioned in the Ka-vacha, and are unprotected, may the Eternal Primeval

Kali protect all such (64).

I have now spoken to Thee of the wonderful heavenly Protective Mantra of the Adya Devi Kalika, which is known as the "Conqueror of the three Worlds" (65).

He who repeats it at his devotions with his mind fixed upon the Adya obtains all his desires, and She becomes propitious unto him (66). He quickly attains Mantra-siddhi. The lesser siddhis become, as it were, his slaves (67). He who is childless gets a son, he who desires wealth gains riches. The seeker of learning attains it, and whatsoever a man desires he attains the same (68).

The Purashcharana of this Protective Mantra is its repetition a thousand times, and this gives the desired fruit (69). If it be written on birch-bark, with the paste of sandal, fragrant aloe, musk, saffron, or red sandal, and encased in a golden ball, worn either on the right arm, round the neck, in the crown lock, or round the waist, then the Adya Kali becomes devoted to its wearer, and grants him whatsoever he may desire (70-71). Nowhere has he fear. In all places he is a conqueror. He becomes ready of speech, free from ailments, long-lived and strong, endowed with all power of endurance (72), and an adept in all learning. He knows the meaning of all Scriptures, has Kings under his control, and holds both pleasure and emancipation in the hollow of his hand (73).

For men affected with the taint of the Kali Age it is a most excellent Mantra for the attainment of final liberation (74).

Shri Devi said:

Thou hast, O Lord! in Thy kindness told me of the Hymn and Protective Mantra; I now desire to hear of the rules relating to Purashcharana (75).

Shri Sadashiva said:

The rules relating to Purashcharana in the worship of the Adya Kalika are the same as those relating to the Purashcharana in the worship with the Brahma-Mantra (76). For Sadhakas who are unable to do them completely, both Japa, Puja and Homa, and Purashcharana may be curtailed (77), since it is better to observe these rites on a small scale than not to observe them at all. Now listen, O Gentle One! the while I describe to Thee the shortened form of worship (78). Let the wise one rinse his mouth with the Mula-Mantra, and then perform Rishi-nyasa. Let him purify the palms of the hands, and proceed to Kara-nyasa and Anga-nyasa (79). Passing

*the hands all over the body, let him practise Pranayama,
and then meditate, worship, and inwardly recite. This is
the ceremonial for the shortened form of worship (80).*

*In this form of worship, in lieu of Homa and other rites,
the Mantras may be recited four times the number
prescribed in the case of each of them respectively (81).
There is also another mode of performance. A person
who, when the fourteenth day of the dark half of the
month falls on a Tuesday or Saturday, worships Jagan-
mayi with the five elements of worship, and recites with
fully attentive mind the Mantra ten thousand times
at midnight and feasts believers in the Brahman has
performed Purashcharana (82-83). From one Tuesday
to another Tuesday the Mantra should every day be
inwardly recited a thousand times. The Mantra thus
recited eight thousand times is equal to the performance
of Purashcharana (84-85).*

*In all Ages, O Devi! but particularly in the Kali Age,
the Mantras of the Sacred Primeval Kalika are of great
efficacy, and yield complete success (85-86). O Parvati!
In the Kali Age, Kali in her various forms is ever watch-
ful, but when the Kali Age is in full sway, then the form
of Kali Herself is for the benefit of the world (87). In
initiation into this Kalika Mantra there is no necessity to
determine whether it be siddha or su-siddha, or the like,*

or favourable or inimical. If japa is made of it, which is both niyama and a-niyama, the Adya Devi is pleased (88). The mortal, by the grace of the glorious Adya, attains a knowledge of the divine essence, and, possessed of such knowledge, is, without a doubt, liberated even while living (89). Beloved, there is no need here for over-exertion or endurance or penances. The religious exercises of the worshippers of the Adya Kali are pleasant to accomplish (90). By the mere purification of the heart the worshipper attains all that he desires (91). So long, however, as the heart is not purified, so long must the worshipper practise the rites with devotion to Kula. (92)

The carrying out of the practices ordained produces purification of the heart. The Mantra should, however, first be received from the mouth of the Guru in the case of the Brahma-Mantra (93). O Great Queen! Purashkriya should be done after the performance of the necessary worship and of other prescribed rites. In the purified heart knowledge of Brahman grows. And when knowledge of Brahman is attained, there is neither that which should, nor that which should not, be done (94).

Shri Parvati said:

O Great Deva! what is Kula, and what is Kulachara? O

*Great Lord! what is the sign of each of the five elements
of worship? I desire to hear the truth relating to these
(95).*

Shri Sadashiva said:

*Thou hast asked well, O Lady of the Kulas. Thou art in-
deed the Benefactress of the worshippers. Listen! For Thy
pleasure I shall accurately describe to Thee these things
(96). The Kula are Jiva, Prakriti, space, time, ether,
earth, water, fire, and air (97). O Primeval One! the
realization that all this is one with Brahman is Kulachara, and produces Dharmma, Artha, Kama, and Moksha
(98). Those whose sins are washed away by merits acquired in various previous births by penances, alms, and
faithful observance of worship, it is they whose minds
are inclined in Kaulika worship (99). When the intelligence realizes the essence of Kaulika worship, it becomes
at once purified, and the mind inclines to the lotus-feet
of the Primeval Kali (100). The excellent worshipper
versed in Kaula doctrine who has received this most
excellent Vidya by the service of a good spiritual teacher,
if he remains firmly attached to Kaulika worship and
to the worship with the five elements of the Primeval
Kalika, the Patron Devi of Kula, will enjoy a multitude
of blessings in this life, and attain final liberation at its
close. (102)*

The characteristic of the first element is that it is the great medicine for humanity, helping it to forget deep sorrows, and is the cause of joy (103). But, O Dearest One! the element which is not purified stupefies and bewilders, breeds disputes and diseases, and should be rejected by the Kaulas (104). Beasts bred in villages, in the air, or forest, which are nourishing, and increase intelligence, energy, and strength, are the second element (105). O Beautiful One! of the animals bred in water, that which is pleasing and of good taste, and increases the generative power of man, is the third element (106). The characteristics of the fourth element are that it is easily obtainable, grown in the earth, and is the root of the life of the three worlds (107). And, O Devi, the signs of the fifth element are that it is the cause of intense pleasure to all living things, is the origin of all creatures, and the root of the world which is without either be-ginning or end (108). Know, Dearest One! that the first element is fire, the second is air, the third is water, the fourth is the earth (109), and, O Beauteous Face! as to the fifth element, know it to be ether, the support of the Universe (110). O Sovereign Mistress of Kula, he who knows Kula, the five Kula-tattvas, and Kula worship, is liberated whilst yet living (111).

End of the Seventh Joyful Message, entitled "Hymn of Praise (Stotra), Amulet (Kavacha), and the descriptin of the Kula-tattva."

CHAPTER 8

The Dharmma and Customs of the Castes and Ashramas

AFTER hearing of the various forms of Dharmma, Bhavani, Mother of the worlds, Destructress of all worldly
bonds, spoke again to Shankara (1).

Shri Devi said:

*I have heard of the different Dharmma, which bring
happiness in this world and the next, and bestow piety,
wealth, fulfilment of desire, ward off danger, and are
the cause of union with the Supreme (2). I wish now to
hear of the castes and of the stages of life. Speak in Thy
kindness, O Omnipresent One! of these, and of the mode
of life which should be observed therein (3).*

Shri Sadashiva said:

*O Thou of auspicious Vows! in the Satya and other Ages
there were four castes; in each of these were four stages
of life, and the rules of conduct varied according to the
caste and stages of life. In the Kali Age, however, there
are five castes–namely, Brahmana, Kshatriya, Vaishya,
Shudra, and Samanya. Each of these five castes, O Great*

Queen! have two stages of life. Listen, then, Adye! whilst I narrate to Thee their mode of life, rites, and duties (4-6). I have already spoken to Thee of the incapacity of men born in the Kali Age. Unused as they are to penance, and devoid of learning in the Vedas, short-lived, and incapable of strenuous effort, how can they endure bodily labour? (7).

O Beloved! there is in the Kali Age no Brahmacharya nor Vanaprastha. There are two stages only, Grihastha and Bhikshuka (8). O Auspicious One! In the Kali Age the householder should in all his acts be guided by the rules of the Agamas. He will never attain success by other ways (9). And, O Devi! at the stage of the mendicant the carrying of the staff is not permitted, since, O Thou of Divine Knowledge! both that and other practices are Vedic (10). In the Kali Age, O Gentle One! the adoption of the life of an Avadhuta, according to the Shaiva rites, is in the Kali Age equivalent to the entry into the life of a Sannyasin (11). When the Kali Age is in full sway, the Vipras and the other castes have equal right to enter into both these stages of life (12) The purificatory rites of all are to be according to the rules ordained by Shiva, though the particular practices of the Vipras and other castes vary (13).

A man becomes a householder the moment he is born.

It is by Sangskara that he enters upon any of the other stages of life. For this reason, O Great Queen! One should first be a householder, following the rules of that mode of life (14). When, however, one is freed of worldly desires by the knowledge of the Real, it is then that one should abandon all and seek refuge in the life of an ascetic (15). In childhood one should acquire knowledge; in youth, wealth and wife. The wise man in middle age will devote himself to acts of religion, and in his old age he should retire from the world (16).

No one should retire from the world who has an old father or mother, a devoted and chaste wife, or young and helpless children (17). He who becomes an ascetic, leaving mothers, fathers, infant children, wives, agnates and cognates, is guilty of a great sin (18). He who becomes a mendicant without first satisfying the need of his own parents and relatives is guilty of the sins of killing his father and mother, a woman, and a Brahmana (19). The Brahmanas and men of other castes should perform their respective purificatory rites according to the ordinances laid down by Shiva. This is the rule in the Kali Age (20).

Shri Devi said:

O Omnipresent One! tell Me what is the rule of life for

*the householder and mendicant, and what are the puri-
ficatory rites for the Vipras and other castes (21).*

Shri Sadashiva said:

*The state of an householder is for all the descendants of
Manu the first duty. I shall, therefore, first speak of it,
and do Thou listen to Me, O Lady of the Kaulas (22). A
householder should be devoted to the contemplation of
Brahman and possessed of the knowledge of Brahman,
and should consign whatever he does to Brahman (23).
He should not tell an untruth, or practise deceit, and
should ever be engaged in the worship of the Devatas
and guests (24). Regarding his father and mother as
two visible incarnate deities, he should ever and by
every means in his power serve them (25). O Shiva!
O Parvati! if the mother and father are pleased, Thou
too art pleased. and the Supreme Being is propitious
to him (26). O Primeval One! Thou art the Mother of
the Worlds, and the Supreme Brahman is the Father;
what better religious act can there be than that which
pleases You both? (27). According to their requirements,
one should offer seats, beds, clothes, drink, and food to
mother and father. They should always be spoken to in
a gentle voice, and their children's demeanour should
ever be agreeable to them. The good son who ever obeys
the behests of his mother and father hallows the family*

(28-29). If one desires one's own welfare, all arrogance, mockery, threats, and angry words should be avoided in the parents' presence (30). The son who is obedient to his parents should, out of reverence to them, bow to them and stand up when he sees them, and should not take his seat without their permission (31). He who, intoxicated with the pride of learning or wealth, slights his parents, is beyond the pale of all Dharmma, and goes to a terrible Hell (32). Even if the vital breath were to reach his throat, the householder should not eat without first feeding his mother, father, son, wife, guest, and brother (33). The man who, to the deprivation of his elders and equals, fills his own belly is despised in this world, and goes to Hell in the next (34). The householder should cherish his wife, educate his children, and support his kinsmen and friends. This is the supreme eternal duty (35). The body is nourished by the mother. It originates from the father. The kinsmen, out of love, teach. The man, therefore, who forsakes them is indeed vile (36). For their sake should an hundred pains be undergone. With all one's ability they should be pleased. This is the eternal duty (37). That man who in this world turns his mind to Brahman and adheres faithfully to the truth is above all a man of good deeds, and knows the Supreme, and is blest in all the worlds (38). The householder should never punish his wife, but should cherish her like a mother. If she is virtuous and devoted to her husband,

he should never forsake her even in times of greatest misfortune (39). The wise man, whilst his own wife is living, should never with wicked intent touch another woman, otherwise he will go to hell (40). The wise man should not, when in a private place, live and sleep or lie down close to other men's wives. He should avoid all improper speech and braggart boldness in their presence (41). By riches, clothes, love, respect, and pleasing words should one's wife be satisfied. The husband should never do anything displeasing to her (42). The wise man should not send his wife to any festival, concourse of people, pilgrimage, or to another's house, except she be attended by his son or an inmate of his own house (43).

O Maheshvari! that man whose wife is both faithful and happy is surely looked upon as if he had performed all Dharmma, and is truly Thy favourite also (44). A father should fondle and nurture his sons until their fourth year, and then until their sixteenth they should be taught learning and their duties (45). Up to their twentieth year they should be kept engaged in household duties, and thenceforward, considering them as equals, he should ever show affection towards them (46). In the same manner a daughter should be cherished and educated with great care, and then given away with money and jewels to a wise husband (47).

The householder should thus also cherish and protect his brothers and sisters and their children, his kinsmen, friends, and servants (48). He should also maintain his fellow-worshippers, fellow-villagers, and guests, whether ascetics or others (49). If the wealthy householder does not so act, then let him be known as a beast, a sinner, and one despised in the worlds (50). The householder should not be inordinately addicted to sleep, idling, care for the body, dressing his hair, eating or drinking, or attention to his clothes (51). He should be moderate as to food, sleep, speech, and sexual intercourse, and be sincere, humble, pure, free from sloth, and persevering (52). Chivalrous to his foes, modest before his friends, relatives, and elders, he should neither respect those who deserve censure nor slight those who are worthy of respect (53). Men should only be admitted to his trust and confidence after association with them and observation of their nature, inclination, conduct, and friendly character (54). Even an insignificant enemy should be feared, and one's own power should be disclosed only at the proper time. But on no account should one deviate from the path of duty (55). A religious man should not speak of his own fame and prowess, of what has been told him in secret, nor of the good that he has done for others (56). A man of good name should not engage in any quarrel with an unworthy motive, nor when defeat is certain, nor with those who are superior or inferior to himself He should diligently earn knowledge, wealth, fame, and religious merit, and avoid all vicious habits, the company of the wicked, falsehood, and treachery (58). Ventures should be undertaken according to the circumstances and one's condition in life, and actions should be done according to their season. Therefore, in everything that a man does he should first consider whether the circumstances and time are suitable (59). The householder should employ himself in the acquisition of what is necessary and in the protection of the same. He should be judicious, pious, good to his friends. He should be moderate in speech and laughter, in particular in the presence of those entitled to his reverence (60). He should hold his senses under control, be of cheerful disposition, think of what is good, be of firm resolve, attentive, far-sighted, and discriminating in the use of his senses (61).

The wise householder's speech should be truthful, mild, agreeable, and salutary, yet pleasing, avoiding both self-praise and the disparagement of others (62). The man who has dedicated tanks, planted trees, built rest-houses on the roadside, or bridges, has conquered the three worlds (63). That man who is the happiness of his mother and father, to whom his friends are devoted, and whose fame is sung by men, he is the conqueror of the three worlds (64). He whose aim is truth, whose cha-

*rity is ever for the poor, who has mastered lust and ang-
er, by him are the three worlds conquered (65). He who
covets not others' wives or goods, who is free of deceit
and envy, by him the three worlds are conquered (66).
He who is not afraid in battle nor to go to war when
there is need, and who dies in battle undertaken for a
sacred cause, by him the three worlds are conquered
(67). He whose soul is free from doubts, who is devoted
to and a faithful follower of the ordinances of Shiva, and
remains under My control, by him the three worlds are
conquered (68). The wise man who in his conduct with
his fellow-men looks with an equal eye upon friend and
foe, by him are the three worlds conquered (69). O Devi!
purity is of two kinds, external and internal. The dedication of oneself to Brahman is known as internal purity
(70), and the cleansing of the impurities of the body by
water or ashes, or any other matter which cleanses the
body, is called external purity (71).*

*O Dearest One! the waters of Ganga, or of any other
river, tank, pond, well, or pool, or of the celestial Ganga,
are equally purifying (72). O Thou of auspicious Vows!
the ashes from a place of sacrifice and cleansed earth are
excellent, and the skin of an antelope and grass are as
purifying as earth (73). O Auspicious One! what need is
there to say more about purity and impurity? Whatever
purifies the mind that the householder may do (74). Let*

there be external purification upon awakening from sleep, after sexual intercourse, making water, voiding the bowels, and at the close of a meal, and whenever dirt of any kind has been touched (75).

Sandhya, whether Vaidika or Tantrika should be performed thrice daily, and according as the worship changes so does its service (76). The worshippers of the Brahma-Mantra have performed their Sandhya when they have made japa of the Gayatri, realizing within themselves the identity of the Gayatri and Brahman (77). In the case of those who are not Brahma-worshippers, Vaidika Sandhya consists of the worship of and offering of oblations to the Sun and the recitation of the Gayatri (78).

O Gentle One! In all daily prayers recitation shouldbe done one thousand and eight or a hundred and eight or ten times (79). O Devi! the Shudras and Samanyas may observe any of the rites proclaimed by the Agamas, and by these they attain that which they desire (80). The three times of performance (of Sandhya) are at sunrise, at noon, and at sunset (81).

Shri Devi said:

Thou hast Thyself said, O Lord! that when the Kali Age

*is in full sway for all castes, commencing with the Brah-
mamas, Tantrika rites are alone appropriate. Why, then,
dost Thou restrict the Vipras to Vedic rites? It behoveth
Thee to explain this fully to Me (82-83).*

Shri Sadashiva said:

*O Thou Who knowest the essence of all things, truly hast
Thou spoken. In the Kali Age all observances bear the
fruit of enjoyment and liberation when done according
to the rites of the Tantras (84). The Brahma-Savitri,
though known as Vaidika, should be called Tantrika
also, and is appropriate in both observances (85). It is,
therefore, O Devi! that I have said that when the Kali
Age is in full sway, the twice-born shall alone be entitled
to the Gayatri, but not the other Mantras (86). In the
Kali Age the Savitri should be said by the Brahmanas,
preceded by the Tara, and by the Kshatriyas and Vaishyas, preceded by the Kamala and Vagbhava Vijas respectively (87). In order, O Supreme Devi! That a distinction
may be drawn between the twice-born and the Shudras,
the daily duties are directed to be preceded by Vaidika
Sandhya (88). Success, however, may also be attained
by the mere following of the ordinances of Shambhu.
This is verily true, and I repeat it is true and very true,
and there is no doubt about it (89). O Adored of the
Devas! even if the stated time for the saying of the daily*

prayer is past, all who desire emancipation and are not prevented by sickness or weakness should say, "Ong the Ever-existent Brahman" (90). The seat, clothes, vessels, bed, carriages, residence, and household furniture of the worshipper should be as clean as possible (91). At the close of the daily prayers the householder should keep himself occupied with household duties or the study of the Vedas; he should never remain idle (92). In holy places, on holy days, or when the Sun or Moon is in eclipse, he should do inward recitation, and give alms, and thus become the abode of all that is good (93).

In the Kali Age life is dependent on the food that is eaten, fasting is therefore not recommended, in lieu of it, the giving of alms is ordained (94). O Great Queen! in the Kali Age alms are efficacious in the accomplishment of all things. The proper objects of such alms are the poor devoted to meritorious acts (95). O Mother! the first days of the month, of the year, of the lunar half-months, the fourteenth day of the lunar half-month, the eighth day of the light half of the lunar month, the eleventh day of the lunar half-month, the new moon, one's birthday, the anniversary of one's father's death, and days fixed as those of festivals, are holy days (96-97).

The River Ganges and all the great Rivers, the house of the religious Teacher, and the places of the Devas are holy places. But for those who, neglecting the study of the Veda, the service of mother and father, and the protection of their wife, go to places of pilgrimage, such holy places are changed to hell (98-99). For women there is no necessity to go on pilgrimage, to fast, or to do other like acts, nor is there any need to perform any devotion except that which consists in the service of their husband (100). For a woman her husband is a place of pilgrimage, the performance of penance, the giving of alms, the carrying out of vows, and her spiritual teacher. Therefore should a woman devote herself to the service of her husband with her whole self (101). She should ever by words and deeds of devotion act for the pleasure of her husband, and, remaining faithful to his behests, should please his relations and friends (102).

A woman whose husband is her vow should not look at him with hard eyes, or utter hard words before him. Not even in her thought should she do anything which is displeasing to her husband (103). She who by body, mind, and word, and by pleasant acts, ever pleases her husband, attains to the abode of Brahman (104). Remaining ever faithful to the wishes of her husband, she should not look upon the face of other men, or have converse with them, or uncover her body before them (105).

In childhood she should remain under the control of her parents, in her youth of her husband, and in her old age of the friends and relatives of her husband. She should never be independent (106).

A father should not marry his daughter if she does not know her duty to a husband and how to serve him, also the other rules of woman's conduct (107).

Neither the flesh of human beings, nor the animals resembling them, nor the flesh of the cow, which is serviceable in various ways, nor the flesh of carnivorous animals, nor such meat as is tasteless, should be eaten (108). Auspicious One! fruits and roots of various kinds whether grown in villages or jungles, and all that is grown in the ground, may be eaten at pleasure (109).

Teaching and the performance of sacrifices are the proper duties of a Brahmana. But if he be incapable of these, he may earn his livelihood by following the profession of a Kshatriya or Vaishya (110). The proper occupation of a Rajanya is that of fighting and ruling. But if he be incapable of these, he may earn his livelihood by following the profession of a Vaishya or Shudra (111). If a Vaishya cannot trade, then for him the following of the profession of a Shudra involves no blame. For a Shudra, O Sovereign Queen! service is the prescribed means of

*livelihood (112). O Devi! members of the Samanya class
may for their maintenance follow all occupations except
such as are specially reserved for the Brahmana (113).
The latter, void of hate and attachment, self-controlled,
truthful, the conqueror of his senses, free of envy and
all guile, should pursue his own avocations (114). He
should ever be the same to, and the well-wisher of, all
men, and teach his well-behaved pupils as if they were
his own sons (115). He should ever avoid falsehood,
detraction, and vicious habits, arrogance, friendship
for low persons, the pursuit of low objects, and the use
of language which gives offence (116). Where peace
is possible, avoid war. Peace with honour is excellent.
O Adorable Face! for the Rajanya it should be either
death or victory in battle (117). A man of the kingly
caste should not covet the wealth of his subjects, or levy
excessive taxes, but, being faithful to his promises, he
should ever in the observance of his duty protect his
subjects as though they were his own children (118). In
government, war, treaties, and other affairs of State the
King should take the advice of his Ministers (119). War
should be carried on in accordance with Dharmma.
Rewards and punishments should be awarded justly and
in accordance with the Shastras. The best treaty should
be concluded which his power allows (120). By stratagem should the end desired be attained. By the same
means should wars be conducted and treaties concluded.*

Victory, peace, and prosperity follow stratagem (121).
He should ever avoid the company of the low, and be
good to the learned. He should be of a calm disposition
judicious of action in time of trouble, of good conduct
and reasonable in his expenditure (122).

He should be an expert in the maintenance of his forts,
well trained in the use of arms. He should ever ascer-
tain the disposition of his army, and teach his soldiers
military tactics (123). O Devil he should not in battle
kill one who is stunned, who has surrendered his arms,
or is a fugitive, nor those of his enemies whom he has
capturedn nor their wives or children (124). Whatever is
acquired either by victory or treaty should be distributed
amongst the soldiers in shares according to merit (125).

The King should make known to himself the character
and courage of each of his warriors, and if he would
care for his interests he should not place a large army
under the command of a single officer (126). He should
not put his trust in any single person, nor place one man
in charge of the administration, nor treat his inferiors
as equals, nor be familiar with them (127). He should
be very learned, yet not garrulous; full of knowledge, yet
anxious to learn; full of honours, yet without arrogance.
In awarding both reward and punishment he should be
discriminating (128). The King should either himself

or through his spies watch his subjects, kinsmen, and servants (129). A wise master should not either honour or degrade anyone in a fit of passion or arrogance and without due cause (130). Soldiers, commanders, ministers, wife, children, and servitors he should protect. If guilty, they should be punished according to their deserts (131). The King should protect, like a father, the insane, incapable, children and orphans, and those who are old and infirm (132). Know that agriculture and trade are the appropriate callings of the Vaishya. It is by agriculture and trade that man's body is maintained (133). Therefore, O Devi! in agriculture and trade all negligence, vicious habits, laziness, untruth, and deceit should be avoided with the whole soul (134). Shiva! when both buyer and seller are agreed as to the object of sale and the price thereof, and mutual promises have been made, then the purchase becomes complete (135). O Dearest One! the sale or gift of property by one who is a lunatic, out of his senses, under age, a captive, or enfeebled by disease, is invalid (136). The purchase of things not seen is concluded by hearing the description thereof. If the article be found to differ from its description, then the purchase is set aside (137). The sale of an elephant, a camel, and a horse is effected by the description of the animal. The sale is, however, set aside if the animal does not answer its description (138). If in the purchase of elephants, camels, and horses a latent vice becomes patent within the course of a year from the date of sale, then the purchase is set aside, but not after the lapse of one year (139). O Devi of the Kulas! the human body is the receptacle of piety, wealth, desires, and final liberation. It should therefore never be the subject of purchase; and such a purchase is by reason of My commands invalid (140).

O Dear One! in the borrowing of barley, wheat, or paddy, the profit of the lender at the end of the year is laid down to be a fourth of the quantity lent, and in the case of the loan of metals one-eighth (141). In monetary transactions, agriculture, trade, and in all other transactions, men should ever carry out their undertakings. This is approved by the laws (142). A servant should be skilful, clean, wakeful, careful and alert, and possess his senses under control (143). He should, as he desires happiness in this and the next world, regard his master as if he were Vishnu Himself, his master's wife; his own mother, and respect his master's kinsmen and friends (144). He should know his master's friends to be his friends, and his master's enemies to be his enemies and should ever remain in respectful attendance upon his master, awaiting his orders (145). He should carefully conceal his master's dishonour, the family dissensions, anything said in private or which would disgrace his master (146). He should not covet the wealth of his mas-

ter, but remain ever devoted to his good. He should not make use of bad words or laugh or play in his masters presence (147). He should not, with lustful mind, even look at the maidservants in his master's house, or lie down with them, or play with them in secret (148). He should not use his master's bed, seat, carriages, clothes, vessels, shoes, jewels, or weapons (149). If guilty, he should beg the forgiveness of his master. He should not be forward, impertinent, or attempt to place himself on an equal footing with his master (150).

Except when in the Bhairavi-chakra or Tattva-chakra persons of all castes should marry in their caste according to the Brahma form, and should eat with their own caste people (151). O Great Queen! in these two circles, however, marriage in the Shaiva form is ordained, and as regards eating and drinking, no caste distinctions exist (152).

Shri Devi said:

What is the Bhairavi-chakra, and what is the Tattva-chakra? I desire to hear, and it kindly behoves Thee to speak of them (153).

Shri Sadashiva said:

*O Devi! in the ordinances relating to Kula worship I
have spoken of the formation of circles by the excellent
worshippers at times of special worship (154). O Dear
One! there is no rule relating to the Bhairavi-chakra.
This auspicious circle may at any time be formed (155).
I will now speak of the rites relating to this circle, which
benefits the worshippers, and in which, if the Devi be
worshipped, She speedily grants the prayers of Her
votaries (156).*

*The Kulacharyya should spread an excellent mat in a
beautiful place, and, after purifying it with the Kama
and Astra Vijas, should seat himself upon it (157). Then
the wise one should draw a square with a triangle in
it with either vermilion or red sandal wood paste, or
simply water (158). Then, taking a painted jar, and
smearing it with curd and sun-dried rice, and placing a
vermilion mark on it, let him put a branch or leaves and
fruit upon it (159). Filling it with perfumed water whilst
uttering the Pranava, the worshipper should place it on
the Mandala, and exhibit before it lights and incense-sticks (160). The jar should then be worshipped with
two fragrant flowers. Ishta-devata should be meditated
upon as being in the jar. The ritual should be according
to the shortened form (161). Listen, O Adored of the
Immortals! whilst I speak to Thee of the peculiar features of this worship. There is no necessity of placing the*

*wine-cups for the Guru and others 162). The worshipper
should then take such of the elements of worship as he
wishes, and place them in front of himself. Then, purifying them with the Weapon Mantra, let him gaze upon
them with steadfast eyes (163).*

*Then, placing scent and flowers in the wine-jar, let
him meditate upon the Ananda-Bhairava and Ananda-Bhairavi in it (164).*

Dhyana

*He should meditate upon the Blissful Devi as in first
bloom of youth, with a body rosy as the first gleam of
the rising Sun. The sweet nectar of Her smiles illumines
Her face as beautiful as a full-blown lotus. Decked with
jewels, clad in beauteous coloured raiment delighting in
dance and song, She with the lotus of her hands makes
the signs which confer blessings and dispel fears (165-
166).*

*After thus meditating on Blissful Devi, let the worship-
per thus meditate upon the Blissful Bhairava (167).*

Dhyana

I meditate upon the Deva Who is white as camphor,

Whose eyes are large and beautiful like lotuses, the lustre of Whose body is adorned with celestial raiments and jewels, Who holds in His left hand the cup of nectar, and in the right a ball of Shuddhi (168).

Having thus meditated upon Them both, and thinking of them in a state of union in the wine-jar, the worshipper should then worship Them therein. With Mantra, beginning with the Pranava and ending with Namah, the names of the Devata being placed between, and with perfume and flower, let him then sanctify the wine (169)

The Kula worshipper should sanctify the wine by repeating over it the Pashadi-trika-vija a hundred and eight times (170). When the Kali Age is in full sway, in the case of the householder whose mind is entirely engrossed with domestic desires, the three sweets should be substituted in the place of the first element of worship (wine) (171). Milk, sugar, and honey are the three sweets. They should be deemed to be the image of wine, and as such offered to the Deity (172). Those born in the Kali Age are by their nature weak in intellect, and their minds are distracted by lust. By reason of this they do not recognize the Shakti to be the image of the Deity (173). Therefore, O Parvati! for such as these let there be, in place of the last element of worship (sexual union), meditation upon the lotus-feet of the Devi and the inward recitation of their Ishta-mantra (174).

Therefore such of the elements of worship as have been obtained should be consecrated by the recitation over each of them of the same Mantra one hundred times (175). Let the worshipper, with closed eyes, meditate upon them as suffused by Brahman, then offer them to Kali, and, lastly, eat and drink the consecrated elements (176). O Gentle One! this is the Bhairavi-chakra, which is not revealed in the other Tantras. I have, however spoken before Thee of it. It is the essence of essences, and more excellent than the best (177). Parvati! In Bhairavi-chakra and Tattva-chakra the excellent worshipper should be wedded to his Shakti, according to the laws prescribed by Shiva (178). The Vira who without marriage worships by enjoyment of Shakti is, without doubt, guilty of the sin of going with another man's wife (179). When the Bhairavi-chakra has been formed, the members thereof are like the best of the twice-born; but when the circle is broken, they revert again to their own respective castes (180). In this circle there is no distinction of caste nor impurity of food. The heroic worshippers in the circle are My image; there is no doubt of that (181). In the formation of the circle there is no rule as to time or place or question as to fitness. The necessary articles may be used by whomsoever they may have been brought (182). Food brought from a long distance, whether it be cooked or uncooked, whether brought by a Vira or a Pashu, becomes pure immediately it is brought within the circle (183).

While the circle is being formed, all dangers flee in confusion, awed by the Brahmanic lustre of its heroes (184). Upon the mere hearing that a Bhairavi circle has been formed at any place, fierce Pishachas, Guhyakas, Yakshas, and Vetalas depart afar off in fear (185). Into the circle come all the holy places, the great and holy places, and with reverence Indra and all the Immortals (186). Shiva! the place where a circle is formed is a great and holy place, more sacred than each and all the other holy places. Even the Thirty desire the excellent offerings made to Thee in this circle (187). Whatever the food be, whether cooked or uncooked, and whether brought by a Mlechchha, Chandala, Kirata, or Huna, it becomes pure as soon as it is placed in the hand of a Vira (188). By the seeing of the circle and of the worshippers therein, who are but images of Myself, men infected with the taint of the Kali Age are liberated from the bonds of the life of a Pashu (189). When, however the Kali Age is in full sway, the circle should not be concealed. The Vira should at all places and at all times practise Kula rites and make Kula worship (190).

In the circle all distinction of caste, frivolous talk, levity, garrulity, spitting, and breaking wind should be avoided (191). Such as are cruel, mischievous, Pashu, sinful, atheists, blasphemers of Kula doctrine, and calumnia-tors of the Kula Scriptures, should not be allowed into the circle (192). Even the Vira who, induced by affection, fear, or attachment, admits a Pashu into the circle falls from his Kula duty, and goes to hell (193). All who have sought refuge in the Kula Dharmma, whether Brahmamas, Kshatriyas, Vaishyas, Shudras, or Samanyas, should ever be worshipped like Devas (194). He who, whilst in the circle, makes, from pride, distinctions of caste, descends to a terrible hell, even though he should have gone to the very end of the Vedanta (195). How within the circle can there be any fear of sin for Kaulas, who are good and pure of heart and who are manifestly the very image of Shiva? (196). Vipras and others who are followers of Shiva should, so long as they are within the circle, follow the ordinance of Shiva and the observances prescribed by Him (197).

Without the circle each should follow his own calling according to his caste and stage of life, and should discharge his duty as a man of the world (198). One Japa made by a devout man, when seated within the circle, bears the fruit attainable by the performance of a hundred Purashcharana and by Shavasana, Mundasana, and Chitasana (199). Who can describe the glory of the Bhairavi-chakra? Its formation, though but once only, frees of all sins (200). The man who for six months worships in such a circle will become a King: he who so worships for a year becomes the conqueror of death, and by the daily performance of such worship he attains to Nirvvana (201).

What is the need, O Kalika! of saying more? Know this for certain: that for the attainment of happiness in this or the next world there is only the Kula-dharmma, and no other (202). When the Kali Age is dominant and all religion is abandoned, even a Kaula merits hell by concealment of the Kula-dharmma (203).

I have spoken of the Bhairavi circle, which is the sole means of attaining enjoyment and final liberation. I will now speak to Thee, O Queen of the Kaulas! of the Tattva circle. Do Thou listen (204).

The Tattva circle is the king of all circles. It is also called the celestial circle. Only worshippers who have attained to a knowledge of Brahman may take part in it (205). Only those servants of the Brahman may take part in this circle who have attained to knowledge of Brahman, who are devoted to Brahman, pure of heart, tranquil, devoted to the good of all things, who are unaffected by the external world, who see no differences, but to whom all things are the same, who are merciful, faithful to their vows, and who have realized the Brahman (206-207).

O Knower of the Supreme Soul! only those who, possessing the knowledge of the Real, look upon this moving and motionless Existence as one with Brahman, such men are privileged to take part in this circle (208). They who regard everything in the Tattva circle as Brahman, they alone, O Devi, are qualified to take part therein (209). In the formation of this circle there is no necessity for placing the wine-jar, no lengthy ritual. It can be formed everywhere in a spirit of devotion to Brahman (210). O Dearest One! the worshipper of the Brahma-Mantra and a devout believer in Brahman should be the Lord of the circle, which he should form of other worshippers who know the Brahman (211). In a beautiful and clean place, pleasant to the worshippers, pure seats should be spread with beautiful carpets (212). There, O Shiva! the Lord of the circle should seat himself with the worshippers of Brahman, and have the elements of worship brought and placed in front of him (213). The Lord of the Circle should inwardly recite the Mantra, beginning with the Tara and ending with the Prana-vija, a hundred times, and then pronounce the following Mantra over the elements (214):

Mantra

The act of offering is Brahman. The offering itself is Brahman. The Fire is Brahman. He by whom the offe-

ring is made is Brahman. By him who is absorbed in the worship of Brahman is unity with Brahman attained (215).

All the elements should be purified by the inward recitation of this Mantra seven or three times (216). Then, with the Brahma-Mantra, making an offering of the food and drink to the Supreme Soul, he should partake thereof with the other worshippers, knowers of the Brahman (217). O Great Queen! there is no distinction of caste in the Brahma circle, nor rule as to place or time or cup. The ignorant who, through want of care, make distinctions of birth or caste go upon the downward path (218-219). And therefore should those excellent worshippers, possessed of the knowledge that the Supreme Brahman pervades all things, perform the rites of the Tattva circle with every care for the attainment of religious merit, fulfilment of desire, wealth, and liberation (220).

Shri Devi said:

Lord! Thou hast spoken in full of the duties of the householder; it now behoves Thee kindly to speak of the duties appropriate to the ascetic life (221).

Shri Sadashiva said:

Devi! the stage of life of an Avadhuta is in the Kali Age called Sannyasa. Now listen while I tell thee what should be done (222).

When an adept in spiritual wisdom has acquired the knowledge of Brahman, and has ceased to care for the things of the world, he should seek refuge in the life of an ascetic (223). If, however, in order to adopt the life of a wandering mendicant, one abandons an old mother or father, infant children and a devoted wife, or helpless dependents, one goes to hell (224). All, whether Brahmana, Kshatriya, Vaishya, Shudra, or Samanya are equally entitled to take part in the purificatory ceremony of the Kula ascetic (225).

After the performance of all the duties of a householder, and after satisfying all dependents, one should go forth from his house indifferent, free from desires, with all his senses conquered (226). He who wishes thus to leave his house should call together his kinsmen and friends, his neighbours and men of his village, and lovingly ask of them their permission (227). Having obtained it, and made obeisance to his Ishta-devata, he should go round his village, and then without attachment set forth from his house (228). Liberated from the bonds of household life, and immersed in exceeding joy, he should approach a Kula ascetic of divine knowledge and pray to him as follows: (229)

"O Supreme Brahman! all this life of mine has been spent in the discharge of household duties. Do Thou O Lord! be gracious to me in this my adoption of the life of an ascetic" (230).

The religious Preceptor should thereupon satisfy himself that the disciple's duties as a householder have all been accomplished, and, on finding him to be meek and full of discernment, initiate him into the second stage (231). The disciple should then, with a well-controlled mind, make his ablutions and say his daily prayer, and then, with the object of being absolved from the threefold debt due to them, worship the Devas, the Rishis, and the Pitris (232).

By the Devas are meant Brahma, Vishnu, and Rudra, with their followers; by the Rishis are meant Sanaka and others, as also the Devarshis and the Brahmarshis (233). Listen, whilst I now enumerate the ancestors which should be worshipped (234). The father, paternal grand-father, paternal great-grandfather, mother, the maternal grandfather, and others in the ascending line, and the maternal grandmother and others in the ascending line (235). Upon the dedication of oneself to the life of an ascetic, the Devas and Rishis should be worshipped in the East, the paternal ancestors in the South, the ma-ternal ancestors in the West (236). Spreading two seats *on each of these sides, beginning from the East, and invoking the Devas and others thereto, they should there be worshipped (237). Having worshipped them in proper form, pindas should be offered to each of them separately according to the rules relating thereto; And then, with folded palms, let the disciple thus supplicate the Devas and Ancestors (238):*

Mantra

O Fathers! O Mothers! O Devas! O Rishis! be you satisfied. Do you absolve me, about to enter upon the path of renunciation from all debts (239).

Having thus prayed to be free from all debts, bowing again and again, and being thus freed of all debts, he should perform his own funeral rites (240). The father and paternal grandfather and great-grandfather are one soul. In offering, therefore, the individual soul to the Supreme Soul, he who is wise should perform his own funeral rites (241). O Devi! sitting with his face to the North, and invoking the spirits of his ancestors upon the seats which he has prepared for them, he should, after doing them homage, offer the funeral cakes (242). In so offering he should spread kusha grass with its end towards the East, South, West, and towards the North for himself (243). After completion, according to the

*directions of the Guru, of the funeral rites, the seeker
after emancipation should, in order to purify his heart
inwardly, recite the following Mantra a hundred times
(244):*

Mantra

*Hring, let us worship the Three-eyed One whose fame
is fragrant, the Augmenter of increase. May I, as the
urvaruka is freed of its stalk, be liberated from death
unto immortality (245).*

*Then the religious Preceptor should draw a figure on the
altar of a shape in accordance with the divinity about to
be worshipped and then place the jar on the altar and
commence worship (246). Then the Guru, possessed
of divine knowledge, should meditate upon the Supreme Spirit in the manner prescribed by Shambhu, and
after worship place fire on the altar (247). The Guru
should then offer unto the fire so sanctified the oblation
according to the Sangkalpa, and then make his disciple
perform the complete homa (248). He should first offer
oblation with the Vyahritis, and then with the vital airs,
prana, apana, samana, udana, vyana (249).*

*For the destruction of the false belief that the body,
whether gross or subtle, is the Atma, the Tattva-Homa*

should be performed, uttering the following words:

Mantra

Earth, water, fire, air, ether, (then) scent, taste, vision, touch, sound, (then) speech, hands, feet, anus and organ of generation, (then) ears, skin, eyes, tongue, and smell, (then) manas, buddhi, ahangkara, and chitta, (and lastly) all the functions of the senses and of life (250-253).

He should then say:

"May they be purified;" (adding) "May I be like unto the universal Chaitanya united with Hring. May I be like the Light beyond and above Rajo-guna, and may I be free of the taint of ignorance" (254).

Having consigned as oblations into the fire the twenty-four tattvas and the functions of the body, he who is now devoid of all action should consider his body as dead (255). Considering his body as dead and devoid of all function, and calling to mind the Supreme Brahman, let him take off his sacred thread (256). He, the possessor of divine knowledge, should take it from his shoulder, uttering the

Mantra

Aing Kling Hangsa.

*Holding it in his hand while he recites the three Vyahri-
tis, ending with Svaha, let him throw it steeped in ghee
into the fire (257). Having thus offered the sacred thread
as an oblation to the fire, he should, whilst uttering the
Kama Vija, cut off his crown-lock and take and place it
in the ghee (258).*

Mantra

*O Crown Lock! Daughter of Brahman! thou art an
ascetic in the form of hair. I am now placing thee in the
Purifying One. Depart, O Devi! I make obeisance to
thee (259).*

*He should then, whilst uttering the Kama, Maya, Kur-
cha, and Astra Vijas, ending with the word Svaha, make
the Homa sacrifice of that lock of hair in the well-sancti-
fied fire (260). The Pitris, Devas, and Devarshis, as also
all acts performed in the stages of life, reside in that lock
and have it as their support (261).*

*Therefore the man who renounces the crown-lock and
sacred thread after the performance of the oblation
becomes one with Brahman (262). The twice-born enter
the stage of an ascetic by renunciation of the crown-lock*

and sacred thread, and the Shudras and Samanyas by the renunciation of the crown-lock only (263). Then he whose crown-lock and sacred thread have been thus removed should make obeisance to the Guru, laying himself full length upon the ground. The Guru should then raise his disciple and say into his right ear: "0 wise one! thou art That." "Think within thyself that I am He and He is I. Free from all attachments and sense of self, do thou go as thou pleasest as moved thereto by thy nature" (264-265). The Guru, full of the knowledge of the Divine essence, should then, after removal of the jar and the fire, bow to the disciple, recognizing in him his own very self (266), and say: "O Thou whose form is this Universe! I bow to Thee and to myself. Thou art 'That' and 'That' is Thou. Again I bow to thee." (267).

The worshippers of the Brahma-Mantra, possessed of divine knowledge, who have conquered themselves, attain the stage of an ascetic by cutting off the crown-lock with their own Mantra (268). What need is there for those purified by divine knowledge of sacrificial or funeral rites or ritual worship? For they, acting as they please, are never guilty of any fault (269). The disciple, image of the absence of all contraries, desireless, and of tranquil mind, may, as he pleases, roam the earth, the visible image of Brahman (270). He will think of everything, from Brahma to a blade of grass, as the image

*of the existent one, and, oblivious of his own name and
form, he will meditate upon the Supreme Soul in himself
(271). Homeless, merciful, fearless, devoid of attachment claiming nothing as his own, devoid of egoism, the
ascetic will move about the earth (272). He is free of all
prohibitions. He shall not strive to attain what he has
not, nor to protect what he has. He knows himself. He is
equally unaffected by either joy or sorrow. He is calm,
the conqueror of himself, and free from all desires (273).*

*His soul is untroubled even in sorrow, desireless even
in prosperity. He is ever joyful, pure, calm, indifferent
and unperturbed. He will hurt no living thing, but
will be ever devoted to the good of all being. He is free
from anger and fear, with his senses under control and
without desire. He strives not for the preservation of his
body. He is not obsessed by any longing (274-275). He
will be free from grief and resentment, equal to friend
and foe, patient in the endurance of cold and heat, and
to him both honour and disgrace are one and the same
(276). He is the same in good or evil fortune, pleased
with whatsoever, without effort, he may obtain. He is
beyond the three attributes, of unconditioned mind free
of covetousness, and (wealth) he will hoard not (277).
He will be happy in the knowledge that, as the unreal
universe exists dependent upon the Truth, so does the
body depend upon the soul (278). He attains liberation*

by the realization that the soul is completely detached from the organs of sense, and is the witness of that which is done (279).

The ascetic should not accept any metal, and should avoid calumny, untruth, jealousy, all play with woman, and all discharge of seed (280). He should regard with an equal eye worms, men, and Devas. The religious mendicant should know that in everything he does, in that is Brahman (281). He should eat without making any distinction of place, time, person, or vessel, and whether from the hand of a Vipra or Chandala, or from any other person whatsoever (282). The ascetic, thouugh passing his time as he pleases, should study the Scriptures relating to the Soul and in meditation upon the nature of That (283). The corpse of an ascetic should on no account be cremated. It should be worshipped with scents and flowers, and then either buried or sunk into water (284). O Devi! the inclination of those men who have not attained union with the Supreme Soul and who ever seek after enjoyment, is by nature turned towards the path of action (285).

They remain attached to the practice of meditation, ritual worship, and recitation. Let them who are strong in their faith therein know that to be the best for them (286). It is on account of them that I have spoken of various rites for the purification of the heart, and have with the same object devised many names and forms (287). O Devi! without knowledge of the Brahman and the abandonment of all ritual worship, man cannot attain emancipation even though he performed countless such acts of worship (288). The householder should consider the Kula ascetic, possessed of divine knowledge, to be the visible Narayana in the form of man, and should worship Him as such (289). By the mere sight of one who has subdued his passions a man is freed of all his sins, and earns that merit which he obtains by journeying to places of pilgrimage, the giving of alms, and the performance of all vows, penances, and sacrifices (290)

End of the Eighth Joyful Message, entitled "The Dharmma and Customs of the Castes and Ashramas."

CHAPTER 9

The Ten Kinds of Purificatory Rites

(Sangskara)

THE Adorable Sadashiva said:

*O Virtuous One! I have spoken to Thee of the custom
and religious duties appropriate to the different castes
and stages of life. Do thou now listen whilst I tell Thee of
the purificatory rites of the different castes (1). Without
such rites, O Devi! the body is not purified, and he who
is not purified may not perform the ceremonies relating to the Devas and the Pitris (2). Therefore it is that
men of every caste, commencing with the Vipras, who
desire their welfare in this life and hereafter, should, in
all things and with care, perform the purificatory rites
which have been ordained for their respective castes (3).*

*The ten purificatory ceremonies are those relating to
conception, pregnancy, and birth of the child; the giving
of its name, its first view of the sun, its first eating of
rice, tonsure, investiture, and marriage (4).*

*The Shudras and mixed castes have no sacred thread,
and but nine purificatory ceremonies; for the twice-born
classes there are ten (5). O Beautiful Lady! all observan-*

ces, whether they be obligatory, occasional, or voluntary, should be performed according to the injunctions of Shambhu (6). O Dearest One! I have already, in My form of Brahma, spoken of the rules appropriate to the purificatory and other observances (7), and of the Mantras appropriate to the various purificatory and other observances, according to the differences in caste (8).

In the Satya, Treta, and Dvapara Ages, the Mantras, O Kalika! were in their application preceded by the Pranava (9); but in the Kali Age, O Supreme Devi! the decree of Shangkara is that man do perform all rites with the aid of the same Mantras, but preceded by the Maya Vija (10). All Mantras in the Nigamas, Agamas, Tantras, Sanghitas and Vedas, have been spoken by Me. Their employment, however, varies according to the Ages (11). For the benefit of men of the Kali Age, men bereft of energy and dependent for existence on the food they eat, the Kula doctrine, O Auspicious One! is given (12).

I will now speak to Thee in brief of the purificatory and other rites, suitable for the weak men of the Kali Age, whose minds are incapable of continued effort (13). Kushandika precedes all auspicious ceremonies. I shall, therefore, O Adored of the Devas! speak firstly of it. Do Thou listen (14). In a clean and pleasant spot, free from husks and charcoal, let the wise one make a square, the *sides of which are of one cubit's length (15). Then draw in it three lines from the West to East (of the square). Let him then sprinkle water over them, uttering the Kurcha Vija the while. Then Fire should be brought to the accompaniment of the Vahni Vija (16). The Fire, when so brought, should be placed by the side of the square, the worshipper breathing the Vagbhava Vija (17). Then, taking up a piece of burning wood with the right hand from the Fire, he should put it aside as the share of the Rakshasas, saying:*

Mantra

Hring, Salutation to the raw-meat eaters: Svaha (18).

The worshipper, lifting up the consecrated Fire with both hands, should place it in front of him on the three lines (above mentioned), inwardly reciting the while the Maya Vija before the Vyahritis (19). Grass and wood should then be thrown upon the Fire to make it blaze, and two pieces of wood should be smeared with ghee and offered as an oblation to it. Thereafter Fire should be named according to the object of worship, and then meditated upon as follows (20):

Dhyana

Ruddily effulgent like the young Sun, with seven tongues and two crowned heads of matted hair, seated on a goat, whose weapon is Shakti. (21)

Having so meditated upon the Carrier of oblations, He should be thus invoked with joined palms (22).

Mantra

Hring, come, O Carrier of Oblations to all the Immortals, come! Come with the Rishis and Thy followers, and protect the sacrifice. I make obeisance to Thee. Svaha (23).

Having thus invoked Him, the worshipper should say, "0 Fire! this is Thy seat," and then worship him, the Seven-tongued, with appropriate offerings (24). The seven licking Tongues of Fire are: Kali, Karali, Ma-no-java, Sulohita, Su-dhumra-varna, Sphulingini, and Vishva-nirupini (25). Then, O Great Devi! the sides of the Fire should be thrice sprinkled with water from the hand, beginning from the East and ending at the North (26). Then the sides of the Fire, from the South to the North, should be thrice sprinkled with water, and following that the articles of sacrifice should be thrice sprinkled (27). Then spread kusha grass on the sides of the square, beginning with the East and ending with the North. The ends of the blades of grass on the North should be turned towards the North, and the rest of the grass should be placed with its ends towards the East (28). The worshipper should then proceed to the seat placed for Brahma, keeping the Fire on his right, and, picking up with his left thumb and little finger a blade of kusha grass from the seat of Brahma, should throw it along with the remaining blades of kusha grass on the South side of the fire, uttering the

Mantra

"Hring, Destroy the abode of the enemy" (29-30).

(The performer of the sacrifice should then say to Brahma:) " O Brahman, Lord of Sacrifices, be thou seated here. This seat is made for thee." The Brahma, saying "I sit," should then sit down, with his face turned towards the North (31). After worshipping Brahma with scent, flowers, and the other articles of worship, let him be supplicated thus (32):

Mantra

O Lord of Sacrifices! protect the sacrifice.O Brihaspati! protect this sacrifice. Protect me also, the performer of this sacrifice.O Witness of all acts! I bow to Thee (33).

Brahma should then say, "I protect," and if there is no person representing Brahma, then the performer of the sacrifice should, for the success of the sacrifice, make an image with darbha grass of the Vipra, and himself say this (34). The worshipper should then invoke Brahma, saying, "0 Brahman, come here, come here!" and, after doing honour to him by offering water for washing his feet and the like, let him supplicate him, saying, "So long as this sacrifice be not concluded, do Thou deign to remain here," and then make obeisance to him (35). He should then sprinkle the space between the North-East corner of the fire and the seat of Brahma three times with water taken in his hand, and should thereafter sprinkle the fire also three times, and then, returning the way he went, take his own seat. Let him then spread on the North side of the square some darbha grass, with the ends of the blades towards the North (36-37). He should then place thereon the articles necessary for the sacrifice, such as the vessel (filled with water) for sprinkling, and the vessel containing ghee, sacrificial fuel, and kusha grass. He should also place the sacrificial ladle and spoon on the darbha grass, and purify them by sprinkling water over them, and then, regarding them with a celestial gaze, uttering the

Mantra

Hrang Hring Hrung (38-39).

Then, with his right knee touching the ground, let him put ghee into the spoon with the ladle, and, with desire for his own well-being, Jet him offer three oblations, saying the

Mantra

Hring to Vishnu. Svaha (4o).

Taking again ghee in the same way, and meditating upon Prajapati, oblations should be offered with ghee streaked across the fire from the corner of Agni to that of Vayu (41). Taking ghee again and meditating on Indra, let him offer oblations from the corner of Nairrita to that of Ishana (42). O Devi! oblations should thereafter be offered to the North, the South, and to the middle of the fire, to Agni, Soma, and to Agni and Soma together (43). Upon that three oblations should be offered, uttering the

Mantras

Hring salutation to Agni,

Hring salutation to Soma,

Hring salutation to both Agni and Soma,

respectively. Having performed these (preliminary) rites, the wise one should proceed to that prescribed for the Homa sacrifice, which is to be performed (44). The offering of oblations (as above described), commencing with the three offerings made to Vishnu and ending with the offering to Agni and Soma, is called Dhara Homa (45).

When making any offering, both the Deva, to which the same is being made, and the thing offered should be mentioned, and upon the conclusion of the principal rite he should perform the Svishti-krit Homa (46). O Beautiful One! in the Kali Age there is no Prayashchitta Homa. The object thereof is attained by Svishti-krit and Vyahriti Homas (47). O Devi! (for Svishti-krit Homa.) ghee should be taken in manner above mentioned, and, whilst mentally reciting the name of Brahma, oblation should be offered with the following:

Mantra

Hring, O Deva of the Devas! do Thou make faultless any shortcomings that there may be in this rite, and anything done needlessly, whether by negligence or mistake. Svaha (48-49).

Then oblation should be offered to Fire, thus:

Mantra

Hring, O Fire! Thou art the Purificator of all things. Thou makest all sacrifices propitious, and art the Lord of all. Thou art the Witness of all sacrificial rites, and the Insurer of their success. Do Thou fulfil all my desires (50).

The sacrificing priest, having thus concluded the Svishti-krit Homa, should thus (pray to the Supreme Brahman):

Mantra

O Supreme Brahman! O Omnipresent One! for the removal of the effects of whatsoever has been improperly done in this sacrifice, and for the success of the sacrifice, I am making this Vyahriti Homa.

Saying this, he should offer three oblations with the three

Mantras

Hring Bhuh Svaha,

Hring Bhuvah Svaha,

Hring Svah Svaha.

Thereafter offering one more oblation with the

Mantra

Hring Bhuh, Bhuvah, Svah Svaha,

*the wise priest should, jointly with the giver of the sacri-
fice, offer the complete oblation (51-53). If the latter has
performed the sacrifice without a priest, he should offer
the oblation himself. This is the rule in Abhisheka and
other observances (54). The Mantra for the complete
oblation is –*

Mantra

*Hring, O Lord of Sacrifice! may this Sacrifice of mine be
complete. May all the Devatas of sacrifices be pleased
and grant that which is desired. Svaha (55).*

*The wise one should then, with the giver of the sacrifice,
stand up, and, with a well-controlled mind, offer oblations with fruit and pan leaves, uttering the while the
aforesaid Mantra (56).*

The learned one should, after offering the complete oblation, perform Shanti-karma. Taking water from the sprinkling vessel, he should with kusha grass sprinkle it over the heads of the persons present (57), reciting the

Mantra

May the water be friendly to me, may water be like a medicament to me, may water preserve me always; water is Narayana Himself (58). Do thou, O water! grant me happiness and my earthly desires, and so forth.

Having said this, and sprinkled water over the heads of those present, throw a few drops on the ground, saying (59):

Mantra

To those who are ever hostile to me, and to those to whom we are ever hostile, may water be their enemy and engulf them (60).

Sprinkling a few drops of water in the North-East corner to the accompaniment of the above-mentioned Mantra, the kusha grass should be put away, and supplication should be made to the Carrier of oblations as follows (61):

Mantra

*O Carrier of Oblations! do Thou grant unto me under-
standing, knowledge, strength, intelligence, wisdom,
faith, fame, fortune, health, energy, and long life (62).*

*Having thus prayed to Fire, he should, O Shiva! be bid-
den to depart with the following (63):*

Mantra

Sacrifice! do thou depart to the Lord of Sacrifice.

Fire! do thou depart to the Sacrifice itself.

*Lord of Sacrifice! do Thou depart to Thine own place
and fulfil my desires (64).*

*Then saying, "Fire, forgive me," the Fire should be
moved to the South by pouring oblations of curd on the
North of Fire (65). Then the worshipper should give a
present to Brahma, and, after bowing to him respectfully, bid him go, and, with the ashes adhering to the ladle,
the officiating priest should then make a mark on his
own forehead and on that of the giver of the sacrifice,
uttering the*

Mantra

*Hring, Kling, do thou bring peace; mayest thou cause
prosperity (66-67). By the grace of Indra, of Agni, of the
Maruts, Brahma, the Vasus, the Rudras, and Praja-pati,
may there be peace, may there be prosperity.*

*Whilst saying this Mantra, he should place a flower
on his own head. Thereafter the giver of the sacrifice
should, as his means allow, offer presents for the success
of the sacrifice and for the Kushandika rite (68-69).*

*I have spoken to Thee, O Devi! of Kushandika, which is
the groundwork of all auspicious ceremonies, and which
all Kula worshippers should with care perform at the
commencement thereof (70).*

*O Auspicious One! I will now speak to Thee of Cha-
ru-karma, in order to insure the ritual success in those
families in which the cooking of charu is a traditional
practice in the performance of all rites (71). The pot for
cooking charu should be made of either copper or mud
(72). In the first place, the articles should be consecrated
according to the rules prescribed in Kushandika, and
then the pot of charu should be placed in front of the
worshipper (73). After careful examination to see that
it is without holes and unbroken, a blade of kusha grass*

of the length of a pradesha should be put in the pot (74).
The rice should be placed near the square and then, O
Adored of the Devas! the names of such of the Devas
as are to be worshipped in each particular ceremony
should be uttered in the dative case, followed by the
words "to please Thee," and then "I take," "I place it in
the pot," and "I put water into it," and put four handfuls of rice in the name of each Deva. He should then
take the rice, put it in the pot, and pour water over it
(75-77). O Virtuous One! milk and sugar should be
added thereto, as is done in cooking. The whole should
then be well and carefully cooked over the consecrated
fire (78). And when he is satisfied that it is well cooked
and soft, the sacrificial ladle, filled with ghee, should
be let into it (79). Thereafter placing the pot on kusha
grass on the northern side of the Fire, and adding ghee
to the charu three times, the pot should be covered with
blades of kusha grass (80). Then, putting a little ghee
into the sacrificial spoon, a little charu should be taken
from the pot. With it Janu Homa is done (81). Then,
after doing Dhara Homa, oblations should be made
with the Mantras of the Devas, who are directed to be
worshipped in the principal rite (82). Completing the
principal Homa after performance of Svishti-krit Homa,
expiatory Homa should be performed, and the rite thus
completed (83). In the sacramental and consecratory
ritual this is the method to be observed. In all auspicious

ceremonies it should be followed for the complete success thereof (84).

Now, O Mahamaya! I will speak of Garbhadhana and other rites. I will speak of them in their order, beginning with Ritusangskara. Do Thou listen (85).

After performing his daily duties and purifying himself, (the priest) should worship the five deities–Brahma, Durga, Ganesha, the Grahas, and the Dikpalas (86). They should be worshipped in the jars on the East side of the square, and then the sixteen Matrikas–namely, Gauri and others–should be worshipped in their order (87). The sixteen Matrikas are Gauri, Padma, Shachi, Medha, Savitri, Vijaya, Jaya, Deva-sena, Svadha, Svaha, Shanti, Pushti, Dhriti, Kshama, the worshipper's own tutelary Devata, and the family Devata (88).

Mantra

May the Mothers that cause the joy of the Devas come and bring all success to weddings, vratas, and yajnas. May they come upon their respective carriers, and in all the fulness of their power, in their benign aspect, and add to the glory of this festival (89-90).

Having thus invoked the Mothers and worshipped them

to the best of his powers, the priest should make five or seven marks with vermilion and sandal paste on the wall, at the height of his navel, and within the space of a pradesha (91).

The wise one should then, whilst breathing the three Vijas–Kling, Hring, and Shring–pour an unbroken stream of ghee from each of the said marks, and there worship the Deva Vasu (92). The wise man, having thus made the Vasu-dhara according to the directions which I have given, and having made the square and placed the Fire thereupon, and consecrated the articles requisite for Homa, should then cook the excellent charu (93). Charu which is cooked in this (Ritu-sangskara) is called Prajapatya, and the name of this Fire is Vayu. After concluding Dhara Homa, the rite of Ritu-sangs-kara should be begun (94). Three oblations of charu should be offered with the

Mantra

Hring. salutation to Prajapati. Svaha.

The one oblation should be offered with the following (95):

Mantra

May Vishnu grant the power to conceive. May Tvashta give the form. May Prajapati sprinkle it, and may Dhata give the power to bear (96).

This oblation should be made with either ghee or charu, or with ghee and charu, and should be offered meditating upon the Sun, Vishnu, and Prajapati (97).

Mantra

May Sinibali give support to thy womb, may Sarasvati give support to thy womb, may the two Ashvins, who wear garlands of lotuses, give support to thy womb (98).

Meditating upon the Devis Sinibali and Sarasvati and the two Ashvins, excellent oblations should be offered with the above Mantra, followed by Svaha (99). Then oblation should be offered to the sanctified Fire, meditating upon Surya and Vishnu with the

Mantra

Kling, String, Hring, Shring, Hung, grant conception to her, who desires a son: Svaha (100).

Then, in the name of Vishnu, oblations should be offered with the following:

Mantra

As this extended Earth ever carries a full womb, do thou likewise carry for ten months until delivery. Svaha (101).

Meditating upon the Supreme Vishnu, let a little more ghee be thrown into the Fire with the following:

Mantra

Vishnu! do Thou in Thy excellent form put into this woman an excellent son: Svaha (102).

And, uttering the following

Mantra

Kling, Hring, Kling, Hring, String, Hring, Kling, Hring,

let the husband touch his wife's head (103). Then the husband, surrounded by a few married women having sons, should place both hands on the head of his wife, and, after meditating on Vishnu, Durga, Vidhi and Surya, place three fruits on the cloth of her lap. Thereupon he should bring the ceremony to a close by making Svishti-krit oblations and expiatory rites (104-105). Or

*the wife and husband may be purified by worshipping
Gauri and Shangkara in the evening, and by giving
oblations to Sun (106).*

*I have now spoken of Ritu-sangskara. Now listen to that
relating to Garbhadhana (107). On the same night, or
on some night having a date of an even number, after
the ceremony, the husband should enter the room with
his wife, and, meditating on Prajapati, should touch his
wife and say:*

Mantra

*Hring, O Bed! be thou propitious for the begetting of a
good offspring of us two (108-109).*

*He should then with the wife get on the bed, and there
sit with his face towards the East or the North. Then,
looking at his wife, let him embrace her with his left
arm, and, placing his right hand over her head, let him
make japa of the Mantra on the different parts of her
body (as follows) (110): Let him make japa over the
head of the Kama Vija a hundred times; over her chin of
the Vagbhava Vija a hundred times; over the throat of
the Rama Vija twenty times; and the same Vija a hundred times over each of her two breasts (111). He should
then recite the Maya Vija ten times over her heart, and*

*twenty-five times over her navel. Next let him place his
hand on her member, and recite jointly the Kama and
Vagbhava Vijas a hundred and eight times, and let him
similarly recite the same Vijas over his own member
a hundred and eight times; and then, saying the Vija
"Hring," let him part the lips of her member, and let him
go into her with the object of begetting a child (112-
113). The husband should, at the time of the spending of
his seed, meditate on Brahma, and, discharging it below
the navel into the Raktikanadi in the Chitkunda, he
should at the same time recite the following (114, 115):*

Mantra

*As the Earth is pregnant of Fire, as the Heaven is preg-
nant of Indra, as the Points of the compass are pregnant
of the Air they contain, so do thou also become pregnant
(by this my seed) (116).*

*If the wife then, or at a subsequent period, conceive, the
householder, O Maheshvari! should perform in the third
month after conception the Pungsavana rite (117). After
the performance of his daily duties, the husband should
worship the five Devas and the heavenly Mothers, Gauri
and others, and should make the Vasu-dhara (118).*

The wise one should then perform Briddhi Shraddha,

*and, as aforementioned, the ceremonies up to Dha-
ra-Homa, and then proceed to the Pungsavana rites
(119). The charu prepared for Pungsavana is called
"Prajapatya," and the fire is called Chandra (120). One
grain of barley and two Masha beans should be put into
curd made from cow's milk, and this should be given
to the wife to drink, and, whilst she is drinking it, she
should be asked three times: "What is that thou art
drinking,O gentle one?" (121). The wife should make
answer: "Hring, I am drinking that which will cause me
to bear a son." In this manner the wife should drink three mouthfuls of the curd (122). The wife should then be
led by women whose husbands and children are living
to the place of sacrifice, and the husband should there
seat her on his left and proceed to perform Charu-Homa
(123).*

*Taking a little charu as aforementioned, and uttering
the Maya Vija and the Kurcha Vija, he should offer it as
oblation, with the following:*

Mantra

*Do thou destroy, do thou destroy all these Bhutas,
Pretas, Pishachas, and Vetalas, who are inimical to
conception and destroyers of the child in the womb, and
of the young. Do thou protect (the child in) the womb,*

do thou protect (the child in) the womb (124-125).

Whilst reciting the above Mantra, meditate upon Fire, as Raksko-ghna, and on Rudra and Prajapati, and then offer twelve oblations (126).

He should then offer five oblations with the

Mantra

Hring, Salutation to Chandra. Svaha.

And then, touching his wife's heart, breathe inwardly the Vijas Hring and Shring one hundred times (127). He should then perform Svishti-krit Homa and Pray-ash-chitta, and complete the ceremony. Panchamrita should be given in the fifth month of pregnancy 128). Sugar, honey, milk, ghee, and curd in equal quantities make Panchamrita. It is needful for the purification of the body (129). Breathing the Vijas Aing, Kling, Shring, Hring, Hung, and Lang, five times over each of the five ingredients, the husband, after mixing them together, should cause his wife to eat it (130). Then, in the sixth or eighth month, the Simantonnayana rite should be performed. It may, however, be performed any time before the child is born (131). The wise one should, after performing the rites as aforementioned, do Dhara-Ho-

ma, and sit with his wife on a seat, and offer three oblations to Vishnu, Surya, and Brahma, saying:

Mantra

To Vishnu Svaha, to the Effulgent One Svaha, to Brahma Svaha (132).

Then, meditating on Chandra, let him offer seven oblations to Soma into Fire under his name of Shiva (133). Then, O Shiva! he should meditate upon the Ashwins, Vasava, Vishnu, Shiva, Durga, Prajapati and offer five oblations to each of them (134). The husband should after that take a gold comb, and comb back the hair on each side of the head and tie it up with the chignon (135). He should, whilst so combing the hair, meditate upon Shiva, Vishnu. and Brahma, and pronounce the Maya Vija (136) and the

Mantra

O Wife! thou auspicious and fortunate one, thou of auspicious vows! do thou in the tenth month, by the grace of Vishva-karma, be safely delivered of a good child. May thou live long and happy. This comb, may it give thee strength and prosperity!

Saying this Mantra, the ceremony should be completed with Svishti-krit Homa and other rites (137-138). Immediately after the birth of the son the wise one should look upon his face and present him with a piece of gold, and then in another room perform Dhara Homa in the manner already described (139). He should then offer five oblations to Agni, Indra, Prajapati, the Vishva-devas, and Brahma (140).

The father should thereafter mix equal quantities of honey and ghee in a bell-metal cup, and, breathing the Vagbhava Vija over it a hundred times, make the child swallow it (141). It should be put into the child's mouth with the fourth finger of the right hand, with the following:

Mantra

Child, may thy life, vitality, strength, and intelligence ever increase (142).

After performing this rite for the longevity of the child, the father should give him a secret name, by which at the time of the investiture with the sacred thread he should be called (143). The father should then finish the Jata-karma by the performance of the usual expiatory and other rites, and then the midwife should with firm-

ness cut the umbilical cord (144). The period of uncleanliness commences only after the cord is cut; therefore all rites relating to the Devas and the Pitris should be performed before the cord is cut (145). If a daughter is born, all the acts as above indicated are to be performed, but the Mantras are not to be said. In the sixth or eighth month the boy should be given the name by which he is usually known (146). At the time of naming of the child the mother should, after bathing him and dressing him in two pieces of fine cloth, come to and place him by the side of her husband, with his face towards the East (147). The father should thereupon sprinkle the head of the child with water taken up upon blades of kusha grass and gold, saying at the time the following:

Mantra

May Jahnavi, Yamuna, Reva, the holy Sarasvati, Narmada, Varada, Kunti, the Oceans and Tanks, Lakes–all these bathe thee for the attainment of Dharmma, Kama, and Artha (149).

O Waters! thou art the Pranava, and thou givest all happiness. Do thou therefore provide for us food in (this) world, and do thou also enable us to see the Supreme and Beautiful (Para-brahman). Water! thou art not different from the Pranava. Grant that we may enjoy in this world thy most beneficent essence. Your wishes arise of themselves spontaneously like those of mothers. Water! thou art the very form of Pranava. We go to enjoy to our fill that essence of thine by which thou satisfieth (this Universe). May thou bring us enjoyment therein (150-152).

The wise one should sprinkle water over the child, with the three preceding Mantras, and then, as aforesaid, consecrate the fire and perform the rites leading up to Dhara Homa in the manner already described, and then should offer five oblations (153). He should make the oblation to Agni, then to Vasava, then to Prajapati, then to the Vishva-Devas, and then to Yahni under his name of Parthiva (154).

Then, taking the son in his lap, the prudent father should speak into his right ear an auspicious name–one that is short, and that can easily be pronounced (155). After whispering the name three times into the son's ear, he should inform the Brahmanas who are present of it, and then conclude the ceremony with Svishtikrit Homa and the other concluding rites (156).

For a daughter there is no Nishkramana, nor is Vriddhi Shraddha necessary. The wise man performs the naming, the giving of the first rice, and tonsure of a daughter without any Mantra (157).

*In the fourth or sixth month after birth the Nishkrama-
na Sangskara ceremony of the son should be performed
(158).*

*After performing his daily duties, the father should, after
bathing, worship Ganesha, and then bathe and adorn
his son with clothes and jewels, and, placing him in
front of himself, pronounce the following (159):*

Mantra

*Brahma, Vishnu, Shiva, Durga, Ganesha, Bhaskara, In-
dra, Vayu, Kuvera, Varuna, Agni, and Brihaspati, may
They always be propitious to this child, and may They
always protect him throughout his going forth from the
house (160).*

*Having said this, he should take the child in his arms,
and, preceded by vocal and instrumental music, and
surrounded by his rejoicing kinsmen, take the son out of
the house (161). Going a little distance, he should show
the Sun to the child, with the following (162):*

Mantra

*Ong, yonder is the Eye (of Heaven) who excels even
Shukra in his effulgence, who is beneficent even to the*

Devas. May we see him a hundred years. May we live a hundred years (163).

Having shown the Sun to his child, the father should return to his own house, and, after making offering to the Sun, feast his kinsmen (164). O Shiva! in the sixth or eighth month either the father's brother or the father himself should give the first rice to the child (165). After worshipping the Devas and purifying fire as aforementioned, and duly performing the ceremonies leading to Dhara Homa, the father should make five oblations to Fire, under his name of Shuchi, to each of the following Devas: He should make the oblations first to Agni, next to Vasava, after him to Prajapati, then to the Vishva-devas, and then the fifth ahuti to Brahma (166-168). He should then meditate upon the Devi Annada, and, after giving Her five oblations in Fire, place the son, adorned with clothes and jewels, in his lap, and give him payasa, either in the same or in another room (169). The payasa should be put into the child's mouth five times, uttering the Mantras for making oblations to the five vital airs; and after that a little rice and curry should be put into the child's mouth (170). The ceremony should be brought to a close by the blowing of conches and horns and other music, and by performing the concluding expiatory rite.

I have done speaking of the rice-eating ceremony. I shall now speak of the tonsure ceremony. Do Thou listen (171).

In the third or fifth year, according to the custom in the family, the tonsure of the boy should be performed for the success of the sacramental rites of the boy (172). The wise father should, after concluding the preliminary rites leading up to Dhara Homa, place on the north side of the Fire, called Satya, a mud platter filled with cow-dung, tila-seeds, and wheat, also a little lukewarm water and a keen-edged razor (173-174).

The father should place the son on his mother's lap, the mother sitting on her husband's left, and, after breathing the Varuna Vija ten times over the water, rub the hair of the boy's head with lukewarm water. He should then tie the hair with two blades of kusha grass into a knot, utte-ring meanwhile the Maya Vija (175-176). Then, saying the Maya and Lakshmi Vijas three times, he should cut off the knot with the steel razor and place it in the hands of the child's mother (177). The boy's mother should then take it with both hands and place it in the platter con-taining the cow-dung, and the father should then say to the barber: "Barber, do thou at thine ease proceed with the shaving of the boy's hair, Svaha." Then, looking at the barber, he should make three oblations to Prajapati, into

Vahni, under his name of Satya (178-179). After the boy has been shaved by the barber he should be bathed and adorned with clothes and jewels, and placed near the fire on the left of his mother, and the father should, after performance of Svishti-krit Homa and the expiatory rites, offer the complete oblation (180-181). Then, uttering the following:

Mantra

Hring, O Child! may the omnipresent Creator of the Universe grant thee well-being,

he should pierce the ears of the boy with gold or silver needles (182). He should then sprinkle the child with water, uttering the

Mantra

O Water! thou art, etc. (aforementioned);

and, after performing Shanti Karma and other rites, and making presents, bring the ceremony to a close (183). The sacramental rites from Garbhadhana to Chudakarana are common to all castes. But for Shudras and Samanyas they must be performed without Mantras (184).

In the case of the birth of a daughter all castes are to perform the rites without Mantras. In the case of a daughter there is no Nishkramana (185).

I will now speak of the Sacred Thread Ceremony of the twice-born classes, by which the twice-born become qualified for performing rites relating to the Devas and Pitris (186).

In the eighth year from conception, or the eighth year after birth, the boy should be invested with the sacred thread. After the sixteenth year the son should not be invested, and one so invested is disqualified for all rites (187).

The learned man should, after finishing his daily duties, worship the five Devas, as also the Matrikas, Gauri, and others, and make the Vasudhara (188). He should thereafter perform Briddhi Shraddha for the satisfaction of the Devas and Pitris, and perform the rites, ending with Dhara Homa, as directed in the performance of Kushandika (189).

The boy should be given a little to eat; then his head, with the exception of the crown lock, should be shaved, and after that he should be well bathed and decked with jewels and silken clothes (190).

The boy should then be taken to the Chhaya-mandapa,
near Fire, under his name of Samudbhava, and there
made to sit on a clean seat to the left (of his father
or Guru) (191). The Guru should say: "My son, dost
thou adopt Brahma-charyya?" The disciple should say
respectfully: "I do adopt it" (192). The Preceptor should
then with a cheerful mind give two pieces of Kashaya
cloth for the long life and strength of mind of the gentle
boy (193). Then when the boy has put on the Kashaya
cloth, he should, without speaking, give him a knotted
girdle made of three strings of munja or kusha grass
(194). On that the boy should say, "Hring, may this
auspicious girdle prove propitious"; and, saying this, and
putting it round his waist, let him sit in silence before
the Guru (195).

Mantra

This sacrificial thread is very sacred; Brihaspati of old
wore it. Do thou wear this excellent white sacrificial
thread which contributes to prolong life. May it be for
thee strength and courage (196).

With this Mantra the boy should be given a sacrificial
thread made of the skin of the black buck, as also a staff
made of bamboo, or a branch of Khadira, Palasha, or
Kshira trees (197). When the boy has put the sacred

thread round his neck and holds the staff in his hand, the Guru should three times recite the

Mantra

"O Water! thou art," etc. (aforementioned),

preceded and followed by Hring, and should sprinkle the boy with water taken with kusha grass, and fill the joined palms of the latter with water (198). After the boy has offered the water to Suryya, the Guru should show the boy the Sun, and recite the

Mantra.

"Yonder is the Sun," etc. (aforementioned) (199).

After the boy has viewed the Sun, the Guru should address him as follows: "My Son! place thy mind on my observances. I bestow upon thee my disposition. Do thou follow the observances with an undivided mind. May my word contribute to thy well-being" (200). After saying this, the Guru, touching the boy's heart, should ask, "My Son! what is thy name?" and the boy should make reply: " . . . Sharmma, I bow to thee" (201). And to the question of the Guru, "Whose Brahma-chari art thou?" the disciple will reverently answer: "I am thy

*Brahma-chari" (202). The Guru should thereupon say:
"Thou art the Brahma-chari of Indra, and Fire is thy
Guru." Saying this, the good Guru should consign him to
the protection of the Devas (203). "My Son! I give thee
to Prajapati, to Savitri, to Varuna, to Prithivi, to the
Vishva-devas, and to all the Devas. May they all ever
protect thee" (204).*

*The boy should thereafter go round the sacrificial fire
and the preceptor, keeping both upon his right, and then
resume his own seat (205). The Guru, O Beloved! should
then, with his disciple touching him, offer five oblations to Five Devas (206)–namely, Prajapati, Shukra,
Vishnu, Brahma, and Shiva (207). When the oblations
are offered into Fire, under his name of Samud-bhava,
the names of each of the Devas should be pronounced
in the dative, preceded by Hring and followed by Svaha.
Where there is no Mantra mentioned, this method is to
be followed in all cases (208). After this, oblation should
be offered to Durga, Mahalakshmi, Sundari, Bhuvaneshvari, Indra, and the other nine regents of the quarters,
and Bhaskara and the eight planets (209). The name of
each of these should be mentioned whilst the offering of
oblations is made. The wise Guru should then cover the
boy with cloth, and ask him, who is desirous of attaining
Brahma-charyya: "What is the ashrama thou desirest,
my son! and what is thy heart's desire?" (210). The disci-*

ple should thereupon hold the feet of the Preceptor, and, with a reverent mind, say: "First instruct me in Divine Knowledge, and then in that of the householder" (211).

O Shiva! when the disciple in this manner has thus beseeched his Guru, the latter should three times whisper into his disciple's right ear the Pranava, which contains all the Mantras in itself, and should also utter the three Vyahritis, as also the Savitri (212). Sadashiva is its Rishi, the verse is Trishtup, the presiding Deva is Savitri, and its object is the attainment of final liberation (213). The Gayatri Mantra is:

Mantra

Ong, let us contemplate the wonderful Spirit of the Divine Creator. May He direct our understanding, Ong.

The Guru should then explain the meaning of the Gayatri (214-215). By the Tara, which contains the letters–i.e., A, U, and M–the Paresh is meant. He Who is the Protector, Destroyer, and Creator. He is the Deva Who is above Prakriti (106).

This Deva is the Spirit of the three worlds, containing in Himself the three qualities. By the three Vyahritis, therefore, the all-pervading Brahman is expressed (217).

*He Who is expressed by the Pranava and the Vyahritis
is also known by the Savitri. Let us meditate upon the
sublime, all-pervading eternal Truth, the great imma-
nent and lustrous energy, adored by the self-controlled;
Savita, effulgent and omnipresent One, Whose manifested form the world is, the Creator. May Bharga, Who
witnesseth all, and is the Lord of all, direct and engage
our mind, intelligence, and senses towards those acts,
which lead to the attainment of Dharmma, Artha,
Kama, and Moksha (218-220).*

*O Devi! the excellent Guru, having thus instructed the
disciple, and explained to him the Divine Wisdom,
should direct him in the duties of a householder (221).
"My Son! do thou now discard the garments of a Brahma-chari, and honour the Devas and Pitris according
to the way revealed by Shambhu" (222). Thy body is
sanctified by the instructions thou hast received in
Divine Wisdom. Do thou, now that thou hast reached
the stage of a householder, engage thyself in thy duties
appropriate to that mode of life (223). Put on two sacred
threads, two good pieces of cloth, jewels, shoes, umbrella,
fragrant garland, and paste (224). The disciple should
then take off his Kashaya cloth and his sacred thread of
black-buck skin and his girdle, and give them and his
staff, begging-bowl, and also what has been received by
him in the shape of customary alms, to his Guru.*

He should then put on two sacred threads and two fine cloths, and wear a garland of fragrant flowers, and perfume himself, and thereafter sit in silence near the Guru, who should address him as follows (225-227):

"Conquer the senses, be truthful and devoted to the acquisition of Divine Knowledge and the study of the Vedas, and discharge the duties of a householder according to the rules prescribed in the Dharmma Shastras" (228).

Having thus instructed the disciple, the Guru should make him offer three oblations into Fire in the name of Samudbhava with the

Mantra

Hring, Earth, Firmament, and Heaven, Ong.

He should then himself perform Svishti-krit Homa, and then, O Gentle One! he should bring the investiture ceremony to a close by offering the complete oblation (229-230).

Beloved! all ceremonies, from the Jivaseka to Upana-yana ceremonies, are performed by the father alone. The ceremony relating to marriage may be performed either by the father or by the bridegroom himself (231).

The pious man should on the day of marriage perform his ablutions and finish his daily duties, and should then worship the five Devas and the Divine Mothers, Gauri and others, and making the Vasu-dhara do Briddhi Shraddha (232). At night the betrothed bridegroom, preceded by vocal and musical instrumental music, should be brought to the chhaya-mandapa and seated on an excellent seat (233). The bridegroom should sit facing the East, and the giver of the bride should face the west, and the latter, after rinsing his mouth, should, with the assisting Brahmanas, say the words "Svasti" and "Riddhi" (234).

The giver of the bride should ask after the bridegroom's welfare, and ask also his permission to honour him, and upon receiving his answer should honour him by the offer of water for his feet and the like (235), and saying, "I give this to you," let him give the bridegroom the gifts. The water should be given at the feet and the oblation at the head (236). Articles for the rinsing of the mouth should be offered at the mouth, and then scents, garlands, two pieces of good cloth, beautiful ornaments and gems, and a sacred thread should be given to the bridegroom (237), The giver should make madhu-parka by mixing together curd, ghee, and honey in a bell-metal cup, and place it in the hand of the bridegroom with the words, "I give you" (238). The bridegroom, after taking *it, should place the cup in his left hand, and, dipping the thumb and ring fingers of his right hand into the madhu-parka, should smell it five times, reciting meanwhile the Pranahuti Mantra, and then place the cup on his north. Having offered the madhu-parka, the bridegroom should be made to rinse his mouth (239-240).*

The giver of the daughter should then, holding durva and akshata, touch the right knee of the bridegroom with his hand, and then, first meditating on Vishnu and saying "Tat Sat," he should mention the name of the month, the paksha, and tithi, and then the names of the gotra and pravara of the bridegroom and his ancestors one by one, from the great-grandfather, beginning with the last, and ending with the father. The bridegroom's name should be in the objective, and the names of the others in the possessive case. Then follow the bride's name and the names of her ancestors, their gotras, etc.; and he should then say: "I honour thee with the object of giving her to thee in Brahma marriage" (241-244).

The bridegroom should then say: "I am honoured." The giver upon this should say, "Perform the ordained marriage rites," and the bridegroom should then say: "I do it to the best of my knowledge" (245). The bride, adorned with beautiful clothes and jewels, and covered with another piece of cloth, should then be brought and placed in front of the bridegroom (246). The giver of the bride should once again show his respect to the bridegroom by the present of clothes and ornaments, and join the right hand of the bridegroom with that of the bride (247). He should place in their joined hands five gems or a fruit and a pan-leaf, and, having saluted the bride, should consign her to his hands (248). At the time of consigning the bride the giver should, as before, mention his name twice in the nominative case, and should state his wish, and should also mention the names of the three ancestors of the bridegroom, with their gotras, all in the possessive case, as before.

He should then mention the name of the bridegroom in the dative singular, and then the names of the three ancestors of the bride, with their gotras, etc., in the possessive case. At the time of mentioning the bride's name in the objective singular he should say after that, "The honoured, adorned, clothed, and Prajapati-devataka," and saying, "to thee I give," he should give away the bride. The bridegroom should, saying "Svasti," agree to take her as his wife (249-251). Let the giver then say, "In Dharmma, in Artha, in Kama, thou should be with thy wife;" and the bridegroom should reply, saying, "So I shall," and then recite the praise of Kama (252).

Mantra

It is Kama who gives and Kama who accepts. It is Kama who has taken the Kamini for the satisfaction of Kama. Prompted by Kama, I take thee. May both our kamas be fulfilled (353).

The giver should then, addressing the son-in-law and the daughter, say: "May, by the grace of Prajapati, the desires of you both be accomplished. May you two fare well. Do you two together perform the religious observances" (254). Then both the bride and bridegroom, to the accompaniment of music and blowing of conch-shells, should be covered with the cloth, so that they may have their first auspicious glance at one another (255).

Then gold and jewels, according to the giver's means, should be offered to the son-in-law as presents. The giver should then think to himself that the ceremony has been faultlessly done (256). The bridegroom either, on the same night or the day following, should establish fire, according to the rules of Kushandika (257).

The fire that is made in this Kushandika is called Yojaka, and the charu which is cooked is called Prajapatya. After performing Dhara Homa in the fire, the bridegroom should offer five oblations (258). The oblation should, after meditation upon Shiva, Durga, Brahma, Vishnu, and the Carrier of Thunder, be made to them one after the other singly in the sanctified fire (259). Taking both his wife's hands, the husband should say: "I take thy hands, O fortunate one! Do thou be devoted to the Guru and the Devatas, and duly perform thy household duties according to the religious precepts" (260). The wife should then, with ghee given by the husband, and fried paddy given by her brother, make four oblations in the name of Prajapati (261). The husband should then rise from his seat with his wife and go round the Fire with her and offer oblations to Durga and Shiva, Rama and Vishnu, Brahmi and Brahma, three times to each couple (262).

Then, without reciting any Mantra, the bride should step on a stone, and, standing thereon, the bride should take seven steps. If the Kushamdika ceremony is performed at night, the bride and bridegroom, surrounded by the ladies present, should gaze upon the stars Dhruva and Arundhati (263). Returning to their seats and seated thereon, the bridegroom should bring the ceremony to a close by performing Svishti-krit Homa and offering complete oblations (264). The Brahma marriage, according to kula-dharmma, in order to be faultless, should take place with a girl of the same caste as the husband, but she should not be of the same gotra, nor should she be a sapinda (265). The wife married according to Brahma rites is the mistress of the house, and without her

*permission another wife should not be married accor-
ding to those rites (266). O Kuleshvari! if the children
of the Brahma wife are living or any of her descendants
be living, then the children of the Shaiva wife shall not
inherit (267).*

*O Parameshvari! the Shaiva wife and her children are
entitled to food and clothing from the heir of her Shaiva
husband in proportion to the property of the latter
(268). Shaiva marriage celebrated in the Chakra is of
two kinds. One kind is terminated with the Chakra and
the other is lifelong (269). At the time of the formation
of the Chakra the Vira, surrounded by his friends, relatives, and fellow-worshippers, should, with a well-controlled mind, by mutual consent, perform the marriage
ceremony (270). He should first of all submit their
wishes, saying to the Bhairavis and Viras there assembled, "Approve our marriage according to Shaiva form"
(271). The Vira should, after obtaining their permission,
bow to the Supreme Kalika, repeating the Mantra of
seven letters (Kalika Mantra) one hundred and eight
times (272).*

*O Shiva! he should then say to the woman: "Dost thou
love me as thy husband with a guileless heart?" (273).*

O Queen of the Devas! the Kaula woman should then

honour her beloved with scents, flowers, and coloured rice, and with a faithful heart place her own hands on his (274). The Lord of the Chakra should then sprinkle them with the following Mantra, and the Kaulas, seated in the Chakra, should approve and say: "It is well" (275)

Mantra

May Raja-rajeshvari, Kali, Tarini, Bhuvaneshvari, Bagala, Kamala, Nitya, Bhairavi, ever protect thee both (276).

The Lord of the Chakra should sprinkle them twelve times with wine or water of oblation, reciting the above Mantra. The two should then bow to him, and he should upon that let them hear the Vijas of Vagbhava and Rama (277). There is no restriction of caste or age in Shaiva marriage. By the command of Shambhu, any woman who is not a sapinda, and has not already a husband, may be married (278).

The wife married for the purposes of Chakra in the Shaiva form should, in the case of the Vira who desires offspring, be released on the dissolution of the Chakra only after the appearance of her menses. The offspring of the Shaiva marriage is of the same caste as the mother if it be an Anuloma marriage, and a Samanya if the mar-

*riage is Viloma (279-281). These mixed castes should, at
the time of their fathers' shraddha and other ceremonies,
give presents of edibles to, and feast the Kaulas only
(282).*

*Eating and sexual union, O Devi! are desired by, and
natural to, men, and their use is regulated for their
benefit in the ordinances of Shiva (283). Therefore, O
Mahe-shani! he who follows the ordinances of Shiva
undoubtedly acquires Dharmma, Artha, Kama, and
Moksha (284).*

*End of the Ninth Joyful Message, entitled "The Ten
Kinds of Purificatory Rites (Sangskara)."*

CHAPTER 10
Rites relating to Vriddhi Shraddha, Funeral Rites, and Purnabhisheka

SHRI DEVI said:

*I have now learned from Thee, O Lord! of the ordinan-
ces relating to Kushandika and the ten Sang-skaras. Do
Thou now,O Deva! reveal to Me the ordinances relating
to Briddhi Shraddha (1). O Shangkara! tell Me in detail,
both for My pleasure and the benefit of all beings, in
which of the sacramental and dedicatory ceremonies
Kushandika and Briddhi Shraddha should be, or be not,
performed. Say this, O Maheshana (2-3).*

Shri Sadashiva said:

*O Gentle One! I have already in detail spoken of all
that should be done in the ten Sangskaras commencing
from Jiva-seka and ending in marriage (4), and of all
that which should be performed by wise men who desire
their own weal.O Beauteous One! I will now speak of
what should be done in other rites. Do Thou listen to it
(5).*

My Beloved! in consecrating tanks, wells, and ponds,

images of Devatas houses, gardens and in vrata, the five Devas and the celestial Mothers should be worshipped, and the Vasu-dhara should be made and Briddhi Shraddha and Kushandika should be performed (6-7). In ceremonies which may be, and are, performed by women alone there is no Briddhi Shraddha, but (in lieu thereof) a present of edibles should be made for the satisfaction of the Devatas and the Pitris (8).

O Lotus-faced One! in such ceremonies the worship of the Deva, Vasu-dhara, and Kushandika should be devoutly performed by the women through the aid of priests (9). If a man cannot perform a rite himself, then his son, the son's son, the daughter's son, agnate relatives, sister's son and son-in-law and the priest, are, O Shiva! the best substitutes (10). I will, O Kalika! now in detail speak of Briddhi Shraddha. Do Thou listen to it (11).

After performing the daily duties, a man should with mind intent worship Ganga, Vishnu–the Lord of Sacrifice, the Divinity of the homestead, and the King (12); and inwardly reciting the Pranava, he should make nine, seven, five, or three Brahmanas of Darbha grass (13). The Brahmanas should be made with ends of the grass which have no knots in them, by twisting the upper ends of the blades from right to left two and a half times (14).

In Briddhi Shraddha and Parvana Shraddha there should be six Brahmanas, but, O Shiva! in Ekoddishta Shraddha there should be only one (15). The wise one should place the Brahmanas made of kusha grass all in one receptacle, with their faces to the north, and bathe them with the following (16)

Mantra

May the Divinity of water, who is like the Maya Vija, be propitious for the attainment of our desire. May He be propitious in that which we drink, May He always stand forward for our good (17).

Then with scents and flowers the Brahmanas made with kusha grass should be worshipped (18). The wise one should then place on the west and the south six vessels in pairs with kusha, sesamum-seed, and Tulasi (19). On the two vessels placed on the west two of the Brahmanas should be seated facing east, and on the four seats on the south the four Brahmanas should be seated facing north (20).

The Divinities should be imagined to be in the two seated on the west and the paternal Ancestors in the two seated on the left of those on the south and the maternal ancestors on the right. Know this, O Parvati (21).

In Abhyudayika Shraddha the Nandimukha fathers and
the Nandimukhi mothers, as also the maternal Ancestors in the male line and in the female line, should be
mentioned by name. Before this, however, one should
turn to his right and face the north, and after the performance of the requisite ceremonies for the worship of the
Devas he should turn to his left and face the south and
perform the rites necessary for the offering of the Pindas
(22-23).

In this Abhyudayika Shraddha, O Shiva! all the rites
should be performed in their order, beginning with the
rites relating to the Devas, and if there be any deviation
the Shraddha fails in its object (24).

The word of supplication addressed to the Devas should
be said whilst facing the north, and when the same
is addressed to the paternal or maternal Ancestors it
should be said whilst facing south. And now, O Thou of
pure Smiles! I will first state the words of entreaty which
should be addressed to the Devas (25).

After mentioning the name of the month and paksha,
the tithi and the occasion, the excellent worshipper
should say "for the prosperous result of the ceremony."
Then he should repeat the names and gotras of the three
fathers and of the three mothers, and of the three mater-

*nal grandfathers and of the three maternal grandmothers, in the possessive case, and he should thereafter say:
"I am performing the Shraddha of the Vishva-Devas represented by the image of the two Brahmanas made of kusha grass." These, O Great Devi! are the words of entreaty" (26-29).*

O Parvati! when the Anujna-vakya is either for paternal or maternal Ancestors, the same words should, with the necessary alterations, be said for the paternal and maternal Ancestors, and the Vishva-Devas left out (30). Then, O Shiva! the worshipper should recite the Brahma-Vidya Gayatri ten times (31). He should next say the following

Mantra

I salute the Divinities, the Fathers–i.e., the Fathers and Mothers–the great Yogis; I salute Pushti and Svaha; may we have such auspicious occasions over and over again.

The excellent worshipper, having repeated the above Mantra three times, and taking water in his hand, should wash the Shraddha articles with the

Mantra

Vang, Hung, Phat (32-33).

O Mistress of the Kula! a vessel should next be placed in the corner of Agni. Then uttering the

Mantra

O Water! Thou art the nectar which killest the Rakshasas, protect this sacrifice of mine.

Water with Tulasi-leaves and barley should be put into it; and the wise one should, after first offering handfuls of water to the Devas and then to the Vipras, give them seats of kusha grass (34-35).

The learned men, O Shiva! should then invoke the Vishva-Devas, the fathers, the mothers, the maternal grandfathers, and the maternal grandmothers (36). Having so invoked them, the Vishva-Devas should first be worshipped; and then the three fathers, the three mothers, the three maternal grandfathers, and the three maternal grandmothers should be worshipped, with offets of Padya, Arghya, Achamaniya, incense, lights, cloths. Then, O Beauteous One! permission should be asked in the first place of the Devas for the spreading of the leaves (37-38).

Then a four-sided figure should be drawn uttering the
Maya Vija, and then in a similar way for the paternal
and maternal sides two figures each should be drawn
(39). After these have been sprinkled with the Varuna
Vija, leaves should be spread over the figures. These
leaves should be sprinkled with the Varuna Vija, and
then drinking-water and different kinds of edibles and
rice should be distributed in their order (40).

After giving honey and grains of barley and sprinkling
the offerings with water, accompanied by the

Mantra

Hrang, Hrung, Phat,

the worshipper possessed of the knowledge of Truth
should dedicate the edibles by the names of the Vishva-Devas, the fathers, the mothers, the maternal grandfathers and the maternal grandmothers, and thereafter
repeat the Gayatri ten times and thrice repeat the

Mantra

"I salute the Divinities," as aforesaid.

After this, O Adya! he should take the directions (of the

officiating Brahmanas) relating to the disposal of the remnants of edibles and of the Pindas (41-43).

Upon receiving the directions of the Brahmana, he should, O Beloved! make twelve Pindas of the size of bael fruits with the remnants of the Akshata and other things (44). He should make one more Pinda equal in size with the others, and then, O Ambika! he should spread some kusha grass and barley on the Nairrita corner of the figure (45).

Mantra

Such of my family as have none to offer Pindas to them whom neither son nor wife survive, who were burnt to death or were killed by tigers or other beast of prey, such kinsmen of mine as themselves are without kinsmen, all such as were my kinsmen in previous births, may they all obtain imperishable satisfaction by the Pinda and water hereby given by me (46-47).

O Adored of the Devas! having with the above Mantra offered the Pinda to those who have no one to offer them Pindas, he should wash his hands and inwardly recite the Gayatri, and repeat the

Mantra

"I salute the Divinities,"

*and so forth, three times, and then make the square
(48).*

*O Devi! the wise man should in front of the vessels con-
taining the remnants of the offerings make such squares
in twos (for his Ancestors), beginning with the paternal
Ancestors (49).*

*O Shive! he should then sprinkle the squares with water
with the Mantra already prescribed, and then spread
kusha grass over them and sprinkle them with the Vayu
Vija (49), beginning with the kusha spread on the square for the paternal (male) Ancestors, and then offer three
Pindas, one at the top, another at the bottom, and one
in the middle, in each of the squares (50).*

*O Maheshvari! the names of each of the Ancestors
should be mentioned, inviting him or her, and then the
Pinda should be given with honey and barley, concluding with Svadha (51). After the Pindas are given (in
manner aforesaid) the Lepa-bhoji Ancestors should
be satisfied by the offer to them of the remnants which
remain on the hand. These should be scattered on all
sides with the*

Mantra

Ong, may the Lepa-bhoji Ancestors be pleased.

*In Ekoddishta Shraddha the offering to the Lepa-bhoji
Ancestors is not made (52).*

*Then for the satisfaction of the Devas and Pitris the
Gayatri should be inwardly recited ten times, and the
Mantra, "I salute the Divinities," as aforesaid should be
similarly recited three times, and then the Pindas should
be worshipped (53). Lighting an incense-stick and a
light, the wise one should, with closed eyes, think of the
Pitris in their celestial forms partaking of their allotted
Pindas, each his own, and should then bow to them,
uttering the following (54)*

Mantra

*My father is my highest Dharmma. My father is my highest Tapas. My father is my Heaven. On my father being
satisfied, the whole Universe is satisfied (55).*

*Taking up some flowers from the remnants, the Pitris
should be asked for their blessings, with the following
(56)*

Mantra

Give me your blessings, O Merciful Pitris. May my knowledge, progeny, and kinsmen always increase. May my benefactors prosper. May I have food in profusion. May many always beg of me, and may I not have to beg of any (57-58).

Then he should remove the Devas and Brahmanas made of kusha grass, as also the Pindas, commencing with the Devas. The wise one should then make presents to all three (59).

He should then make japa of the Gayatri ten times, and the Mantra, "I salute the Divinities," five times, and, after looking at the fire and the Sun, should, with folded palms, ask the Vipra the following question (60):

"Is the Shraddha complete?" and the Brahmana should make reply:

"It has been completed according to the injunctions" (61).

Then, for the removal of the effects of any error or omission, the Pranava should be inwardly recited ten times, and the ceremony should be brought to a close, uttering the following

Mantra

"May the Shraddha rite be faultless";

*and then the food and drink in the vessels should be
offered to the officiating Brahmana (62).*

*In the absence of a Vipra, it should be given to cows
and goats, or should be thrown into water. This is called
"Vriddhi Shraddha," enjoined for all obligatory sacramental rites (63). Shraddha performed on the occasion
of any Parvvan is called "Parvvana Shraddha" (64).*

*In ceremonies relating to the consecration of emblems or
images of Devas, or while starting for or returning from
pilgrimage, the Shraddha should be according to the
injunctions laid down for Parvvana Shraddha (65). On
the occasion of Parvvana Shraddha the Pitris should not
be addressed with the prefix "Nandimukha," and for the
words "Salutation to Pushti" should be substituted the
words "Salutation to Svadha" (66).*

*O Beautiful One! if any of the three Ancestors be alive,
then the wise one should make the offerings to another
Ancestor of higher degree (67). If the father, grandfather,
and great-grandfather be alive, then, O Queen of the
Devas! no Shraddha need be performed. If they are*

pleased, then the object of the funeral rite and sacrifice is attained (68).

If his father be living, then a man may perform his mother's Shraddha, his wife's Shraddha, and Nandi-mukha Shraddha; but he is not entitled to perform the Shraddha of anyone else (69).O Queen of the Kula! at the time of Ekoddishta Shraddha the Vishva-Devas are not to be worshipped. The word of entreaty should be addressed to one Ancestor only (70).

At the time of Ekoddishta Shraddha cooked rice and Pinda should be given whilst facing south. The rest of the ceremony is the same as that which has been already described, with the exception that sesamum should be substituted for barley (71).

The peculiarity in Preta Shraddha is that the worship of Ganga and others is omitted, and in the framing of the Mantra the deceased should be spoken of as Preta whilst rice and Pindas are offered to him (72).

The Shraddha performed for one man is called "Ekoddishta." In offering Pinda to the Preta, fish and meat should be added (73). O Mistress of the Kula! know this, that the Shraddha which is performed on the day following the end of the period of uncleanliness is Preta

Shraddha (74). If there is a miscarriage, or if the child dies immediately on birth, or if a child is born or dies, then the period of uncleanliness is to be reckoned according to the custom of the family (75).

The period of uncleanliness in the case of the twice-born is ten days (for Brahmanas), twelve (for Kshatriyas), and a fortnight (for Vaishyas); for Shudras and Samanyas the period is one month (thirty days) (76).

On the death of an Agnate who is not a Sapinda, the period of uncleanliness is three days, and on the death of a Sapinda, should information of it arrive after the period prescribed, one becomes unclean for three days (77).

The unclean man, O Primordial One! is not entitled to perform any rite relating to the Devas and the Pitris, excepting Kula worship and that which has been already commenced (78).

Persons over five years of age should be burnt in the burning-ground, but, O Kuleshani! a wife should not be burnt with her dead husband (79). Every woman is Thy image–Thou residest concealed in the forms of all women in this world. That woman who in her delusion ascends the funeral pyre of her lord shall go to hell (80).

Kalika! the corpses of worshippers of Brahman should be either buried, thrown into running water, or burnt, according as they may direct (81).

Ambika! death in a holy place or a place of pilgrimage, or near the Devi, or near the Kaulikas, is a happy one (82).

He who at the time of his death meditates on the one Truth, forgetful of the three worlds, attains to his own Essential Being (83).

After death the corpse should be taken to the burning-ground, and when it has been washed it should be smeared with ghee and placed on the pyre, with the face to the north (84).

The deceased should be addressed by his name, and Gotra and as Preta. Giving the Pinda to the mouth of the corpse, the pyre should be lighted by applying the torch to the mouth of the corpse, inwardly the while reciting the Vahni Vija (85).

Beloved! the Pinda should be made of boiled or unboiled rice, or crushed barley, or wheat, and should be of the size of an emblic myrobalam (86). To the eldest son of the Preta is given the privilege of performing the

Shraddha; in his absence to the other sons, according to
the order of their seniority (87).

The day after the day upon which the period of uncleanliness expires, the mourner should bathe and purify
himself, and give away gold and sesamum for the liberation of the Preta (88).

The son of the Preta should give away cattle, lands,
clothes, carriages, vessels made of metals, and various
kinds of edibles, in order that the Preta may attain
Heaven (89).

He should also give away scents, garlands, fruits, water,
a beautiful bed, and everything which the Preta himself
liked to insure his passage to Heaven (90).

Then a bull should be branded with the mark of a trident, and decorated with gold and ornaments, and then
let loose, with the object that the deceased may attain
Heaven (91).

He should then with a devout spirit perform the Shraddha, according to the injunctions laid down for the
performance of Preta Shraddha, and then feed Brahmanas and Kaulas possessed of Divine knowledge, and the
hungry (92).

The man who is unable to make gifts should perform the Shraddha to the best of his ability, and feed the hungry, and thus liberate his father from the state of existence of a Preta (93).

This Preta Shraddha is known as Adya or Ekod-dishta Shraddha, and it liberates the deceased from the state of Preta. After this every year on the tithi of his death edibles should be given to the deceased (94).

There is no necessity for a multitude of injunctions nor for a multitude of rituals. Man may attain all siddhi by honouring a Kaulika. The object of all Sangskaras is completely attained if, in lieu of the prescribed Homa, Japa, and Shraddha, even a single Kaulika is duly hono-ured (96), at the time of the ceremony.

The injunction of Shiva is that all auspicious ceremonies should be performed between the period beginning with the fourth day of the light half of the lunar half-month, and ending on the fifth of the dark half-month (97).

He, however, who is desirous of performing any rite which must be performed may perform it even on an in-auspicious day, provided he be so directed by his Guru, by a Ritvij, or a Kaulika (98).

A Kaulika should commence the building of a house, should first enter a house, start on a journey, wear new jewels, and the like, only after worshipping the Primordial One with the five Elements (99).

Or the excellent worshipper may shorten the rite. He may thus, after meditating on the Devi, and inwardly reciting the Mantra and bowing to the Devi, go wherever he may desire (100).

In the worship of all Devatas, such as the Autumnal Festival and others, dhyana and puja should be performed according to the ordinances laid down in the Shastras relating to such worship (101).

According to the ordinances relating to the worship of the Primordial Kali, animal sacrifice and Homa should be performed, and the rite should be brought to an end by the honouring of Kaulikas and making of offerings (102).

The general rule is that Ganga, Vishnu, Shiva, Suryya, and Brahma should first be worshipped, and then the Deva the special object of worship (103).

The Kaulika is the most excellent Dharmma, the Kaulika is the most excellent Deva, the Kaulika is the most excellent pilgrimage, therefore should the Kaula be always worshipped (104).

The three and a half kotis of Places of Pilgrimage, all the Devas beginning with Brahma Himself, reside in the body of the Kaula. What, therefore, is there which is not attained by worshipping him? The land in which the good and fully initiated Kaula resides is blessed and deserving of honour. It is most holy, and is coveted even by the Devas (105-106). Who can in this world understand the majesty of the fully initiated Sadhaka, who is Shiva Himself, and to whom there is nothing either holy or sinful? (107).

Such a Kaula, possessing merely the form of man, moves about this earth for the salvation of the entire world and the instruction of men in the conduct of life (108).

Shri Devi said:

Thou hast, O Lord! spoken of the greatness of the Soul of the fully initiated Kaula. Do Thou in Thy mercy speak to Me of the ordinances relating to such initiation (109).

Shri Sadashiva said:

In the three Ages this rite was a great secret.; men then

used to perform it in all secrecy, and thus attain liberation (110).

When the Kali Age prevails, the followers of Kula rite
should declare themselves as such, and, whether in the
night or the day, should openly be initiated (111).

By the mere drinking of wine, without initiation, a man
does not become a Kaula. The Kula worshipper becomes
the Lord of the Kula Chakra only after full initiation
(112).

The Guru should, the day before the initiation, worship
the Deva of Obstacles with offerings, according to his
ability for the removal of all obstacles (113).

If the Guru is not qualified to officiate at a full initiation
ceremony, then it should, O Beloved! be performed by a
duly initiated Kaula (114). Gang is the Vija of Ganapati
(Ganesha) (115). Ganaka is the Rishi, the Chhanda
is Nivrit, the Lord of Obstacles is the Devata, and the
Mantra is applicable for the removal of obstacles to the
performance of the rite (116).

Adding successively six long vowels to the Mula Mantra,
Shadanga-nyasa should be performed, and O Shiva!
after doing Pranayama let Ganapati be meditated upon
(117).

Dhyana

Meditate on Gana-pati as of the colour of vermilion, having three eyes, a large belly, holding in His lotus-hands the conch, the noose, the elephant-goad, and the sign of blessing. His great trunk adorned with the jar of wine which it holds. On His forehead shines the young Moon. He has the head of the King of elephants; His cheeks are constantly bathed in wine. His hody is adorned with the coils of the King of servants. He is dressed in red raiment, and His body is smeared with scented ointments (118).

Having thus meditated upon Ganapati, he should be worshipped with mental offerings, and then the protecting power of the seat should be worshipped. These are Tibra, Jvalini, Nanda, Bhoga-da, Kama-rupini, Ugra, Tejasvati, Satyi, and Vighna-vinashini. The first eight should be worshipped in their order, beginning from the east, and the last should be worshipped in the middle of the Mandala. Having thus worshipped them all, the lotus-seat itself should be worshipped (119-120).

Meditating on Ganesha once again, He should be worshipped with offerings of the five elements. On each of His four sides should the excellent Kaulika worship Ganesha, Gana-nayaka, Gana-natha, Gana-krida,

Eka-danta, Rakta-tunda, Lambodara, Gajanana, Mahodara, Vikata, Dhumrabha, and Vighna-nashana (121-123).

Then the eight Shaktis, Brahmi, and others, and the ten Dikpalas and their weapons, should be worshipped, and after that Vighna-raja should be bidden to depart (124).

Having thus worshipped the King of Obstacles, the worshipper should perform the preliminary ceremony, and then entertain the Kaulas versed in divine knowledge with the five elements (125).

The next day, having bathed and performed his ordinary daily duties as already enjoined, he should, O Beloved! give away sesamum-seed and gold for the destruction of all sins from his birth, and a bhojya for the satisfaction of the Kaulas (126). Then, giving arghya to Suryya, and having worshipped Brahma, Vishnu, Shiva, and the nine Planets, as also the sixteen divine Mothers, he should make a Vasu-dhara (127).

He should then perform Vriddhi Shraddha for the good result of the rite, and, going up to the Guru, bow to him, and pray to him as follows (128):

(Prayer to the Guru)

Save me, O Lord! thou that art the Sun of the Kaulas. Protect my head, O Ocean of Mercy! with the shade of thy lotus-foot (129). Grant us leave, O Exalted One! in this auspicious Purnabhisheka that by thy grace I may attain the success of my undertaking without any hindrance (130).

(The Guru should then reply:)

My son! be thou, by the permission of the Shiva-Shakti, initiated with the full initiation. May thou attain the object of thy desire by the command of Shiva (131).

Having thus obtained the permission of the spiritual Preceptor, he should make the Sangkalpa for the removal of all obstacles and for the attainment of long life, prosperity, strength, and good health (132).

The Sadhaka, having solemnly formed his resolve, should worship the Guru, by presenting him with clothes and jewels, and karana with Shuddhi, and do honour to him (133).

The Guru should then make with earth an altar four fingers in height and measuring one and a half cubit either way in a beautiful room painted with red earth, etc., decorated with pictures, flags, fruits, and leaves, and strings of small bells.

The room should have a beautiful ceiling-cloth, lighted with lines of lamps fed with ghee to dispel all traces of darkness, and should be scented with burning camphor, incense-sticks, and incense, and ornamented with fans, fly-whisks, the tail feathers of the peacock, and mirrors, etc., and then he should with rice powdered and coloured yellow, red, black, white, and dark blue draw Mandala called Sarvato-bhadra, beautiful and auspicious in every way (134-138).

Then each person should perform the rite preparatory to mental worship, according to his Sangkalpa, and then, having made mental worship, should purify the five elements with the Mantra previously mentioned (139). After the Pancha-tattvas have been purified, the jar, which must be either of gold or silver or copper or earth, should be placed with the Brahma Vija on the Mandala. It should be washed with the Weapon Mantra and smeared with curd, Akshata, and then a vermilion mark should be placed on it with the Mantra "Shring" (140-141).

He should then recite three times the letters of the alphabet, with the Vindu superposed from Ksha to A, and recite inwardly the Mula Mantra, and fill the jar with wine or water from some holy place, or with ordinary pure water, and then throw into the jar nine gems or gold (142-143).

*The merciful Guru should then place over the mouth
of the jar a leafy branch of a Jack-tree, a Fig-tree, an
Ashvattha-tree, and of a Vakula and Mango-tree, with
the Vagbhava Vija (144).*

*He should then place on the leafy branch a gold, silver,
copper, or earthen platter, uttering the Rama Vija and
Maya Vija (145). Then, O Beauteous One! two pieces
of cloth should be tied to the neck of the jar. When
worshipping Shakti the cloth should be of a red colour,
and in the worship of Shiva and Vishnu it should be
white (146).*

Inwardly reciting the

Mantra

Sthang, Sthing, Hring, Shring,

*the jar should be fixed in its place, and after putting into
it the Pancha-tattvas the nine cups should be placed in
their order (147). The Shakti Patra should be of silver,
the Guru Patra of gold, the Shri Patra should be made
of the human skull, the rest of copper (148). Cups made
of stone, wood, and iron should be rejected; the material
of the cups in the worship of the Maha-Devi should be
according to the means of the worshipper (149).*

After placing the cups, libations should be offered to the four Gurus and the Devi, and the wise one should then worship the jar filled with nectar (150). Lights and incense should then be waved and sacrifices made to all beings, and after worshipping the divinities of the pitha he should perform Shadangganyasa (151). He should then do Pranayama, and, meditating on the Great Devi, invoke Her, and thereafter worship Her, the Object of his worship, to the best of his ability and without niggardliness (151). The excellent Guru, O Shiva! should perform all the rites ending with Homa, and then honour the Kumaris and worshippers of Shakti by presenting them with flowers, sandal-paste, and clothes (153).

The Guru should then ask the permission of those present with the following words:

O you Kaulas! who are vowed to Kula-worship, be kind to my disciple. Do you give your permission to his Sangskara of Purnabhisheka (154).

The Lord of the Chakra, having thus asked those present, should respectfully say: "By the grace of Maha-maya and the majesty of the Supreme Soul, may thy disciple be perfect and devoted to the Supreme Essence" (155).

The Guru should then make the disciple worship the Devi in the jar, which has been worshipped by himself, and then, mentally repeating the

Mantra

Kling, Hring, Shring

over it, move the immaculate jar, with the following

Mantra

Rise, O Brahma-kalasha, thou art the Devata and grantest all success. May my disciple, being bathed with thy water and leaves, be devoted to Brahman (156-157).

Having moved the jar in this manner, the Guru should mercifully sprinkle the disciple seated with his face to the North with the Mantra about to be spoken (158).

The Rishi of the Mantra of this auspicious Purnabhisheka rite is Sadashiva, the presiding Devata is the Adya Devata, the Vija is "Ong," and its applicability is for the auspicious sprinkling on the occasion of the Purnabhisheka ceremony (158-159).

Mantra

*May the Gurus sprinkle thee. May Brahma, Vishnu,
and Maheshvara sprinkle thee; may the Mothers Durga,
Lakshmi, Bhavani, sprinkle thee; may Shodashi, Tarini,
Nitya, Svaha, Mahisha-mardini, all these sprinkle thee
with the water that has been sanctified by the Mantra;
may Jaya-durga, Vishalakshi, Brahmani, Sarasvati, may
all These sprinkle thee; may Bagala, Varada, and Shiva
sprinkle thee; may the Shaktis, Narasinghi, Varahi,
Vaishnavi, Vana-malini, Indrani, Varuni, Raudri,
sprinkle thee; may Bhairavi, Bhadra-kali, Tushti, Pushti,
Uma, Kshama, Shraddha, Kanti, Daya, Shanti, always
sprinkle thee; may Maha-kali, Maha-lakshmi, Maha-nila-sarasvati, Ugra-chanda, Prachanda, constantly
sprinkle thee; may Matsya, Kurma, Varaha, Nrising-
ha, Vamana, Rama, Bhrigu-Rama, sprinkle thee with
water; may Asitanga, Ruru, Chanda, Krodhonmatta,
Bhayangkara, Kapali, Bhishana, sprinkle thee; may
Kali, Kapalini, Kulla, Kurukulla, Virodhini, Viprachitta,
Mahogra, ever sprinkle thee; may Indra, Agni, Shama-
na, Raksha, Varuna, Pavana, Dhana-da, Maheshana,
who are the eight Dikpalas, sprinkle thee; may Ravi,
Soma, Mangala, Budha, Jiva, Sita, Shani, Rahu, Ketu,
with all their Satellites, sprinkle thee; may the stars, the
Karanas, the Yogas, the Days of the Week, and the two
Divisions of the Month, the Days, Seasons, Months, and
the Year anoint thee always; may the Salt Ocean, the
Sweet Ocean, the Ocean of Wine, the Ocean of Ghee, the*

Ocean of Curd, the Ocean of Milk, the Ocean of Sweet Water sprinkle thee with their consecrated waters; may Ganga, Yamuna, Reva, Chandra-bhaga, Sarasvati, Sarayu, Gandaki, Kunti, Shveta-ganga, Kaushiki, may all these sprinkle thee with their consecrated waters; may the great Nagas beginning with Ananta, the birds beginning with Garuda, the trees beginning with the Kalpa tree, and the great Mountains sprinkle thee; may the beneficent Beings residing in Patala, on the earth, and in the air, pleased at this hour of thy Purnabhisheka, sprinkle thee with water (160-175). May thy ill-luck, bad name, illness, melancholy and sorrows be destroyed by the Purnabhisheka, and by the glory of the Supreme Brahman (176). May Alakshmi, Kala-karni, the Dakinis, and the Yoginis, being driven away by the Kali Vija, be destroyed by the Abhisheka (177). May the Bhuta, Preta, Pishachas, and the maleficent Planets be driven out, put to flight, and destroyed by the Rama Vija; may all misfortune caused thee by magic and by the incantations of thy enemies, may all thy transgressions of mind, word, and body be destroyed as the result of this initiation; may all thy adversities be destroyed, may thy prosperity be undisturbed, may all thy desires be fulfilled as the result of this Purnabhisheka (178-180).

With these twenty-one Mantras the disciple should be sprinkled with water; and if he has obtained already the

Mantra from the mouth of a Pashu, the Guru should make him hear it again (181).

The Kaulika Guru should, having informed the worshippers of Shakti, call his disciple by his name and give him a name ending with Anandanatha (182).

Being thus initiated in the Mantra by the Guru, the disciple should worship his Ishta-devata in the Yantra (of the Guru), and then honour the Guru by presenting him with the Pancha-tattvas (183).

The disciple should also give as Dakshina cows, land, gold, clothes, drinks, and jewels to the Guru, and then honour the Kaulas, who are the very embodiments of Shiva (184).

The self-possessed, purified, and humble disciple, having honoured the Kaulas, should touch the sacred feet of the Guru with veneration, and, bowing to him, pray to him as follows (185):

Prayer to Guru

Holy Lord! Thou art the Lord of the world. Lord! thou art my Lord.O Ocean of Mercy! do Thou gratify my heart's desire by the gift of the excellent nectar (186).

The Guru should then say:

*"Give me leave, O Kaulas! you who are the visible
images of Shiva Himself, that I may give to my good and
humble disciple the excellent nectar" (187).*

The Kaulas will then say:

*"Lord of the Chakra! thou art the Supreme Lord Him-
self, Thou art the Sun of the Kaula lotus. Do Thou gratify this good disciple, and give him the Kaula nectar"
(188).*

*The Guru, having obtained the leave of the Kaulas,
should place in the hand of the disciple the drinking-cup
filled with the excellent nectar, as also the Shuddhi
(189).*

*The Guru should then, devoutly meditating on the Devi
in his heart, place the tilaka on the forehead of the disciple, as also of the Kaulas, with the ashes adhering to the
sacrificial spoon (190).*

*Let the Guru then distribute the Tattvas offered to the
Devi, and partake of the food and drink as directed
in the injunctions relating to the formation of Chakra
(191).*

O Devi! I have spoken to Thee of the auspicious rites relating to Purnabhisheka. By this one attains divine knowledge and becomes Shiva Himself (192).

The Purnabhisheka should be performed for nine or seven or five or three or one night (193).

There are, O Kuleshani! five different forms in this purificatory rite. In the rite which lasts nine nights the Mandala known as Sarvato-bhadra should be made (194).

Beloved! in the rite which lasts seven nights the Mandala Nava-nabha, in the rite which lasts five nights the Mandala Panchabja, in the rite which lasts three nights and in the rite which lasts one night the Mandala of eight-petalled lotus should be respectively made (195).

O Devi! the injunction is that on the Sarvato-bhadra and Nava-nabha Mandalas nine jars should be placed, on Panchabja Mandala five, and on Ashta-dalabja Mandala one jar, and the Angga-Devatas and the Avarana-Devatas should be worshipped in the filaments and other parts of the lotuses (196-197).

The Kaulas who have been fully initiated are pure of soul. All things are purified by their looking, touching,

*and by their smelling them (198). All men, whether they
are Shaktas, Vaishnavas, Shaivas, Sauras, or Gana-
patas, should worship the Kaula Sadhu with devotion
(199).*

*It is good for a Shakta to have a Guru who is a Shakta,
for a Shaiva a Shaiva Guru is commendable, and for a
Vaishnava a Vaishnava, for a Saura a Saura as Guru
is advised, and a Ganapata is the proper Guru for a
Ganapata, but a Kaula is excellent as Guru in the case
of all; therefore the wise one should with all his soul be
initiated by a Kaula (200-201). Those who worship the
Kaulas with Pancha-tattva and with heart uplifted cause the salvation of their Ancestors, and themselves attain
the highest end (202).*

*The man who has obtained the Mantra from the mouth
of a Pashu is of a certainty a Pashu, and he who has
obtained the Mantra from a Vira is a Vira, and he who
obtains it from a Kaula knows the Brahman (203).
One who has been initiated according to Shakta rites
is a Vira; he may purify the Pancha-tattvas only in the
worship of his own Ishta-devata, he may never be the
Chakreshvara (204).*

*He who kills a Vira, he who drinks wine which has not
been consecrated, he who seduces the wife of or steals*

*the property of a Vira, these four are great sinners, and
the man who associates with any of these is the fifth
sinner (205). Those evil-natured men who disparage the
Kula Way, Kula articles, and the Kula worshipper go
down the low and vile path (206).*

*The Rudra-dakinis and Rudra-bhairavis dance in joy
(at the thought of) chewing the bones and flesh of men
who hate wine and the Kaulas (207). They are merciful
and truthful, and ever desire the good of others, for such
as slander them there is no escape from Hell (208).*

*I have in the various Tantras spoken of various ceremo-
nies and of many repetitions of practices; but in the case
of a Kaula who is devoted to the Brahman, it is a matter
of indifference whether he practises or omits them (209).*

*There is one Supreme Brahman Who exists, spread
throughout the Universe (or any part of it). He is
worshipped, because there is nothing which exists apart
from Him (210).*

*Beloved! even those who look to the fruit of action and
are governed by their desires and by the worship of different Devas, and addicted to worldly pursuits, go to and
become united with Him (211). He who sees everything
in Brahman, and who sees Brahman everywhere, is*

undoubtedly known as an excellent Kaula, who has attained liberation while yet living (212).

End of the Tenth Joyful Message, entitled "Rites relating to Vriddhi Shraddha, Funeral Rites, and Purnabhisheka."

CHAPTER 11

The Account of Expiatory Rites

LISTENING to the injunctions of Shambhu relating to the different castes and stages of life, Aparna was greatly pleased, and questioned Shangkara thus (1):

Shri Devi said:

Thou hast, O Lord! out of Thy kindness for Me and in Thy omniscience, spoken of the customs and the rules of religious conduct and sacraments for the well-being of the world (2). But the men of the Kali Age, being wicked, and blinded by anger and lust, atheists, of wavering minds and addicted to the gratification of their senses, will not in their ignorance and folly follow the way laid down by Thee; it behoves Thee, O Ishana! to say what will be the means of their liberation (3-4).

Shri Sadashiva said:

Thou hast asked well, O Devi! Thou who art the Benefactress of the world, the Mother of the world, Thou art Durga, Thou liberatest people from the bonds of birth and the toils of this world (5). Thou art the Primordial

One, Thou fosterest and guardest this world, Thou art beyond the most excellent; Thou, O Devi! supportest the moving and the motionless Universe (6). Thou art Earth, Thou art Water, Thou art Fire, Thou art Air,

Thou art the Void, Thou art consciousness itself, Thou art the mahat-tattva (7). Thou art life in this world;

Thou art the knowledge of self, and Thou art the Supreme Divinity. Thou art the senses; Thou art the mind, Thou art the intellect; Thou art the motion and existence of the Universe (8).

Thou art the Vedas, Thou art the Pranava, Thou art the Smritis, the Sanghitas, the Nigamas, the Agamas, and the Tantras, Thou pervadest all the Shastras, and art the Abode of all that is good (9). Thou art Mahakali,

Mahalakshmi, Maha-nila-sarasvati, Mahodari, Mahamaya, Maharaudri, and Maheshvari; Thou art Omniscient and full of knowledge, there is nothing which Thou knowest not; yet, O Wise One! since Thou askest Me, I will speak of it for Thy pleasure (10-11).

Thou hast truly spoken, O Devi! of the ways of men, who, knowing what is for their welfare, yet, maddened by sinful desire for things which bring immediate enjoyment, and devoid of the sense of right and wrong, will desert the True Path. I speak now of that which will contribute to their salvation (12-13).

In the doing of what is forbidden and in the omitting of what is enjoined men sin, and sins lead to pain, sorrow, and disease (14).

O Kula-nayika! know that there are two kinds of sin – that which contributes merely to the injury of one's own self, and that which causes injury to others (15). Man is released of the sin of injuring others by the punishment inflicted by the King, and from other sins by expiatory rites and Samadhi (16).

Those sinful men who are not purified by either punishment or expiation cannot but go to hell, and are despised both in this world and the next (17).

O Adya! I shall first of all speak of the Rules relating, O Maheshvari! to punishment by the King. The King who deviates from these himself goes upon the downward path (18).

In the administration of justice, servants, sons, mendicants, friends, and foes should all be treated alike (19).

If the King is guilty of any sin himself, or if he should have wronged one who is not guilty, then he may purify himself by fasting and by placating those he has wronged by gifts (20). If the King should consider that he is guilty of any sin which is punishable by death, he should then abdicate his kingdom and go to a forest, and there labour for his liberation and penances (21). The King should not, without sufficient reason, inflict heavy punishment on persons guilty of a light offence, nor should he inflict light punishment on persons guilty of a great offence (22). But the punishment by which many offenders may be deterred from ill-doing, and (punishment) in the case of an offender who is fearless of crimes, should be heavy, although the offence be a light one (23).

In the case of one who has committed the offence but once only and is ashamed of his ill-deed, or of one who fears crime and is a respectable man, a light punishment should be inflicted, even if the offence be a grave one (24).

If a Kaula or a Brahmana is guilty of a slight offence, they should even, though highly honourable, be punished by the King by a rebuke (25).

The King who does not bestow adequate rewards and

*punishments after consultation with his ministers is a
great sinner (26).*

*A son should not leave his mother and father, the
subjects should not leave their King, nor the wife her
husband, even though they are greatly guilty (27).*

*The subjects should actively protect the kingdom, pro-
perty, and life of the just King; otherwise they will go
upon the downward path (28).*

*Shiva! those who knowingly go with their, mother,
daughter, or sister, those who have killed their Maha-gurus, those who have, after having taken refuge in the
Kula Faith, abandoned it, and those who have broken
the trust placed in them, are great sinners (29-30).*

*Shiva! the punishment of those that go with their
mother, sister, and daughter is death, and if the latter
are wilful participants the same punishment should be
inflicted upon them (31).*

*The sinful man who with a lustful mind goes to the bed
of his mother or father's sister, or daughters-in-law, or
mothers-in-law (wife's mother), the wife of his preceptor,
the wife of his maternal or paternal grandfather, the
daughter or wife of his mother or father's brother, the*

wife or daughter of his brother, the sister's daughter, the master's wife or daughter, or with an unmarried girl, should be punished by castration, and these women also if they are wilful participants in the crime should be punished by the cutting of their noses and turning them out of the house that they may be released from sin (32-34).

The punishment of the man who goes with the wife or daughter of a sapinda, or with the wife of a man who has trusted him, is to be deprived of all his property and to have his head shaved (35).

If through mistake (by ignorance) one should happen to marry any of these, either in Brahma or Shaiva form, then she should at once be disespoused (36).

A man who goes with the wife of another man of the same caste as himself, or of a caste inferior to his own, should be punished by the imposition of a fine and by being kept on a diet of grains for one month (37).

If a Kshatriya, Vaishya, Shudra, or Samanya, O Thou of Beauteous Face! goes with a Brahmana woman knowing her to be such, then his punishment is castration, and the Brahmana woman should be disfigured and banished from his kingdom by the King. For such as go with the wives of Viras, and for such wives, the punishment should be the same (38-39).

The wicked man who enjoys the wife of one of a higher caste should be heavily fined, and kept on a diet of grains for three months (40).

And if the woman is a wilful party, she should be punished as above mentioned. If the wife is the victim of a rape, then she should be separated from, but maintained by, her husband (41).

A wife, whether married according to Brahma or Shaiva form, should in all cases be renounced if she has gone with another even if it be only once, and then whether of her own desire or against it (42).

Those who have intercourse with public women, or with cows or other animals, should, O Deveshi! be purified by being kept on a diet of grains for three nights (43).

The punishment of those wicked men who have unnatural intercourse with a woman is death; this is the injunction of Shambhu (44).

A man who ravishes a woman, even if she be the wife of a Chandala, should be punished by death, and should never be pardoned (45).

A man should consider as wife only that woman who has been married to him according to Brahma or Shaiva form. All other women are the wives of others (46).

A man who with lust looks at another man's wife should fast for a day to purify himself. He who accosts her in a secret place should fast for two days. He who touches her should fast for four days; and he who embraces her should fast for eight days to purify himself (47).

And the woman who with a lustful mind behaves in the same manner should purify herself by following the same rules of fasting (48).

The man who uses offensive language towards a woman, who sees the private parts of a woman who is not his wife, and laughs derisively at her, should fast for two days to purify himself (49).

A man who shows his naked body to another, or who makes another person naked, should cease eating for two days to purify himself (50).

If the husband proves that his wife has had intercourse with another, then the King should punish her and her paramour according to the injunction laid down (51).

If the husband (has good cause to believe and yet) is unable to prove the faithlessness of his wife, then he should separate from her, but he should maintain her if she remains under his control (52).

If the husband, on seeing his wife enjoying with her paramour, kills her with her paramour, then the King should not punish him with death (53).

If the husband prohibits the wife to go to any place or to talk with anyone, then the wife should neither go to that place nor talk with that person (54).

If, on the death of the husband, the widow lives with the relatives of the husband under their control, following the customs of a widow's life, or in their absence she lives with the relatives of her father, then she deserves to inherit her husband's property (55).

The widow should not eat twice a day, nor should she eat food cooked by one who is not her husband's Agnate; she should renounce sexual enjoyment, animal food, jewels, sleeping on soft beds, and coloured clothes (56).

The widow faithful to her Dharmma should not anoint herself with fragrant ointments, she should avoid village gossip, and should spend her time in the worship of the

Deities and in the performance of Vratas (57).

In the case of the boy who has neither father, mother, nor paternal grandfather, the mother's relatives are the best guardians (58). The mother's mother, mother's father, mother's brother, mother's brother's son, mother's father's brother, these are the relatives on the mother's side (59).

Father's mother, father, brother, father's brother's and sister's sons, father's father's brother, are known as paternal relatives (60).

The husband's mother, father, brother, the husband's brother's and sister's sons, and the husband's father's brothers, all these are known as the relatives of the husband (61).

Ambika! the King should compel a man, according to his means, to give food and clothes to his father, mother, father's father, father's mother, the wife whose son cannot support her, and to the maternal grandfather and grandmother, who are poor and have no son (62-63).

If a man speaks rudely to his wife he must fast for a day, if he beats her he must go without food for three days, and if he causes her bloodshed then he must fast for seven days (64).

If a man in his anger or folly calls his wife his mother, his sister, or daughter, then he should purify himself by fasting seven days (65).

If a girl be married to an impotent man, then the King should cause her to be married again, even if the fact is discovered after the lapse of some time. This is Shiva's injunction (66).

If a girl becomes a widow before consummation of marriage, she also ought to be remarried. This also is the command of Shiva (67).

The woman who is delivered of a child within six months of her marriage, or after the lapse of a year following her husband's death, is not a wife, nor is the child legitimate (68).

The woman who causes a miscarriage before the completion of the fifth month, as well as the person who helps her thereto, should be heavily punished (69).

The woman who after the fifth month destroys the child in her womb, and the person who helps her thereto, are guilty of killing a human being (70).

The cruel man who wilfully kills another man should

always be sentenced to death by the King (71).

The King should correct the man who kills another man through ignorance, or in a fit of passion, or by mistake, either by taking his property from him or by giving him a severe beating (72).

The man who tries to compass his own death, whether by himself or by the aid of another, should be awarded the same punishment as the man who kills another through ignorance (73).

The man who kills another in a duel, or kills an enemy who attempts to kill him, is not guilty of any offence (74).

The King should punish the man who has maimed another by maiming him, and the man who has beaten another by having him beaten (75).

The wicked man who flings any missile, or lifts his hand to strike a Vipra, or one who should be honoured, or who strikes either of them, should be punished by a pecuniary fine for the first offence, and by the burning of his hand for a second offence (76).

If a man dies consequent upon a wound inflicted by any

*weapon or otherwise after six months, then the offender
should be punished for the assault, and shall not be
punished with death by the King (77).*

*If the King kills subverters of his government, men who
plot to usurp his kingdom, servants secretly befriending
the King's enemies, men creating dissatisfaction against
the King among the troops, subjects who wish to wage
war against the King, or armed highway robbers, he
shall not be guilty of any sin (78-79).*

*The man who kills another, compelled by his master's
order, is not himself guilty of the killing, for it is the master's killing. This is the command of Shiva (80).*

*If a man's death is caused by a beast belonging to, or
weapons in the hand of, a careless man, then the latter
should be punished by a pecuniary or bodily punishment (81).*

*Those detestable persons who disobey the King's com-
mand, who are arrogant in their speech in the King's
presence, or who decry the Kula faith, should be punished by the King (82).*

*He who misappropriates property entrusted to him,
the malicious man, the cheat, he who creates ill-feeling*

between men, or who makes people quarrel with one another, should be banished from the kingdom by the King (83).

The King should banish from his kingdom those abandoned and wicked-minded men who give away their sons and daughters in marriage for money, and who give their daughters (in marriage) to impotent husbands (84).

Persons who attempt to harm others by the spreading of baseless calumnies should be punished by the just King in accordance with their offence (85).

The King should compel the calumniator to pay the sufferer money commensurate with the harm done (86).

For such persons as steal gems, pearls, gold, and other metals, the punishment should be either the cutting off of the hand or the entire arm, according to the value of the stolen property (87).

Those who steal buffaloes, horses, cattle, jewels, etc., and infants, should be punished by the King as thieves (88).

Thieves who steal food and articles of small value should be corrected by being kept on a diet of grains for a week or a fortnight (89).

O Adored of the Devas! the traitor and the ingrate can never attain liberation by sacrifices, votive observances, penances, acts of charity, and other expiatory rites (90).

The King should, after severely punishing them, exile from his dominion men who give false evidence, or who are partial as arbitrators (91).

The testimony of six, four, or even three witnesses is sufficient to prove a fact; but, O Shiva! the testimony of two witnesses of well-known piety is enough (92).

Beloved! if witnesses contradict one another on questions of place, time, and other details of fact, then their testimony should be rejected (93).

O Beloved! the word of the blind and the deaf should be accepted as evidence, and the signs and writing of a dumb man and of one who is both deaf and dumb should also be accepted (94).

Of all evidence and in all cases, and particularly in litigation, documentary evidence is the best, as it does not perish and always endures (95).

The man who fabricates a writing for his own use or for the use of another should be punished with double the punishment of a false witness (96).

The statement on oath, on his own behalf, of a careful and unerring man is of a higher probative value than the word of many witnesses (97).

O Parvvati! as all virtues find their support in Truth, so do all vices find their support in untruth (98).

Therefore, the King shall incur no blame by chastizing those who are devoid of Truth and are the receptacle of all vices. This is the command of Shiva (99).

Devi! if a man says, "I tell the truth," at the same time touching any of the following – a Kaula, the Guru, a Brahmana, water of Ganga, an image of a Devata, a Kula religious Book, Kulamrita, or the offerings made to a Deity, he has taken an oath. If after that he speaks an untruth, then he will go to hell for one Kalpa (100-101).

An oath that an act which is not sinful will be or will not be done, should always be kept by men (102).

The man who has broken his oath should purify himself by a fortnight's fast; and one who has broken it by mistake should live on grains for twelve days (103).

Even the Kula-dharmma, if not followed according to Truth and the injunctions, not only fails to secure final liberation and beatitude, but leads to sin (104).

Wine is Tara Herself in liquid form, is the Saviour of beings, the Mother of enjoyment and liberation, who destroys danger and diseases, burns up the heaps of sins, and purifies the world. O Beloved! She grants all success, and increases knowledge, intellect, and learning, and, O Adya! She is ever worshipped by those who have attained final liberation and those who are desirous of attaining final liberation, by those that have become and those striving to be adepts, and by Kings and Devas for the attainment of their desires (105-107).

Mortals who drink wine with their minds well under control and according to the injunctions (of Shiva) are, as it were, Immortals on earth (108).

By partaking, in accordance to the injunctions, of any of the tattvas, man becomes like unto Shiva. What, then, is the result of partaking of all the five Tattvas? (109).

But the drinking of this Devi Varuni in disregard of the injunctions destroys the intellect (understanding), life, fame, and wealth of men (110).

By the excessive drinking of wine the drunkard destroys the understanding, which is the means for the attainment of the fourfold end of human existence (111).

Only harm at every step, both to himself and to others, comes out of a man whose mind is distracted and who knows not what should and what should not be done (112).

Therefore, the King or the Lord of the Chakra should correct by bodily and pecuniary punishments those who are over-addicted to wine and intoxicating drugs (113).

The understanding of men is clouded by the drinking of wine, whether in small or large quantities, according to the difference in the quality of the wine, to the temperament of the individuals, to the place where and the time when it is taken (114).

Therefore, excessive drinking is to be judged, not from the quantity drunk, but from the result as shown in difficulty of speech and from the unsteadiness of hands, feet, and sight (115).

The King should burn the tongues and confiscate the money of, and inflict corporal punishments on, men who hold not their senses under control, whose minds are distracted by drink, who deviate from the duty they owe to Devas and Gurus, who are fearful to behold, who are the source of all folly, who are sinful, and transgressors of the injunctions of Shiva, and bring ruin on themselves (116-117).

*The King should severely chastise and fine the man who
is unsteady in hands, feet, or in speech, who is bewilde-
red, maddened, and beyond himself with drink (118).*

*The King, who labours for the happiness of his subjects,
should inflict pecuniary punishment on the drunkard
who is guilty of evil language and is devoid of fear and
shame (119).*

*O Kuleshvari! a Kaula, even if he has been initiated
a hundred times, should be regarded as a Pashu, and
expelled from the Kula community (120).*

*The Kaula who drinks excessively of wine, be it conse-
crated or not, should be renounced by all Kaulas and
punished by the King (121).*

*The drunken twice-born man who makes his Brahmi
wife drink wine should purify both himself and his wife
by living on a diet of grains for five days (122).*

*The man who has drunk wine which has not been
sanctified should purify himself by fasting for three days,
and who has eaten meat which has not been sanctified
should fast for two days (123).*

If a man partakes of fish and parched food which have

not been sanctified, he should fast for a day, but who participates in the fifth tattva without conforming to the rites should be corrected by the King's punishment (124).

He who knowingly eats human flesh or beef should purify himself by a fortnight's fast. This is the expiation for this sin (125).

Beloved! a man who has eaten the flesh of animals of human shape, or of carnivorous animals, should purify himself by a three days' fast (126).

The man who partakes of food cooked by Mlechchhas, Chandalas, and Pashus, who are the enemies of the Kula creed, is purified by a fortnight's fast (127).

And, O Kuleshvari! if anyone knowingly partakes of the leavings of these, then he should fast for a month to purify himself, and if he has done so unknowingly he should fast for a fortnight (128).

The injunction is that if a man partakes of food cooked by a man of a caste inferior to his own, he should, to purify himself, fast for three days (129).

By the partaking of food of a Pashu, Chandala, and Mlechchha, which has been placed in the Chakra or in the hands of a Vira, no sin is incurred (130).

One who partakes of forbidden food at a time when food is scarce, in times of famine and danger, or when life is at stake, is guiltless of any transgression (131).

If food is eaten on the back of an elephant, or on a block of stone, or on a piece of wood, which can be carried only by several men, or in places where nothing objectionable is actually perceived, there is no fault (132).

Animals the flesh of which is forbidden, as also diseased animals, should not be killed even for the purpose of sacrifice to the Devas. By killing such animals sin is incurred (133).

If anyone knowingly kills a bull, then he shall do penance (as described below), and if he does so unknowingly he shall do half of such penance. This is the command of Shangkara (134).

So long as the penance is not performed he shall not shave or pare his nails nor wear clean raiments (135).

Shiva! he should fast for a month, and should live on grains for another month, and should live eating food which he has begged during the third month. This is called Krichchhra-Vrata (136).

At the end of the penance he should shave his head and free himself from the sin of wilful killing of the bull by feasting Kaulas, relatives (Agnates), and Bandhavas (137).

If the death of a cow or bull is caused by want of care, the expiation is an eight days' fast for a Brahmana, and for a Kshatriya or inferior castes fasting for six, four, and two days (138).

O Kaulini! the sin of wilfully slaughtering an elephant or a camel, or a buffalo, or a horse is expiated by a three days' fast (139).

Expiation for killing a deer, sheep, goat, or a cat, is a fast for one whole day and a night, and one who has killed a peacock, a parrot, or a gander should abstain fom food till sunset of the day on which the sin is committed (140).

If anyone kills any other inferior animal which possesses bones, he should live on vegetable food for a night. The killing of a boneless animal is expiated by repentance (141).

There is no blame upon Kings who kill beasts, fish, and oviparous creatures when hunting; for hunting, O Devi! is an immemorial practice among Kings (142).

Killing should always be avoided, O Gentle One! except if it be for the purpose of sacrifice to a Deva. The man who kills according to the injunctions sins not (143).

Should a man be unable to complete a religious devotion which he has undertaken, if he walks across the remnants after the worship of any Devata, or if he touches an image of a Deva when he is unclean, then in all such cases he should recite the Gayatri (144).

The father, the mother, and the giver of the Brahman are the Maha-gurus. He who speaks ill of, or towards, them should, in order to purify himself, fast for five days (145).

Similarly, O Beloved! if anyone speaks ill of other persons entitled to respect, Kaulas and Vipras, then he should purify himself by fasting two days and a half (146).

A man may for the acquisition of wealth go to any country, but he should avoid such countries and Shastras as prohibit Kaulika rites (147).

The man who of his own free-will goes to a country where the Kaula-dharmma is prohibited falls from his status, and should be purified by Purnabhisheka (148).

*In expiatory penance, that which is recognized as a
fast is going without food for eight yamas from sunrise
(149).*

*The fast is, however, not broken should one drink a
handful of water or eat the air for the preservation of his
life (150).*

*If one is unable, by reason of old age or disease, to fast,
then, in lieu of each fast, he should feast twelve Brahmanas (151).*

*The sins of speaking ill of others, self-laudation, evil ha-
bits, impropriety in speech or action, should be expiated
by repentance (152).*

*All other sins, whether committed knowingly or unk-
nowingly, are destroyed by repeating the Gayatri of the
Devi and feeding the Kaulas (153).*

*These general rules are applicable to men, women, and
the sexless; the only difference is that in the case of the
women the husband is their Maha-guru (154).*

*Men who are suffering from very great disease and those
who are always ailing become purified and entitled to
perform rites relating to the Devas and the Pitris by
giving away gold (155).*

A house which has been defiled by unnatural death, or which has been struck by lightning, should be purified by one hundred Vyahriti Homas (156).

If the dead body of an animal possessing bones be found in a lake, tank, or well, then it should be at once taken out, and the same should be purified (157).

The method of purifying such places is as follows: Twenty-one jars of pure water should, after being consecrated with Purnabhisheka Mantra, be poured into it (158).

If such places contain but a small quantity of water, and this has been polluted by the stench of the dead body, then they should be dewatered and the loose mud removed therefrom, and when this has been done water should be poured in the manner described (159).

If they contain water of sufficient quantity to drown an elephant, then a hundred jars of water should be removed, and then consecrated water should be poured into them (160).

If not so purified, then the waters of the reservoirs polluted by the touch of the dead body become undrinkable, and the reservoir cannot be consecrated (161).

Bathing in these reservoirs is useless, and any rite performed with their waters becomes fruitless, and any person using the water for any purpose whatever should remain without food for a day and take Panchamrita to purify himself (162).

Should anyone perchance see a wealthy man who begs, a warrior averse to battle, a detractor of the Kula dharmma, a lady of the family who drinks wine, a man who is a traitor, or a learned man addicted to sin, then in any of these cases he should view the Sun, utter the name of Vishnu, and bathe in the clothes which he is wearing at the time (163-164).

Men of the twice-born classes should, if they sell donkeys, fowls, or swine, or if they engage in any low pursuits, purify themselves by observing the three days' vrata (165).

The Tri-dina-vrata, O Ambika! is thus performed: the first day is to be spent in fasting, the second day is to be spent in eating grain meals only, and the third in drinking water only (166).

The man who, without being asked, enters a room the door of which is closed, and one who speaks of things which he has been asked to keep secret, should go without food for five days (167).

*The man who from pride fails to rise when he sees anyo-
ne worthy of veneration coming towards him, or when
he sees the Kula Scriptures being brought in, should go
without food for a day in order to purify himself (168).*

*In this Shastra spoken by Shiva the meanings of the
words used are plain; those who put far-fetched meanings upon them go the downward path (169).*

*I have spoken to thee, O Devi! of that which is the
Essence of essences, of that which is above the most
excellent, of that which conduces to the well-being (of
men) in this world and the next, as also of that which is
both purifying and beneficent and according to Dharmma (170).*

*End of the Eleventh Joyful Message, entitled "The Ac-
count of Expiatory Rites."*

CHAPTER 12

An Account of the Eternal and Immutable Dharmma

SHRI SADASHIVA said:

O Primordial One! I am speaking to Thee again of the everlasting laws; the wise King may easily rule his subjects if he follows them (1).

If Kings did not establish rules, men in their covetousness would quarrel among themselves, even with their friends, relatives, and their superiors (2).

These self-seeking men, O Devi! would for the sake of wealth kill one another, and be full of sin by reason of their maliciousness and desire to thieve (3).

It is therefore for their good that I am laying down the rule in accordance with Dharmma, by following which men will not swerve from the right (path) (4).

As the King should punish the wicked for the removal of their sins, so should he also divide the inheritance according to the relationship (5).

Relationship is of two kinds–by marriage and by birth; of these, relationship by birth is stronger than relationship by marriage (6).

In inheritance, O Shiva! descendants have a stronger claim than ascendants, and in this order of descendants and ascendants the males are better qualified for inheritance than females (7).

But among these, again, the proximate relation is entitled to the inheritance; the wise ones should divide the property according to this rule and in this order (8):

If the deceased leaves son, grandson, daughters, father, wife, and other relations, then the son is entitled to the whole of the inheritance, and not the others (9).

If there are several sons, they are all entitled to equal shares. (In the case of a King) the kingdom goes to the eldest son, but that is in accordance to the custom of the family (10).

If there be any paternal debt which should be paid out of the paternal property, such property should not be divided (11).

If men should divide and take paternal property, then

*the King should take it from them, and discharge the
paternal debt (12).*

*As men go to hell by reason of their own sins, so they are
bound by their individually incurred debts, and others
are not (13).*

*Whatever general property there may be, either im-
movable or of other kinds, sharers shall get the same
according to their respective shares (14).*

*The division is complete on the co-partners agreeing to
it. If they do not agree, then the King should divide it
impartially (15).*

*The King should divide the value or profits of property
which is incapable of division, whether the same be
immovable or movable (16).*

*If a man proves his right to a share after the property is
divided, then the King should divide the property over
again, and give the person entitled his share (17).*

*O Shiva! the King should punish the man who, after
property is once divided by the consent of the co-partners, quarrels again with respect to it (18).*

If the deceased dies leaving behind him grandson, wife, and father, then the grandson is entitled to the property by reason of his being a descendant (19).

If the childless man leaves (surviving him) father, brother, and grandfather, then the father inherits the property by reason of the closeness of consanguinity (20).

Beloved! if the deceased leaves daughters (surviving him), although they are closer to him, yet the grandsons (sons' sons) are entitled to his property, because man is prior (21).

From the grandfather the property goes to the grandson by the deceased son, and thus it is that men proclaim that the father's self is in the image of the son (22).

In marital relationship the Brahmi wife is the superior, and the sonless man's property should go to the wife, who is half his body (23).

The sonless widow, however, is not competent to sell or give away property inherited from her husband, except what is her own by her own right (24).

Anything given by the fathers and fathers-in-law app-

roved by Dharmma, whatever is earned by her personal efforts, is to be recognized as "Woman's property" (25).

On her death it goes to the husband, and to his heirs according to the grades of descendants and ancestors (26).

If the woman remains faithful to her Dharmma, and lives under the control of the relations of her husband, and in their absence under the control of her father's relations, then only is she entitled to inherit (27).

The woman who is even likely to go astray is not entitled to inherit the husband's property. She is merely entitled to a living allowance from the heirs of her husband (28).

If the man who has died has many wives, all of whom are pious, then, O Thou of pure Smiles! they are entitled to the husband's property in equal shares (29).

If the woman who inherits her husband's property dies leaving daughters, then the property is taken to have gone back from the husband and from him to the daughter (30).

In this way, if there is a daughter and the property goes to the son's widow, then, on the death of the latter, it would go back to the husband, and from the father-in-law descend to the daughter of the latter (31).

Similarly, O Shiva! if property goes to the mother in the lifetime of the paternal grandfather, then, on her death, it goes to her father-in-law through her son and husband (32).

As the property of the deceased ascends to the father, so it also ascends to the mother if she is a widow (33).

But the stepmother shall not inherit if the mother is living, but on the death of the mother it goes to the step-mother through the father (34).

Where, in the absence of descendants, the inheritance cannot descend, it would ascend the same way by which it would descend (35).

Therefore, even when the father's brother is alive, the daughter inherits the property, and if she dies childless then such property goes to the father's brother (36).

As inheritance descends in the male line, the stepbrother inherits even when there is a uterine sister (37).

And when there is a uterine sister and sons of step-brother, it is the latter who inherit the property (38).

If the deceased leaves (surviving him) both uterine and

stepbrother, then, by reason of the property descending through the father, they are entitled to inherit in equal shares (39).

In the lifetime of their daughters their sons are not entitled to inherit until the obstruction is removed by the death of the daughters (40).

In the absence of sons, the daughters divide among themselves the paternal property, after deducting the marriage expenses of an unmarried daughter (if any) out of the general estate (41).

On the death of a childless woman the stri-dhana goes to her husband, and the property which she inherited from anyone else goes back to the line of the person from whom she inherited (42).

The woman may spend property inherited by her on her own maintenance, and she may spend profits of it on acts of religious merit, but she is not able to sell or make gifts of it (43).

Where the daughter-in-law of the grandfather (father's father) is living, or the stepmother of the father is living, the inheritance goes to the grandfather, and through his son to the (grandfather's) daughter-in-law (44).

Where the grandfather, the father's brother, and the brother are living, the brother succeeds by reason of the priority in claim of the descendant (45).

If a man dies leaving him surviving his grandfather, brother, and uncle, both of the former are nearer in degree – than the last, and the property descends through the father to the deceased's brother (46).

If the deceased leaves a daughter's son and father (surviving him), then the daughter's son inherits, because property in the first place descends (47).

If both the father and the mother of the deceased be living (at his death), then, O Kalika! by reason of the superior claim of the male, the father takes his property (48).

If the mother's brother is living, the sapindas of the father take the property of the deceased by reason of the superior claim of the paternal relationship (49).

Property failing to go downwards has (here) gone upwards, but, O Shiva! by reason of the superior claim of the male line it has gone to the father's family. The mother's brother, in spite of the nearness of his relationship, does not inherit (50).

The grandson by a deceased son inherits from his grandfather's estate the share which his father would have inherited along with his (the father's) brothers (51).

Similarly, the granddaughter who has no brother and whose parents are dead, inherits, if she be well conducted, her grandfather's (father's father) property with her father's brothers (52).

On the death of the grandfather leaving him surviving his wife, his daughter, and granddaughter, the last, O Devi! is the heiress of the property, since she takes it through her father (53).

In property which descends the male among the descendants, and in property which ascends, the male among the ascendants, are pre-eminently qualified (to inherit) (54).

Therefore, O Beloved! if the deceased has daughter-in-law, granddaughter, and daughter surviving him, then his father cannot take the property (55).

If there is no one in the family of the father of the deceased entitled to inherit his property, then in manner above indicated it goes to the family of his mother's father (56).

Property which has gone to the maternal grandfather shall ascend and descend, and go both to males and females through the maternal uncle and his sons and others (57).

If the line of Brahmi marriage, or if the sapindas of the father or of the mother, be in existence, then the issue of the Shaiva marriage are not entitled to inherit the father's property (58).

The wife and children of the Shaiva marriage, O Gentle One! are entitled to receive, from the person who inherits the property of the deceased, their food and clothes in proportion to the property left (59).Beloved! the Shaiva wife, if well conducted, is entitled to be maintained by the Shaiva husband alone. She has no claim to the property of her father and others (60).

Therefore, the father who marries his well-born daughter according to Shaiva rites by reason of anger or covetousness will be despised of men (61).

In the absence of issue of the Shaiva marriage, the Sodaka, the Guru, and the King shall, by the injunctions of Shiva, take the property of the deceased (62).

Beloved! men within the seventh degree are sapindas,

and beyond them to the seventh degree are sodakas, and beyond them are Gotra-jas merely (63).

Where property which has been divided is again wilfully mixed together, it should be divided again as if it had not been divided (64).

The heirs of a deceased are on his death entitled to such share of property, whether partitioned or not partitioned, as the deceased himself was entitled to (65).

Those who inherit the property of another should offer him pindas as long as they live; it is otherwise in the case–of a son by Shaiva marriage (66).

Just as the rules relating to uncleanliness should, in this world, be observed by reason of birth-connection, so they should be observed for three nights by reason of connection by heirship (67).

The twice-born and other classes shall purify themselves by observing the rules as to uncleanliness from the day they hear the cause of it until the end of the period prescribed; this is so both in the case of Purnashaucha and of Khandashaucha (68).

If the period has expired when one hears the cause of

it, then there is no Khandashaucha. And as regards Purnashaucha, it should be observed for only three days, but if one hears of the cause of the uncleanliness after the lapse of a year there is no period of uncleanliness to be observed (69).

If a son hears of his father's or mother's death, or if the faithful wife hears of her husband's death after one year, then the son or the widow shall observe the period of uncleanliness for three nights (71).

If during the continuance of a period of uncleanliness another new period begins, then the period comes to an end with the end of the Garu-ashaucha (71).

The degree of different kinds of uncleanliness depends on the greater or lesser length of the period which should be observed. Of the various kinds of uncleanliness, that which is extensive in point of time is greater than that which is less extensive (72).

If on the last day of a period of uncleanliness another period commences, then the uncleanliness is removed on the last day of the first period of uncleanliness; but if the cause of uncleanliness be such as to necessitate the observance of the full period, then the pre-existing period should be extended by two days (73).

The unmarried female shall observe the period of uncleanliness of the father's family, but after she is married she is to observe impurity for three days on the death of her parents (74).

After her marriage the wife becomes of the same gotra as her husband; the adopted son similarly becomes of the same gotra as the person who adopts him (75).

A son should be adopted with consent of his father and mother, and at the time of adoption the adopted should, with his kinsmen, perform the sacramental rites, mentioning his own gotra and name (76).

The adopted son shall have the same right to the property of his adoptive mother and father, and the same rights to offer pindas to them as the natural-born son has, since they are his mother and father (77).

A boy of less than five years of age and of one's own caste should be adopted and brought up; a boy of over five years of age is not eligible (78).

O Kalika! if a brother adopts his brother's son, then the brother adopting becomes the father, and the natural father becomes the uncle of the boy so adopted (79).

He who inherits the property of another should observe the Dharmma of the person he inherits; he should also follow his family custom and please his kinsmen (80).

In the case of the death of kaninas, golakas, kundas, and persons guilty of great sins, there is no uncleanliness to be observed, and they are not qualified to inherit (81).

In the case of the death of a man who has been punished by castration, or of a woman who has been punished by the cutting of her nose, or of persons guilty of very great sins, there is no period of uncleanliness to be observed (82).

The King should for twelve years protect the family and property of those of whom no news is known, and who have disappeared without any trace of their whereabouts (83).

On the expiration of twelve years the image of such a person should be made with kusha grass and cremated. His children and others should observe a period of uncleanliness for three days, and liberate him from the condition of a Preta (84).

The King should then divide his property among the members of his family in their order, beginning with the son; otherwise he (the King) incurs sin (85).

The King should protect the man who has no protector, who is powerless, who is in the midst of adversity, because the King is the Lord of his subjects (86).

Kalika! if the man who has disappeared returns after the lapse of twelve years, then he shall recover his wife, children, and property; there is no doubt of that (87).

Even a man is not competent to give away ancestral, immovable property, either to his own people or to strangers, without the consent of his heirs (88).

A man may, at his pleasure, give away self-acquired property, be it movable or immovable, and may also give away ancestral movable property (89).

If there be a son or wife living, or daughter or daughter's son, or father or mother, or brother or sister, even then one may give away self-acquired property, both movable and immovable, and inherited movable property (90-91).

If a man gives away or dedicates such property to any religious object, then his sons and others cannot affect such gift or dedication (92).

Property dedicated to any religious object should be

looked after by the giver. The latter is, however, not competent to take it back, because the ownership of such property is Dharmma (93).

Ambika! the property or the profits thereof should be employed by the dedicator himself, or his agent, for the religious object to which it was dedicated (94).

If the proprietor out of affection gives away half his self-acquired property to anyone, then his heirs shall not be able to annul the gift (95).

If the proprietor gives half his self-acquired wealth to any of his heirs, in such a case the other heirs shall not be able to avoid such gift (96).

If one of several brothers earns money with the help of the paternal property, then, while the other brothers are entitled to proportionate shares of the paternal property, no one but the acquirer is entitled to the profits (97).

If one brother acquires ancestral property which was lost, then he shall receive two shares, and the other brothers shall together receive one share (98).

Religious merit, wealth, and learning are all dependent on the body, and inasmuch as this body comes from the father, then (in such sense) what is there which is not paternal property? (99).

If whatever men earn, even when separate in mess and separate in property, is to be considered paternal property, then what is there that is self-acquired? (100).

Therefore, O Great Devi! whatever money is earned by one's own individual labour shall be self-acquired; the person acquiring it shall be the owner thereof, and no one else (101).

O Devi! the man who even lifts his hand against his mother, father, Guru, paternal and maternal grandfathers, shall not inherit (102).

The man who kills another shall not inherit his property; but the other heirs of the person killed shall inherit his property (103).

Ambika! eunuchs and persons who are crippled are entitled to food and clothes so long as they live, but they are not entitled to inherit property (104).

If a man finds property which belongs to another, on the road or anywhere else, then the King shall, after due deliberation, make the finder restore it to the owner (105).

If a man finds property, or a beast of which there is no owner, then the finder becomes the owner of the same, but should give the King a tenth share of such property or beast (or of the value thereof) (106).

If there be a competent buyer for immovable property, who is a near relation, then it is not competent for the owner of the immovable property to sell the same to another (107).

Among buyers who are near, the agnate and one of the same caste are specially qualified, and in their absence friends, but the desire of the seller should prevail (108).

If immovable property is about to be sold at a price fixed, and a neighbour pays the same price, then the latter is entitled to purchase it and no other (109).

If the neighbour is unable to pay the price and consents to the sale (to another), then only may the householder sell the property to another (110).

O Devi! if immovable property be bought without the knowledge of the neighbour, the latter is entitled to have it upon the condition of his paying the price immediately he hears of such sale (111).

Should, however, the buyer, after purchasing it, have converted the place into a garden, or built a house thereon, or if he has pulled down any building, the neighbour is not entitled in such a case to obtain the immovable property by the payment of its price (112).

A man may, without permission, without payment, and without obstruction, bring under cultivation any land which rises from the water, which is in the middle of a forest, or otherwise difficult of access (113).

Where land has been brought under cultivation by considerable labour, the King, since he is the Lord of the soil, should be given a tenth of the profits of the land, and the rest should be enjoyed by him who has reclaimed it (114).

One should not excavate tanks, reservoirs, or wells, nor plant trees, nor build houses in places where they are likely to injure other people (115).

All have the right to drink the water of tanks and wells dedicated to Devas, as also the water of rivers, but the neighbours alone have the right to bale it out (116).

The water should not be baled out of tanks, etc., even by neighbours, if to do so would cause a water famine (117).

The mortgage and sale of property which is undivided without the consent of the co-sharers, as also when the right of the parties therein is not determined, is invalid (118).

If property mortgaged or deposited with another is destroyed wilfully or by negligence, then the King should make the mortgagee or depositee restore the value thereof to the owner (119).

If any animal or any other thing is used with the consent of the depositor by the person with whom they are placed, then the depositee should bear the expense of food and keep (120).

Where immovable or movable property is made over to another for profit, such transaction will be invalid if it be not for a definite time, or if the amount of profits is indeterminate (121).

Common (joint) property should not, on the father's death, be employed for profit without the consent of all the co-sharers (122).

If articles are sold at improper prices, then the King may set aside such sale (123).

As a body is born and dies only once, and property can be given away only once, so there can be but one Brahma marriage of the daughter (124).

The man, devoted to his ancestors, who has an only son, should not give him away (in adoption), and, similarly, he should not give away an only wife or an only daughter in Shaiva marriage (125).

In rites relating to the Devas and the Pitris, in mercantile transactions, and in Courts of law, whatever the substitute (Agent) does is the act of the employer (126).

The immutable rule is that the Agent or emissary should not be punished for the guilt of the employer (127).

In monetary dealings, in agriculture, in mercantile transactions, as also in all other dealings, whatever is undertaken, the same should be performed if in agreement with Dharmma (128).

The Lord protects this universe. Whoever wish to destroy it will be themselves destroyed, and whosoever protect it them the Lord of the Universe Himself protects. Therefore should one act for the good of the world (129).

End of Twelfth Joyful Message, entitled, "An Account of the Eternal and Immutable Dharmma."

CHAPTER 13

Installation of the Devata

PARVATI, the Mother of the three worlds, Her mind engrossed with thoughts for the purification of men polluted with the impurities of the Kali Age, humbly asked Mahesha, the Deva among Devas, who had thus spoken of the essence of all the Nigamas, which is the seed of heaven and final liberation (as follows) (1):

Shri Devi said:

How should the form of Mahakali be thought of, She who is the Great Cause, the Primordial Energy, the Great Effulgence, more subtle than the subtlest elements? (2).

It is only that which is the work of Prakriti which has form. How should She have form? She is above the most high. It behoves thee, O Deva! to completely remove this doubt of mine (3).

Shri Sadashiva said:

Beloved! I have already said that to meet the needsof the

worshippers the image of the Devi is formed according to Her qualities and actions (4).

As white, yellow, and other colours all disappear in black, in the same way, O Shailaja! all beings enter Kali (5).

Therefore it is that by those who have attained the knowledge of the means of final liberation, the attributeless, formless, and beneficent Kalashakti is endowed with the colour of blackness (6).

As the eternal and inexhaustible One image of Kala and soul of beneficence is nectar itself, therefore the sign of the Moon is placed on her forehead (7). As She surveys the entire universe, which is the product of time, with Her three eyes – the Moon, the Sun, and Fire – therefore she is endowed with three eyes (8).

As She devours all existence, as She chews all things existing with her fierce teeth, therefore a mass of blood is imagined to be the apparel of the Queen of the Devas (at the final dissolution) (9).

As time after time She protects all beings from danger, and as She directs them in the paths of duty, her hands are lifted up to dispel fear and grant blessings (10).

*As She encompasses the universe, which is the product
of Rajoguna, she is spoken of, O Gentle One! as the Devi
who is seated on the red lotus, gazing at Kala drunk
with intoxicating wine and playing with the universe.
The Devi also, whose substance is intelligence, witnesseth all things (11-12).*

*It is for the benefit of such worshippers as are of weak
intelligence that the different shapes are formed according to the attributes (of the Divinity) (13).*

Shri Devi said:

*What merit does the worshipper gain who makes an
image of the Great Devi of mud, stone, wood, or metal,
in accordance with the representation described by Thee
for the salvation of humanity, and who decks the same
with clothes and jewels, and who, in a beautifully decorated house, consecrates it? (14-15).*

*O Lord! out of Thy kindness for me, reveal this also, with
all the particular rules according to which the image of
the Devi should be consecrated (16).*

*Thou hast already spoken of the consecration of Tanks,
Wells, Houses, Gardens, and the images of Devas, but
Thou didst not speak in detail (17).*

I wish to hear the injunctions relating to them from thy lotus-mouth. Out of thy kindness, speak, O Para-meshana! if it pleases Thee (18).

Shri Sadashiva said:

O Parameshvari! this supreme essence about which Thou hast asked is very mysterious. Do thou, therefore, listen attentively (19).

There are two classes of men – those who act with, and without, a view to the fruits of action. The latter attain final liberation. I am now speaking of the former (20).

Beloved! the man who consecrates the image of a Deva goes to the region of such Deva, and enjoys that which is there attainable (21).

He who consecrates an image of mud stays in such region for ten thousand kalpas. He who consecrates an image of wood stays there ten times that period. In the case of the consecration of a stone image the length of stay is ten times the latter period, and in the case of the consecration of a metal image it is ten times the last-mentioned period (22).

Listen to the merit which is acquired by the man who,

in the name of any Deva, or for the attainment of any desire, builds and consecrates and gives away a temple made of timber and thatch and other materials, or renovates such a temple, decorated with flags and images of the carriers of the Deva (23).

He who gives away a thatched temple shall live in the region of the Devas for one thousand koti years (24).

He who gives away a brick-built temple shall live a hundred times that period, and he who gives away a stone-built temple, ten thousand times the last-mentioned period (25).

Adya! the man who builds a bridge or causeway shall not see the region of Yama, but will happily reach the abode of the Suras, and will there have enjoyment in their company (26).

He who dedicates trees and gardens goes to the region of the Devas, and lives in celestial houses surrounded by Kalpa trees in the enjoyment of all desired and agreeable enjoyments (27).

Those who give away ponds and the like for the comfort of all beings are washed of all sins, and, having attained the blissful region of Brahma, reside there a hundred years for each drop of water which they contain (28).

Devi! the man who dedicates the image of a Vahana for the pleasure of any Deva shall live continually in the region of such Deva, protected by Him (29).

Ten times the merit which is acquired on earth by the gift of a Vahana made of mud is acquired by the gift of one made of wood, and ten times the latter is acquired by the gift of one made of stone. Should one made of brass or bell-metal or copper, or any other metal, be given, then the merit is multiplied in each case tenfold (30-31).

The excellent worshipper should present a great lion to the temple of Devi, a bull to the temple of Shangkara, and a Garuda to the temple of Keshava (32).

The geat lion has sharp teeth, a ferocious mouth, and mane on his neck and shoulder. The claws of his four feet are as hard as the thunderbolt (33).

The bull is armed with horns, is white of body, and has four black hoofs, a large hump, black hair at the end of his tail, and a black shoulder (34).

The Garuda is winged, has thighs like a bird, and a face

like a man's, with a long nose. He is seated on his haunches, with folded palms (35).

By the present of flags and flag-staffs the Devas remain pleased for a hundred years. The flag-staff should be thirty-two cubits long (36), and should be strong, without defects, straight, and pleasant to look at. It should be wrapped round with a red cloth, with a chakra at its top (37)

The flag should be attached to the top of the staff, and should be marked with the image of the carrier of the particular Devata. It should be broad at the part nearest the staff and narrow at the other end. It should be made of fine cloth. In short, whatever ornaments the top of the flag-staff is a flag (38).

Whatever a man presents with faith and devotion in the name of a Deva, be it clothes, jewels, beds, carriages, vessels for drinking and eating, pan plates, spittoon, precious stones, pearl, coral, gems, or anything else with which he is pleased, such a man will reach the region of such Deva and receive in turn a Koti times the presents he made (39-40).

Those who worship with the object of attaining a particular reward gain such reward which (however) is as destructible as a kingdom acquired in a dream. Those, however, who rightly act without hope of reward attain nirvana, and are released from rebirth (41).

In ceremonies relating to the dedication of a reservoir of water, a house, a garden, a bridge, a causeway, a Devati, or a tree, the Vastu Spirit should be carefully worshipped (42).

The man who performs any of these ceremonies without worshipping the Vastu-Daitya is troubled by the Vastu-Daitya and his followers (43).

The twelve followers of the Vastu Daitya are Kapi-lasya, Pingakesha, Bhishana, Raktalochana, Kotara-raksha, Lambakarna, Dirghajanggha, Mahodara, Ashvatunda, Kakakantha, Vajravahu, and Vratantaka, and these followers of Vastu should be propitiated with great care (44-45).

Now, listen! I am speaking of the Mandala where the Vastu-Purusha should be worshipped (36).

On an altar or on a level space, which has been well washed with pure water, a straight line should be drawn, one cubit in length, from the Vayu to the Ishana corner.

In the same manner another line should be drawn from the Ishana to the Agni corner, and another from the Agni to the Nairita corner, and then from the Nairita to the Vayu corner (47-48).

By these straight lines a square mandala should be drawn (49). Then two lines should be drawn from corner to corner (diagonally) to divide the mandala into four parts, like four fish-tails (50).

The wise man should then draw two lines, one from the West to the East, and the other from the North to the South, through the point where the diagonal lines cut one another, so as to pass through the tip of the fish-tails (51).

Then four diagonal lines should be drawn connecting the corners of the four inner squares so formed by the lines at each of the corners (52).

According to these rules, sixteen rooms should be drawn with five different colours, and an excellent yantra thus made (53).

In the four middle rooms draw a beautiful lotus with four petals, the pericarp of yellow and red colour, and the filaments of red (54).

*The petals may be white or yellow, and the interstices
may be coloured with any colour chosen (55).*

*Beginning with the corner of Shambhu, the twelve
rooms should be filled up with the four colours – viz.,
white, black, yellow, and red (56).*

*In filling up the rooms one should go towards one's right,
and in the worship of the Devas therein one should go to
the left (57).*

*The Vastu Spirit should be worshipped in the lotus,
and the twelve daityas, Kapilasya and others, should
be worshipped in the twelve rooms, beginning with the
Ishana corner (58).*

*Fire should be consecrated according to the injunctions
laid down for Kushandika, and after offer of oblations
to the best of one's ability, the Vastu-yajna should be
concluded (59).*

*I have thus described, O Devi! the auspicious Vastu
worship, by the performance of which a man never suf-
fers dangers from Vastu (and his followers) (60).*

Shri Devi said:

Thou hast described the mandala of, and the injunctions relating to, the worship of Vastu, but thou hast not spoken of the Dhyana, my husband; do thou now reveal it (61).

Shri Sadashiva said:

I am speaking of Dhyana of the Vastu-Rakshasa, by constant and devoted repetition of which all dangers are destroyed. O Maheshani! do thou listen (62).

The Deva Vastu-pati should be meditated upon as four-armed, of great body, his head covered with matted hair, three eyed, of ferocious aspect, decked with garlands and earrings, with big belly and long ears and hairy body, wearing yellow garments, holding in his hand the mace, the trident, the axe, and the Khatvanga. Let him be pictured as (red) like the rising Sun and like the God of Death to one's enemies, seated in the padmasana posture on the back of a tortoise, surrounded by Kapilasya and other powerful followers, carrying swords and shields (63-66).

Whenever there is panic caused by pestilence or epidemics, an apprehension of any public calamity, danger to one's children, or fear arising from ferocious beasts or Rakshasas, then Vastu with his followers should be meditated upon as above, and then worshipped, and thus all manner of peace may be obtained by the offer of oblations of sesamum-seeds, ghee, and payasa (67-68).

O Suvrata! in these rites the Grahas and the ten Dikpalas should be worshipped in the same way as Vastu is worshipped (69).

Brahma, Vishnu, Rudra, Vani, Lakshmi, the celestial mothers, Ganesha, and the Vasus, should also be worshipped (70).

O Kalika! if in these rites the Pitris are not satisfied, then all which is done becomes fruitless, and there is danger in every stage (71).

Therefore, O Maheshi! in all these rites Abhyudayika. Shraddha should be performed for the satisfaction of the Pitris (72).

I shall now speak of the Graha-yantra, which is the cause of all kinds of peace. If Indra and all the planets are worshipped, then they grant every desire (73).

In order to draw the yantra three triangles should be drawn with a circle outside them, and outside, but touching the circle, eight petals should be drawn (74).

Then should a beautiful Bhupura be drawn (outside the yantra) with four entrances, and (outside the Bhupura) between the East and North-East corners a circle should be drawn with its diameter the length of a pradesha, and between the West and the South-West corners another similar circle should be drawn (75-76).

Then the nine corners should be filled up with colours of the nine planets, and the left and right sides of the two inner triangles should be made white and yellow, and the base should be black. The eight petals should be filled up with the colours of the eight regents of the quarters (77-78).

The walls of the Bhupura should be decorated with white, red, and black powders, and, O Devi! the two circles outside the Bhupura should be coloured red and white, and the intervening spaces of the yantra may be coloured in any manner the wise may choose (79-80).

Listen now to the order in which each planet should be worshipped in the particular chambers, and in which each Dikpati should be worshipped in the particular petals, and as to the names of the Devas who are present at each particular entrance (81).

In the inner triangle the Sun should be worshipped, and

in the angles of the two sides Aruna and Shikha. Behind him with the garland of rays the two standards of the two fierce ones (Shikha and Aruna) should be worshipped (82).

Worship the maker of nights in the corner above the Sun on the East, in the Agni corner Mangala, on the South side Budha, in the Nairrita corner Vrihaspati, on the West Shukra, in the Vayu corner Shani, in the corner on the North Rahu, and in the Ishana corner Ketu, and, lastly, round about the Moon the multitude of stars (83-84). Sun is red, Moon is white, Mangala is tawny, Budha is pale or yellowish-white, Vrihaspati is yellow, Shukra is white, Shani is black, and Rahu and Ketu are of variegated colour; thus I have spoken of the different colours of the Grahas (85-86).

The Sun should be meditated upon as having four hands, in two of which he is holding lotuses; and of the other two, one hand is lifted up to dispel fear, and the other makes the sign of blessing. The Moon should be meditated upon as having nectar in one hand, and the other hand in the attitude of giving. Mangala should be meditated upon as slightly bent and holding a staff in his hands. Budha, the son of Moon, should be meditated upon as a boy, the locks of whose hair play about upon his forehead. Guru should be meditated upon with a sacred thread, and holding a book in one hand and a string of Rudraksha beads in the other; and the Guru of Daityas should be meditated upon as blind of one eye, and Shani as lame, and Rahu as a trunkless head, and Ketu as a headless trunk, both deformed and wicked (86-87).

Having worshipped each of the planets in this manner, the eight Dikpalas, Indra and others, beginning from the East, should be worshipped (89).

He of a thousand eyes, of a yellow colour, should first be worshipped. He is dressed in yellow silk garments, and, holding the thunder in his hand, is seated on Airavata (90).

The body of Agni is of red hue. He is seated on a goat; in his hand is the Shakti. Yama is black, and, holding a staff in his hand, is seated on a bison. Nirriti is of dark green colour, and, holding a sword in his hand, is seated on a horse. Varuna is white, and, seated on an alligator, holds a noose in his hand. Vayu should be meditated on as possessed of a black radiance, seated on a deer and holding a hook. Kuvera is of the colour of gold, and, seated on a jewelled lion-seat, holding the noose and hook in his hands. He is surrounded by Yakshas, who are singing his praises. Ishana is seated on the bull; he holds the trident in one hand, and with the other bestows blessings, He is dressed in raiments of tiger-skin, and his effulgence is like that of the full moon (91-95).

Having thus meditated upon and worshipped them in their order, Brahma should be worshipped in the upper circle, which is outside the mandala, and Vishnu in the lower one. Then the Devatas at the entrances should be worshipped (96).

Ugra, Bhima, Prachanda, and Isha, are at the eastern entrance; Jayanta, Kshetra-pala, Nakulesha, and Vrihat-shirah, are at the southern entrance; at the door on the west are Vrika, Ashva, Ananda, and Durjaya; and Trishirah, Purajit, Bhimanada, and Mahodara are at the northern entrance. As protectors of the entrances, they are all armed with weapons, offensive and defensive (97-98).

Suvrata! listen to the meditation on Brahma and Ananta. Brahma is of the colour of the red lotus, and has four hands and four faces. He is seated on a swan. With two of his hands he makes the signs which dispel fear and grant boons, and in the others he holds a garland and a book. Ananta is white as the snow, the Kunda flower, or the Moon. He has a thousand hands and a thousand faces, and he should be meditated upon by Suras and Asuras (99-101).

Beloved! I have now spoken of the meditation, the mode of worship, and the yantra. Now, my beloved, listen to their Mantras in their order, beginning with the Vastu Mantra (102).

Mantras

When Ksha-kara is placed on the Carrier of Oblations. and the long vowels are then added to it, and ornamented with the nada-vindu, the six-lettered Vastu Mantra is formed (103).

The Suryya Mantra is thus formed: first the tara should be said; then the Maya; then the word tigma-rashme; then the word arogya-daya (in the dative singular); and, last of all, the wife of Fire (104).

The recognized or approved Mantra of Soma is formed by saying the vijas of Kama, Maya and Vani, then Amrita-kara, amritam plavaya plavaya svaha (105).

The Mantra of Mangala is proclaimed to be Aing hrang hring sarva-dushtan nashaya nashaya svaha (106).

The Mantra of the son of Soma is Hrang, Shring, Saumya sarvan kaman puraya svaha(107).

The Mantra of the Sura-Guru is formed thus: Let the tara precede and follow the Vija of Vani, and then say, Abhishtam yachchha yachchha, and lastly svaha (108).

The Mantra of Shukra is Shang, Shing, Shung, Shaing, Shaung, Shngah (109).

The Mantra of the Slowly Moving One is Hrang hrang hring hring sarva-shatrun vidravaya vidravaya Mar-tan-dasunave namah – Destroy, destroy all enemies – I bow to the son of Martanda (110).

The Mantra of Rahu is Rang, Hraung, Bhraung, Hring – Soma-shatro shatrun vidhvangsaya vidhvangsaya Rahave namah--O Enemy of Soma (Moon)! destroy, destroy all enemies. I bow to Rahu (111).

Krung, Hrung, Kraing to Ketu – is proclaimed to be the Mantra of Ketu (112).

Lang, Rang, Mring, Strung, Vang, Yang, Kshang, Haung, Vring, and Ang are in their order the ten Mantras of the ten Dikpalas, beginning with Indra and ending with Ananta (113).

The names of the other attendant Devas are their Mant-ras; in all instances where there is no Mantra mentioned this is the rule. (114).

Sovereign Mistress of the Devas! the wise man should not add Namah to Mantras that end with the word Namah, nor should he put the wife of Vahni to a Mantra that ends with Svaha (115).

To the Planets and others should be given flowers, clothes, and jewels, but the colour of the gifts should be the same as that of the respective Planets; otherwise they are not pleased (116).

The wise man should place fire in the manner prescribed for Kushandika, and perform homa either with flowers of variegated colours or with sacred fuel (117).

In rites for the attainment of peace or good fortune, or nourishment or prosperity, the Carrier of Oblations is called Varada; in rites relating to consecration he is called Lohitaksha; in destructive rites he is called Shatruha (118).

Maheshani! in Shanti, Pushti, and Krura rites the man who sacrifices to the Planets will obtain the desired end (119).

As in the rites relating to the consecration the Devas should be worshipped and libations offered to the Pitris, so also should there be the same sacrifices to Vastu and the Planets (120).

Should one have to perform two or three consecratory and sacrificial rites on the same day, then the worship of the Devas, the Shraddha of the Pitris, and consecration of fire are required once only (121).

One who desires the fruit of his observances should not give to any Deva reservoirs of water, houses, gardens, bridges, causeways, carriers, conveyances, clothes, jewels, drinking-cups, and eating-plates, or whatever else he may desire to give, without first sanctifying the same (122-123).

In all rites performed with an ultimate object the wise one should in all cases perform a sangkalpa, in accordance with directions, for the full attainment of the good object (124).

Complete merit is earned when the thing about to be given is first sanctified, worshipped, and mentioned by name, and then the name of him to whom it is given is pronounced (125).

I will now tell you the Mantras for the consecration of reservoirs of water, houses, gardens, bridges, and cau-se-ways. The Mantras should always be preceded by the Brahma-Vidya (126).

Mantras

*Reservoir of Water! thou that givest life to all beings!
thou that art presided over by Varuna! may this consecration of thee (by me) give satisfaction to all beings that
live and move in water, on land, and in air (127).*

*House made of timber and grass! thou art the favourite
of Brahma; I am consecrating thee with water; do thou
be always the cause of pleasure (128).*

*When consecrating a house made of bricks and other
materials, one should say: "House made of bricks," etc.
(129).*

Mantras

*Garden! thou art pleasant by reason of thy fruits, leaves,
and branches, and by thy shadows. I am sprinkling thee
with the sacred water (of sacred places); grant me all my
wishes (130).*

*Bridge! thou art like the bridge across the Ocean of
Existence, thou art welcome to the wayfarer; do thou,
being consecrated by me, grant me the fitting reward
thereof (131).*

Causeway! I am consecrating thee, as thou helpest people in going from one place to another: do thou likewise help me in my way to Heaven (132).

The wise ones shall use the same Mantra in consecrating a tree as is prescribed for the sprinkling of a garden (133).

In consecrating all other things, the Pranava, Varuna, and Astra should be used (134).

Those vahanas that can (or ought to be) bathed should be bathed with the Brahma-gayatri; others should be purified by arghya-water taken up with the ends of kusha grass (135).

After performing prana-pratishtha, calling it by its name, the vahana called by its name should be duly worshipped, and when decked out should be given to the Devata (136).

Whilst consecrating a reservoir, Varuna, the lord of aquatic animals, should be worshipped. In the case of a house, Brahma, the lord of all things born, should there be worshipped. Whilst consecrating a garden, a bridge a causeway, Vishnu, who is the protector of the universe, the soul of all, who witnesseth all and is omnipresent, should be worshipped (137).

Shri Devi said:

Thou hast spoken of the different injunctions relating to the different rites, but thou hast not yet shown the order in which man should practise them (138).

Rites not properly performed according to the order enjoined do not, even though performed with labour, yield the full benefit to men who follow the life of Karmma (139).

Shri Sadashiva said:

O Parameshani! thou art beneficent like a mother. What thou hast said is indeed the best for men whose minds are occupied with the results (of their efforts) (140).

The practices relating to the aforementioned rites are different. Devi! I am relating them in their order, beginning with the Vastu-yaga. Do thou listen attentively (141).

(He who wishes to perform the Vastu-yaga) should the day previous thereto live on a regulated or a restricted diet. After bathing in the early auspicious hour of morning, and performing the ordinary daily religious duties, he should worship the Guru and Narayana (142).

The worshipper should then, after making sangkalpa, worship Ganesha and others for the attainment of his own object, according to the rules shown in the ordinances (143).

Dhyanam

Worship Ganapati who is of the colour of the Bandhuka flower, and has three eyes; whose head is that of the best of elephants; whose sacred thread is made of the King of Snakes; who is holding in his four lotus hands the conch, the discus, the sword, and a spotless lotus; on whose forehead is the rising young moon; the shining effulgence of whose body and raiments is like that of the Sun; who is decked with various jewels, and is seated on a red lotus (144).

Having thus meditated upon and worshipped Ganesha to the best of his ability, he should worship Brahma, Vani, Vishnu, and Lakshmi (145).

Then, after worshipping Shiva, Durga, the Grahas, the sixteen mothers, and the Vasus in the Vasudhara, he should perform the Vriddhishraddha (146).

Then the mandala of the Vastu-daitya should be drawn, and there the Vastu-daitya with his followers should be worshipped (147).

Then there make a sthandila and purifying fire as before; first perform Dhara-homa, and then commence Vastu-homa (148).

Oblations should be offered to the Vastu-purusha and all his followers according to the best of one's ability. The sacrifice should be brought to a close by the gift of oblations to the Devas worshipped (149).

When Vastu-yajna is separately performed, this is the order which is prescribed, and in this order also the sacrifice to the planets should be performed (150).

Moreover, the Planets being the principal objects of worship, they should not be subordinately worshipped. The Vastu should be worshipped immediately after the sangkalpa (151).

Ganesha and the other Devas should be worshipped as in Vastu-yaga. I have already spoken to you of the Yantra and Mantra and Dhyana of the Planets (152).

I have, O Gentle One! during my discourse with thee spoken of the order to be observed in the yajnas of the planets and of Vastu. I shall now speak to thee of the various praiseworthy acts, beginning with the consecration of wells (153).

After making sangkalpa in the proper manner, Vastu should be worshipped either in a mandala, or a jar, or a Shilagrama, according to inclination (154).

Then Ganapati should be worshipped, as also Brahma and Vani, Hari, Rama, Shiva, Durga, the Planets, the Dikpatis (155).

Then the Matrikas and the eight Vasus having been worshipped, Pitrikriya should be performed. Since Varuna is principal Deva (for the purposes of this ceremony), he should then be worshipped with particular care (156).

Having worshipped Varuna with various presents to the best of his ability, Varuna Homa should then be performed in Fire duly consecrated (157). And after offering oblations to each of the Devas worshipped, he should bring the Homa rite to an end by giving the Purnahuti (158).

Then he should sprinkle the excellent well, decorated with flagstaffs and flags, garlands, scents, and vermilion, with the Prokshana Mantra, spoken of before (159).

Then he should, in the name of the Deva, or for the attainment of the object of his desire, give away the well or tank for the benefit of all beings (160).

Then the most excellent worshipper should make supplication with folded palms as follows:

"Be well pleased, all beings, whether living in the air or on earth or in water; I have given this excellent water to all beings; may all beings be satisfied by bathing in, drinking from, or plunging into this water; I have given this common water to all beings. Should anyone by his ownmisfortune be endangered in this, may I not be guilty of that sin, may my work (good work) bear fruit!" (161-163).

Then presents should be made, and Shanti and other rites performed, and thereafter Brahmanas, Kaulas, and the hungry poor should be fed. Shive! this is the order to be observed in the consecration of all kinds of reservoirs of water (164-165).

In the consecration of a Tadaga and other kinds of reservoirs of water there should be a Nagastambha and some aquatic animals (166).

Aquatic animals, such as fish, frogs, alligators, and tortoises, should be made of metal, according to the means of the person consecrating (167). There should be made two fish and two frogs of gold, two alligators of silver, and two tortoises, one of copper and another of brass (168).

After giving away the Tadaga or Dirghika or Sagara with these aquatic animals, Naga should, after having been supplicated, be worshipped (169).

Ananta, Vasuki, Padma, Mahapadma, Takshaka, Kulira, Karkata, and Shankha – all these are the protectors of water (170).

These eight names of the Nagas should be written on Ashvattha leaves, and, after making japa of the Pranava and the Gayatri, the leaf should be thrown into a jar (171).

Calling upon Sun and Moon to witness, the leaves should be mixed up together, and one-half should be drawn therefrom, and the Naga whose name is drawn should be made the protector of water (172).

Then a wooden pillar, auspicious and straight, should be brought and smeared with oil and turmeric, and bathed in consecrated water, to the accompaniment of the Vyahriti and the Pranava, and then the Naga who has been made the protector of the water should be worshipped with the Shaktis Hri, Shri, Kshama, and Shanti (173-174).

Mantra

O Naga! Thou art the couch of Vishnu, Thou art the adornment of Shiva; do Thou inhabit this pillar and protect my water (175).

Having thus made supplication to Naga, the pillar should be set in the middle of the reservoir, and the dedicator should then go round the Tadaga, keeping it on his right (176).

If the pillar has been already fixed, then the Naga should be worshipped in a jar, and, throwing the water of the jar into the reservoir, the remainder of the rites should be performed (177).

Similarly, the wise man who has taken a vow to consecrate a house should perform the rites, beginning with the worship of Vastu, and ending with that of the Vasus, and perform the rites relating to the Pitris as prescribed for the consecration of a well, and the excellent devotee should worship Prajapati and do Prajapatya homa (178-179).

The house should be sprinkled with the Mantra already mentioned, and then worshipped with incense, etc.; after that, with his face to the Ishana corner, he should pray as follows (180):

Mantra

"O Room (or House)! Prajapati is thy Lord; decked with flowers and garlands and other decorations, be thou always pleasant for our happy residence." (181).

He should then offer presents, and, performing Shanti rites, accept blessings. Thereafter he should feed Vipras, Kulinas, and the poor to the best of his ability (182).

O Daughter of the Mountain! if the house is being consecrated for someone else, then in the place "our residence" should be said "their residence"; and now listen to the ordinances relating to the consecration of a house (or room) for a Deva (183).

After consecrating the house in the above manner, the Deva should be approached with the blowing of conch-shells and the sound of other musical instruments, and he should be supplicated thus (184):

Mantra

Rise, O Lord of the Deva among Devas! thou that grantest the desires of thy votaries! come and make my life blessed, O Ocean of Mercy! (185).

Having thus invited (the Deva) into the room, he should be placed at the door, and the Vahana should be placed in front of Him (186).

Then on the top of the house a trident or a discus should be placed, and in the Ishana corner a staff should be set with a flag flying from it (187).

Let the wise man then decorate the room with awnings, small bells, garlands of flowers, and mango-leaves, and then cover the house up with celestial cloth (188).

The Deva should be placed with his face to the North, and in the manner to be described he should be bathed with the things prescribed. I now am speaking of their order; do thou listen (189).

After saying Aing, Hring, Shring, the Mula Mantra should be repeated, and then let the worshipper say:

Mantra

I am bathing thee with milk; do thou cherish me like a mother (190).

Repeating the three Vijas and the Mula Mantra aforesaid, let him then say:

Mantra

I am bathing thee to-day with curds; do thou remove the heat of this mundane existence (191).

Repeating again the three Vijas and the Mula Mantra, let him say:

Mantra

O Giver of Joy to all! being bathed in honey, do Thou make me joyful (192).

Repeating the Mula Mantra as before, and inwardly reciting the Pranava and the Savitri, he should say:

Mantra

I am bathing Thee in ghee, which is dear to the Devas, which is longevity, seed, and courage; do Thou, O Lord! keep me free from disease (193).

Again repeating the Mula Mantra, as also the Vyahriti and the Gayatri, let him say:

Mantra

O Devesha ! bathed by me in sugar water, do Thou grant me (the object of) my desire (194).

Repeating the Mula Mantra, the Gayatri, and the Varuna Mantra, he should say:

Mantra

I am bathing thee with cocoanut-water, which is the creation of the Vidhi, which is divine, which is welcome to Devas, and is cooling, and which is not of the world; I bow to thee (195).

Then, with the Gayatri and the Mula Mantra, the Deva should be bathed with the juice of sugar-cane (196).

Repeating the Kama Vija and the Tara, the Savitri, and the Mula Mantra, he should, whilst bathing the Deva, say:

Mantra

Be thou well bathed in water scented with camphor, fragrant aloe, saffron, musk, and sandal; be thou pleased to grant me enjoyment and salvation (197).

After bathing the Lord of the World in this manner with

eight jarfuls (of water, etc.), He should be brought inside the room and placed on His seat (198).

If the image be one which cannot be bathed, then the Yantra, or Mantra, or the Shalagrama-shila, should be bathed and worshipped (199).

If one be not able to bathe (the Deva) in manner above, then he should bathe (Him) with eight, seven, or five jars of pure water (200).

The size and proportions of the jar has been already given whilst speaking of Chakra worship. In all rites prescribed in the Agmas that is the jar which is appropriate (201).

Then the Great Deva should be worshipped according to the injunctions to be followed in His worship. I shall speak of the offerings. Do thou, O Supreme Devi! Listen (202).

A seat, welcome, water to wash the feet, offerings, water for rinsing the mouth, Madhuparka, water for sipping, bathing water, clothes and jewels, scents and flowers, lights and incense-sticks, edibles and words of praise, are the sixteen offerings requisite in the worship of the Devas (203-204).

*Padya, Arghya, Achamana, Madhuparka, Achamya,
Gandha, Pushpa, Dhupa, Dipa, Naivedya – these are
known as Dashopachara (ten requisite offerings) (205).*

*Gandha, Pushpa, Dhupa, Dipa, and Naivedya, are
spoken of as the Panchopachara (five offerings) in the
worship of a Deva (206).*

*The articles should be sprinkled with water taken from
the offering with the Weapon Mantra, and be worshipped with scents and flowers, the names of separate
articles being mentioned. (207)*

*Mentally repeating the Mantra that is about to be said,
as also the Mula Mantra, and the name of the Deva
in the dative case, the words of gift should be repeated
(208).*

*I have told you of the way in which the things to be gi-
ven to the Devas should be dedicated. The learned man
should in this manner give away an article to a Deva
(209).*

*I have shown (whilst describing) the mode of worship
of the Adya Devi how Padya, Arghya, etc., should be
offered, and how Karana should be given (210).*

To such of the Mantras as were not spoken then, do thou, O Beloved ! listen to them here; these should be said when Asana and other requisites are offered (211).

Mantra

(O Deva!) Thou who residest within all beings! who art the innermost of all beings! I am offering this seat for Thee to sit. I bow to Thee again and again (212).

O Deveshi! after giving the excellent asana in this way, the giver of the asana sbould with folded arms bid him welcome as follows (213):

Mantra

(O Deva!) Thou art He whom even the Devas seek for the accomplishment of their objects, yet for me Thy auspicious visit has easily been obtained. I bow to Thee, O Supreme Lord! (214).

My life's aim is accomplished to-day; all my efforts are crowned with success; I have obtained the fruits of my tapas – all this by Thy auspicious coming (215).

Ambika! the Deva should thus be invited, prayed to, and questioned as to His auspicious coming, and then, *taking padya, the following Mantra should be repeated (216):*

Mantra

By the mere touch of the washings of Thy feet the three worlds are purified; I am offering Thee padya for washing Thy lotus feet (217). He by whose grace is attained all manner of supreme bliss, to Him who is the Soul of all beings I offer this Anandarghya (218).

Then pure water which has been scented with nutmeg, cloves, and kakkola, should be poured out, and taken and offered with the following (219):

Mantra

(O Lord!) By the mere touch of that which Thou hast touched the whole of this impure world is purified; for washing that lotus mouth I offer thee this achamaniya (220).

Then, taking madhuparka, offer it with devotion and with the following (221):

Mantra

For the destruction of the three afflictions, for the attainment of uninterrupted bliss, I give Thee to-day, O Parameshvara! this madhuparka; be Thou propitious (222).

By the mere touch of anything which has touched Thy mouth things impure become pure: this punaracha-ma-niyam is for the lotus mouth of Thine (223).

Taking water for the bath, and pouring it and consecrating it as before, it should be placed before the Deva, and the following Mantra should be repeated (224):

Mantra

To Thee whose splendour envelops the world, from whom the world was born, who is the support of the world, do I offer this water for Thy bath (225).

When offering bathing water, clothes, and edibles, achamaniya should be given as each is offered, and, after offering other articles, water should be given only once (226).

Bringing the cloth consecrated as aforementioned, holding it up with both hands, the wise man should repeat the following (227):

Mantra

Without any raiments as Thou art, Thou hast kept Thy splendour or glory concealed by Thy maya. To Thee I offer these two pieces of cloth. I bow to Thee (228).

Taking different kinds of ornaments made of gold and silver and other materials, and sprinkling and consecrating them, he should offer them to the Deva, uttering the following (229):

Mantra

To Thee who art the ornament of the Universe, who art the one cause of the beauty of the universe, I offer these jewels for the adornment of Thy illusion-image (230).

Mantra

To Thee who by the subtle element of smell hast created the earth which possesses all scents, to Thee, the Supreme Soul, I offer this excellent scent (231).

Mantra

By me have been dedicated with devotion beautiful flowers, and charming and sweet scents prepared by

Devas: do Thou accept this flower (232).

Mantra

This incense-stick is the sap of the trees; it is Divine, and possesses a delicious scent, and is charming, and is fit to be inhaled by all beings. I give it to Thee to smell (233).

Mantra

Do Thou accept this light which illumines and has a strong flame, which removes all darkness, and which is brightness itself, and makes bright that which is around it (234).

Mantra

This offering of food is of delicious taste, and consists of various kinds of edibles. I offer it to Thee in a devout spirit; do Thou partake of it (235).

Mantra

O Deva! this clear drinking-water, perfumed with camphor and other scents which satisfies all, I offer to Thee – Salutation to Thee (236).

*The worshipper should then offer pan made with camp-
hor, catechu, cloves, cardamums, and, after offering
achamaniya, bow to Him (237).*

*If the offerings are presented along with the vessels in
which they are contained, then the names and description of the offerings may jointly be repeated when
making the present, or the names (or description) of the
vessels may separately be said and the same given (238).*

*Having worshipped the Deva in this manner, three
double handfuls of flowers should be given to the Deva.
Then, sprinkling the temple and its awnings with water,
the following Mantra should be said with folded palms
(239):*

Mantra

*Temple! thou art adorable of all men; thou grantest vir-
tue and fame. In affording a resting-place to this Deva,
do thou be like unto Sumeru (240). Thou art Kailasa,
thou art Vaikuntha, thou art the place of Brahma, since
thou art holding the Deva, who is the adored of the
Devas within thee (241).*

*Since thou holdest within thyself the image of Him
whose body is produced by Maya, and within whose*

belly exists this universe, with all that is movable and immovable therein (242). Thou art the equal of the Mother of the Devas; all the holy places are in thee; do thou grant all my desires, and do thou bring me peace. I bow to thee (243).

Having thus praised the temple decorated with the discus, flag, etc., and worshipped it three times, the worshipper should give it to the Deva, mentioning the object of his desire (444).

Mantra

To Thee, whose abode is the universe for Thy residence, I dedicate this temple.O Maheshana! do Thou accept it and in Thy mercy abide here (245).

Having said this and having made presents, the Deva to whom the temple has been dedicated should be placed on the altar to the accompaniment of the music of conches, horns, and other instruments (246).

He should then touch the two feet of the Deva and utter the Mula Mantra, and say, Sthang! Sthing! be Thou steady; this temple is made by me for Thee, and, having fixed the Deva there, he should pray again to the temple thus (247):

Mantra

Temple! be thou always in every way pleasant for the residence of the Deva; thou hast been dedicated by me; may the Lokas be lasting and without danger for me (248).

Help my fourteen generations of ancestors, my fourteen generations of successors, and me and the rest of my family to find places to reside in the abode of the Devas (249).

May I, by thy grace, attain the fruits attainable by performing all forms of yajnas, by visiting all the places of pilgrimage (250).

May my line continue so long as this world, so long as these mountains, so long as the Sun and Moon endure (251).

The wise man, after having thus addressed the temple and worshipped the Deva, should dedicate mirrors and other articles and the flag to Him (252).

Then the Vahana appropriate to the Deity should be given. To Shiva should be given a bull. Then pray to Him thus (253):

Mantra

O Bull! thou art large of body, thy horns are sharp, thou killest all enemies, thou art worshipped even by the Tridashas, as thou carriest on thy back the Lord of the Devas (254).

In thy hoofs are all the holy shrines, in thy hair are all the Vedic Mantras, in the tip of thy teeth are all the Nigamas, Agamas, and Tantras (255).

May the husband of Parvati, pleased with this gift of thee, give me a place in Kailasa, and do thou protect me always (256).

O Maheshani! do Thou listen to the manner of prayer upon giving a lion to Mahadevi or a Garuda to Vishnu (257).

Mantra

Thou didst display thy great strength in the wars between the Suras and the Asuras; thou didst give victory to the Devas, and didst destroy the Demons. Thou formidable one, thou art the favourite of the Devi, thou the favourite of Brahma, Vishnu, and Shiva; with devotion I am dedicating thee to the Devi; do thou destroy my enemies. I bow to thee (258-259).

O Garuda! most excellent bird! Thou art the favoured one of the husband of Lakshmi; Thy beak is hard like adamant; Thy talons are sharp, and golder are Thy wings. I bow to Thee, O Indra among birds! I bow to Thee, O King of birds! (260).

As Thou abidest near Vishnu with folded palms, do Thou, O Destroyer of the pride of enemies! help me to be there as Thou art (261). When Thou art pleased, the Lord of the Universe is pleased, and grants success (262).

When a gift is made to any Deva, an additional present should be made to the Deva for His acceptance of such gifts, and the merit of such rites should also be given to Him in a spirit of devotion (263).

He should then, with dancing, singing, and music, go round the temple, accompanied by his friends and kinsmen, keeping the temple on his right, and, having bowed to the Deva, feed the twice-born! (264).

This is the way in which a temple to a Deva should be dedicated, and the same rule is to be observed in the dedication of a garden, a bridge, a causeway, or a tree (265).

With this difference only: that in these rites the ever-ex-

*isting Vishnu should be worshipped; but Puja and
Homa, etc., are the same as in the case of the dedication
of a temple (266).*

*No temple or other thing should be dedicated to a Deva
whose image has not been consecrated. The rules laid
down above are for the worship of and dedication to a
Deva who has been worshipped and consecrated (267).*

*I shall now speak of the manner in which the auspicious
Adya should be installed, and by which the Devi grants
quickly all desires (268).*

*On the morning of the day (of Pratishtha) the worship-
per should, after bathing and purifying himself, sit
facing the North, and, having taken Sangkalpa, worship
the Vastu-devata (269).*

*After performing the worship of the planets, the Pro-
tectors of the Quarters, Ganesha and others, and having
performed the Shraddha of his Pitris, he should approach the image with a number of devout Vipras (270).*

*The excellent worshipper should then bring the image to
the temple which has been dedicated, or to some other
place, and there duly bathe it (271).*

It should first be bathed with water, then with sandy earth, then with mud thrown up by the tusk of the boar or elephant, then with mud taken from the door of a Veshya, and then with mud from the lake of Pradyumna (272).

The wise man should then bathe the image with Pan-cha-kashaya and Pancha-pushpa, and three leaves, and then with scented oil (273).

The decoctions of Vatyala, Vadari, Jambu, Vakula, and Shalmali, are called the five Kashayas for bathing the Devi (274).

Karavira, Jati, Champaka, Lotus, and Patali, are the five flowers (275).

By three leaves are meant the leaves of Varvvara, Tulasi, and Vilva (276).

With the above-mentioned articles water should be mixed, but no water should be put into scented oil and the five nectars (277).

He should, after repeating the Vyahriti, the Pranava, the Gayatri, and the Mula Mantra, say, "I bathe thee with the water of these articles" (278).

The wise man should then bathe the image with the eight jars filled with milk and other ingredients in manners aforementioned (279).

The image should then be rubbed with powdered white wheat or sesamum cakes, or powdered shali rice, and thus cleansed (280).

After bathing the image with eight jars of holy water, and rubbing it with cloth of fine texture, it should bc brought to the place of worship (281).

Should one be unable to perform all these rites, then he should in a devout spirit bathe the image with twenty-five jars of pure water (282).

On each occasion that the Great Devi is bathed she should, to the best of one's ability, be worshipped (283).

Then, placing the image on a well-cleaned seat, She should be worshipped by offering padya, arghya, etc., and then prayed to (as follows) (284):

Mantra

O Image! thou that art the handicraft of Vishvakarmma, I bow to thee; thou art the abode of the Devi, I bow *to thee; thou fulfillest the desire of the votary, I bow to thee (285).*

In thee I worship the most excellent primordial Supreme Devi; if there be any defect in thee by reason of the want of skill of him who has fashioned thee, do thou make it good; I bow to thee (286).

He should then restrain his speech, and, placing his hand over the head of the Image, inwardly do japa of the Mula Mantra one hundred and eight times, and thereafter do Anga-nyasa (287).

He should then perform Shadanga-nyasa and Matri-ka-nyasa on the body of the Image, and, when performing Shadanga-nyasa, add one after the other the six long vowels to the Vija (288).

The eight groups of the letters of the alphabet preceded by the Tara, Maya, and Rama, with the Vindu, added to them, and followed by Namah, should be placed in different parts of the body of the Deva (289).

The wise man should place the vowels in the mouth; kavarga in the throat; chavargaon the belly; tavarga on the right and tavarva on the left arm; pavarga on the right thigh, and yavarga on the left thigh, and shavarga on the head (290-291).

*Having placed these groups of the letters of the alphabet
on different parts of the image (the worshipper) should
perform Tattva-nyasa (as follows): (292)*

*Place on the two feet Prithivi-tattva; on the Linga
Toya-tattva; on the region of the navel Tejas-tattva;
on the lotus of the heart Vayu-tattva; on the mouth
Gagana-tattva; on the two eyes Rupa-tattva; on the two
nostrils Gandha-tattva; on the two ears Shabda-tattva;
on the tongue Rasa-tattva; on the skin Sparsha-tattva.
The foremost of worshippers should place Manas-tattva
between the eyebrows, Shiva-tattva, Jnana-tattva, and
Para-tattva on the lotus of a thousand petals; on the
heart Jiva-tattva and Prakriti-tattva. Lastly, he should
place Mahat-tattva and Ahangkara-tattva all over the
body. The tattvas should, whilst being placed, be preceded by Tara, Maya, and Rama, and should be uttered
in the dative singular, followed by namah (293-297).*

*Repeating the Mula Mantra, preceded and followed
by each of the Matrika-varnas, with vindu added to
them, and followed by the word namah, Matrika-nyasa
should be performed at the Matrikasthanas (298). (The
worshipper should then say):*

Mantra

*(Although) Thy radiance embraces all the sacrifices, and
although Thy body embraces all being, this is the image
that has been made of Thee. I place Thee here (299).*

*Thereafter the Devi should be meditated upon and
invoked, according to the rules of worship, and after Prana-pratishtha the Supreme Devata should be
worshipped (300).*

*The Mantras which are prescribed for the dedication of
a temple to a Deva should be used in this ceremony, the
necessary changes in gender being made (301).*

*The Devi should then be invoked into the fire, which has
in due form been consecrated by the offer of oblations to
the Devatas who are to be worshipped; and thereafter
the Devi should be worshipped, and jata-karmma, etc.,
should be performed (302).*

*The Sangskaras are six in number – viz., Jatakarmma,
Namakarana, Nishkramana, Annaprashana, Chudi-
karana, and Upanayana – this has been said by Shiva
(303).*

Repeating the Pranava, the Vyahritis, the Gayatri, the

Mula Mantra, the worshipper used in the injunctions should say, "thine," and then the name of (the sangskara) jatakarmma, and others, and uttering, "I perform, Svaha," offer five oblations at the end of each sangskara (304-305).

Thereafter repeating the Mula Mantra and the name (given to the Devi), one hundred oblations should be offered, and the remnants of each oblation should be thrown over the head of the Devi (306).

The wise man, after having brought the ceremony to a close by Prayashchitta and other rites, should feed and thus please Sadhakas and Vipras and the poor and the helpless (307).

Should anyone be unable to perform all these rites, he should bathe (the Deva) with seven jars of water, and, having worshipped to the best of his ability, repeat the name of the Devi (308).

Beloved! I have now spoken to Thee of the Pratishtha of the illustrious Adya. In a similar way should men versed in the regulations carefully perform the Pratishtha of Durga and other Vidyas, Mahesha, and other Devatas, and of the Shiva-lingas that may be moved (309-310).

End of the Thirteenth Joyful Message, entitled "Installa-tion of the Devata."

CHAPTER 14

The Consecration of Shiva-linga and

Description of the Four Classes of

Avadhutas

SHRI DEVI said:

I am grateful to Thee, O Lord of Mercy! in that Thou hast in Thy discourse upon the Worship of the Adya Shakti, spoken, in Thy mercy, of the mode of Worship of various other Devas (1).

Thou hast spoken of the Installation of a Movable Shiva-linga, but what is the object of installing an immovable Shiva-linga, and what are the rites relating to the installation of such a Linga? (2).

Do Thou, O Lord of the Worlds! now tell Me all the particulars thereof; for say, who is there but Thee that I can honour by My questions anent this excellent subject? (3).

Who is there that is Omniscient, Merciful, All-knowing, Omnipresent, easily satisfied, Protector of the humble, like Thee? Who makes My joys increase like Thee? (4).

Shri Sadashiva said:

What shall I tell Thee of the merit acquired by the installation of a Shiva-linga? By it a man is purified of all great sins, and goes to the Supreme Abode (5).

There is no doubt that by the installation of a Shiva-linga a man acquires ten million times the merit which is acquired by giving the world and all its gold, by the performance of ten thousand horse-sacrifices, by the digging of a tank in a waterless country, or by making happy the poor and such as are enfeebled by disease (6-7).

Kalika! Brahma, Vishnu, Indra, and the other Devas reside where Mahadeva is in His linga form (8).

Thirty-five million known and unknown places of pilgrimage and all the holy places abide near Shiva. The land within a radius of a hundred cubits of the linga is declared to be Shiva-kshetra (9-10).

This land of Isha is very sacred. It is more excellent than the most excellent of holy places, because there abide all the Immortals and there are all the holy places (11).

He who in a devout spirit lives there, be it even for but a little while, becomes purged of all sins, and goes to the heaven of Shangkara after death (12).

*Anything great or small (meritorious or otherwise)
which is done in this land of Shiva becomes multiplied
(in its effect) by the majesty of Shiva (13).*

*All sins committed elsewhere are removed (by going)
near Shiva, but sins committed in Shiva-kshetra adhere
to a man with the strength of a thunderbolt (14).*

*The merit acquired by the performance there of Purash-
charana, japa, acts of charity, Shraddha, tarpana, or
any other pious acts is eternal (15).*

*The merit acquired by the performance of a hundred
Purashcharana at times of lunar or solar eclipse is acquired by merely performing one japa near Shiva (16).*

*By the offering of Pinda once only in the land of Shiva, a
man obtains the same fruit as he who offers ten million
pindas at Gaya, the Ganges, and Prayaga (17).*

*Even in the case of those who are guilty of many sins or
of great sins attain the supreme abode if Shraddha be
performed in their names in the land of Shiva (18).*

*The fourteen worlds abide there where abides the Lord
of the Universe in His Linga form with the auspicious
Devi Durga (19).*

I have spoken a little about the majesty of the immovable Mahadeva in His linga form. The mahima of the Anadi-linga is beyond the power of words to express (20).

O Suvrat! even in Thy worship at the Mahapithas the touch of an untouchable is unclean, but this is not so in the worship of Hara in His linga image (21).

O Devi! as there are no prohibitions at the time of Chakra worship, so know this, O Kalika! that there are none in the holy shrine in Shiva's land (22).

What is the use of saying more? I am but telling Thee the very truth when I say that I am unable to describe the glory, majesty, and sanctity of the linga image of Shiva (23).

Whether the Linga is placed on a Gauri-patta or not, the worshipper should, for the successful attainment of his desires, worship it devoutly (24).

The excellent worshipper earns the merit of (performing) ten thousand horse-sacrifices if he performs the Adhivasa of the Deva in the evening previous to the day of installation (25).

*The twenty articles to be used in the rite of Adhiva-
sa are: Earth, Scent, a Pebble, Paddy, Durvva grass,
Flower, Fruit, Curds, Ghee, Svastika, Vermillion, Conch-shell, Kajjala, Rochana, White Mustard Seed, Silver,
Gold, Copper, Lights, and a Mirror (26-27).*

*Taking each of these articles, the Maya Vija and the
Brahma-Gayatri should be repeated, and then should be
said "Anena" (with this) and "Amushya" (of this one's or
his or hers) – "may the auspicious Adhivasa be" (28).*

*And then the forehead of the worshipped divinity should
be touched with the earth and all other articles aforesaid. Then Adhivasa should be performed with the Pras-
hasti-patra – that is, the receptacle should be lifted up,
and with it the forehead of the image should be touched
three times (29).*

*The worshipper conversant with the ordinances, having
thus performed the Adhivasa of the Deva, should bathe
the deity with milk and other liquids, as directed in the
ceremony relating to the dedication of a temple (30).*

*Rubbing the linga with a piece of cloth and placing it on
its seat, Ganesha and other Deities should be worshipped according to the rules prescribed for their worship
(31).*

Having performed Kara-nyasa and Anga-nyasa and Pranayama with the Pranava, the ever-existent Shiva should be meditated upon.

Dhyana

As tranquil, possessed of the effulgence of ten million Moons; clothed in garments of tiger-skins; wearing a sacred thread made of a serpent; His whole body cove-red with ashes; wearing ornaments of serpents; His five faces are of reddish-black, yellow, rose, white, and red colours, with three eyes each; His head is covered with matted hair; He is Omnipresent; He holds Ganga on His head, and has ten arms, and in His forehead shines the (crescent) Moon; He holds in His left hand the skull, fire, the noose, the Pinaka, and the axe, and in His right the trident, the thunderbolt, the arrow, and blessings; He is being praised by all the Devas and great Sages; His eyes half-closed in the excess of bliss; His body is white as the snow and the Kunda flower and the Moon; He is seated on the Bull; He is by day and night surrounded on every side by Siddhas, Gandharvas, and Apsaras, who are chanting hymns in His praise; He is the husband of Uma; the devoted Protector of His worshippers (32-38).

Having thus meditated upon Mahadeva and worship-ped Him with articles of mental worship, He should be invoked into the Linga, and worshipped to the best of one's powers, and as laid down in the ordinances relating to such worship (39).

I have already spoken of the Mantras for the giving of Asana and other articles of worship. I shall now speak of the Mula Mantra of the Great Mahesha (40).

Maya, Tara, and the Shabda Vija, with Au and Ardhen-du-Vindu added to it, is the Shiva Vija – that is, "Hring Ong Haung." (41).

Covering Shangkara with clothes and garland of sweet-smelling flowers, and placing Him on a beautiful couch, the Gauri-patta should be consecrated in manner above-mentioned (42).

The Devi should be worshipped in the Gauri-patta according to the following rites: with the Maya Vija, Anga-nyasa, Kara-nyasa, and Pranayama should be performed (43).

The Great Devi should, to the best of the worshipper's ability, be worshipped after meditation upon Her as follows:

Dhyana

I meditate upon the stainless One, Whose splendour isthat of a thousand rising Suns, Whose eyes are like Fire, Sun and Moon, and Whose lotus face in smiles is adorned with golden earrings set with lines of pearls. With her lotus hands She makes the gestures which grant blessings and dispel fear, and holds the discus and lotus; Her breasts are large and rounded; She is the Dispeller of all fear, and She is clothed in saffron-coloured raiments.

Having thus meditated upon Her, the ten Dikpalas and the Bull should be worshipped to the best of one's powers (44-45).

I will now speak of the Mantra of the Bhagavati, by which the World-pervading One should be worshipped (46).

Repeating the Maya, Lakshmi Vijas, and the letter which follows Sa with the sixth vowel, with the Vindu added to it, and thereafter uttering the name of the Wife of Fire, the Mantra is formed (which is as follows):

Mantra

Hring Shring Hung Svaha (47).

Placing the Devi as aforementioned, offerings should be made to all the Devas with a mixture of Masha beans, rice, and curds, with sugar, etc., added to it (48).

These articles of worship should be placed in the Ishana corner, and purified with the Varuna Vija, and should be offered after purification with scents and flowers and the following (49)

Mantra

O Devas, Siddhas, Gandharvas, Uragas, Rakshasas, Pishachas,' Mothers, Yakshas, Bhutas, Pitris, Rishis, and other Devas! do you quietly take this offering, and do you stay surrounding Mahadeva and Girija (50-51).

Then japa should be made of the Mantra of the Great Devi as often as one may, and then with excellent songs and instrumental music let the festival be celebrated (52).

Having completed the Adhivasa in manner above, the following day after performance of the compulsory daily duties, and having taken the vow, the Five Devas should be worshipped (53).

After worshipping the Matris and making the Vasudha-

*ra, and performing Vriddhi-Shraddha, the Door-keepers
of Mahesha should, in a calm and devout frame of
mind, be worshipped (54).*

*The Door-keepers of Shiva are – Nandi, Maha-bala, Kis-
havadana, and Gana-nayaka; they are all armed with
missiles and other weapons (55).*

*Bringing the Linga and Tarini, as represented by the
Gauri-patta, they should be placed on a Sarvato-bhadra
Mandala, or on an auspicious seat (56).*

*Shambhu should then be bathed with eight jars of water
with the Mantra "Tryambaka," etc., and worshipped
with the sixteen articles of worship (57).*

*After bathing the Devi in a similar way with the Mula
Mantra, and worshipping Her, the good worshipper
should pray to Shangkara with joined palms (58).*

Mantra

*Come, O Bhagavan! O Shambhu! O Thou before Whom
all Devas bow! I bow to Thee, Who art armed with the
Pinaka, Thee the Lord of all, O Great Deva (59).*

O Deva! Thou Who conferrest benefits on Thy votaries!

*do Thou in Thy mercy come to this temple with Bhaga-
vati: I bow to Thee again and again (60).*

*O Mother! O Devi! O Mahamaya! O All-beneficent
One! be Thou along with Shambhu pleased: I bow to
Thee, O Beloved of Hara (61).*

*Come to this house, O Devi! Thou Who grantest all
boons, be Thou pleased, and do Thou grant me all
prosperity (62).*

*Rise, O Queen of Devas! and Each with Thy followers
abide happy in this place; may Both of You be pleased,
You Who are kind to your devotees (63).*

*Having thus prayed to Shiva and the Devi, They should
first be carried three times round the Temple, keeping
the latter on the right to the accompaniment of joyful
sounds, and then taken inside (64).*

*Repeating the Mula Mantra, one-third of the Linga
should be set in a hollow made in a piece of stone or in a
masonry hole (65). (With the following Mantra):*

Mantra

O Mahadeva! do Thou remain here so long as the Moon

*and the Sun endure, so long as the Earth and the Oce-
ans endure: I bow to Thee (66).*

*Having firmly fixed Sadashiva with this Mantra, the
Gauri-patta, with its tapering end to the North, should
be placed on the Linga, that it may be entered by the
latter (67).*

Mantra

*Be still, O Jagad-dhatri! Thou That art the Cause of cre-
ation, existence, and destruction of things; abide Thou
here so long as the Sun and the Moon endure (68).*

*Having firmly fixed it, the Linga should be touched and
the following (Mantra) should be repeated (69):*

Mantra

*I invoke that Deva Who has three eyes, the Decayless,
Ishana, around whose lion-seat are tigers, Bhutas,
Pishachas, Gandharvas, Siddhas, Charanas, Yakshas, Nagas, Vetalas, Loka-palas, Maharshis, Matris,
Gana-nathas, Vishnu Brahma, and Vrihaspati, and all
beings which live on earth or in the air; come, O Bhagavan! to this Yantra, which is the handiwork of Brahma,
for the prosperity, happiness, and Heaven of all (70-72).*

Beloved! Shiva should then be bathed according to the injunctions relating to the consecration of a Deva, and, having been meditated upon as before-mentioned, should be worshipped with mental offerings (73).

After placing a special arghya,' and having worshipped the Gana-devatas, and meditated upon Mabesha again, flowers should be placed on the Linga (74).

Repeating the Shakti Vija between Pasha and Ang-kusha, and the letters from Ya to Sa with the nasal point, and then " Haung Hangsa," the life of Sadashiva should be infused into the Linga (75).

Then, smearing the Husband of the Daughter of the Mountain with sandal, aguru, and saffron, He should be worshipped with the sixteen articles of worship according to the injunctions laid down after performing the jata, the nama, and other rites (76).

After concluding everything according to the injunctions, and after worshipping the Devi in the Gauri-patta, the eight images of the Deva should be carefully worshipped (77).

By the name Sharva the Earth is meant; by Bhava is meant Water; by Rudra, Fire; by Ugra, Wind; by Bhuna,

Ether; by Pashu-pati is meant the Employer of a priest
for sacrifice; by Mahadeva, the Source of Nectar, and
by Ishana, the Sun: these are declared to be the Eight
Images (78-79).

Each of these should be invoked and worshipped in
their order (in the corners), beginning with the East and
ending with the North-East, uttering the Pranava first
and Namah last (80).

After having worshipped Indra and the other Dikpalas,
the eight Matris, Brahmi, and others, the worshipper
should give to Isha the Bull, awning, houses, and the like
(81).

Then, with joined palms, he should with fervour pray to
the Husband of Parvati (as follows) (82):

Mantra

O Ocean of Mercy! O Lord! Thou hast been placed in
this place by me; be Thou pleased (with me). O Shambhu! Thou Who art the Cause of all causes, do Thou abide in this room, O Supreme Deva! so long as the Earth
with all its Oceans exist, so long as the Moon and the
Sun endure. I bow to Thee. Should there occur the death
of any living being, may I, O Dhurjjati! by Thy grace, be
kept from that sin (83-85).

The dedicator should go round the image, keeping it on his right, and, having bowed before the Deva, go home. Returning again in the morning, he should bathe Chandra-Shekhara (86).

He should first be bathed with consecrated Panchamrita with a hundred jars of scented water, and the worshipper, having worshipped Him to the best of his powers, should pray to Him (as follows) (87-88):

Mantra

O Husband of Uma,! if there has been any irregularity, omission, want of devotion in this worship, may they all, by Thy grace, be rectified, and may my fame remain incomparable in this world so long as Moon, the Sun, the Earth, and its Oceans endure (89-90).

I bow to the three-eyed Rudra, Who wields the excellent Pinaka, to Him Who is worshipped by Vishnu, Brahma, Indra, Suryya, and other Devas, I bow again and again (91).

The worshipper should then make presents, and feast the Kaulika-dvijas, and give pleasure to the poor by gifts of food, drink, and clothes (92).

The Deva should be worshipped every day according to one's means. The fixed Shiva-linga should on no account be removed (93).

Parameshvari! I have in brief spoken to you of the rites relating to the consecration of the immovable Shiva-linga, gathering same from all the Agamas (94).

Shri Devi said:

If, O Lord! there be an accidental omission in the worship of the Devas, then what should be done by their votaries – do Thou speak in detail about this (95).

Say, on account of what faults are images of Devas unfit for worship, and should thus be rejected, and what should be done? (96).

Shri Sadashiva said:

If there be an omission to worship an image for a day, then (the next day) the worship should be twice performed; if for two days, then the worship should be four times performed; if for three days, then it should be celebrated eight times (97).

If the omission extends three days, but does not exceed

six months, then the wise man should worship after bathing the Deva with eight jars of water (98).

If the period of omission exceeds six months, then the excellent worshipper should carefully consecrate the Deva according to the rules already laid down, and then worship Him (99)

The wise man should not worship the image of a Deva which is broken or is holed, or which has lost a limb, or has been touched by a leper, or has fallen on unholy ground (100).

The image of a Deva with missing limbs, or which is broken or has holes in it, should be consigned to water. If the image has been made impure by touch, it should be consecrated, and then worshipped (101).

The Mahapithas and Anadi-lingas are free from all deficiencies, and these should always be worshipped for the attainment of happiness by each worshipper as he pleases (102).

Mahamaya! whatever Thou hast asked for the good of men who act with a view to the fruits of action, I have answered all this in detail (103).

Men cannot live without such actions even for half amoment. Even when men are unwilling, they are, in spite of themselves, drawn by the whirlwind of action (104).

By action men enjoy happiness, and by action again they suffer pain. They are born, they live, and they die the slaves of action (105).

It is for this that I have spoken of various kinds of action, such as S,dhana and the like, for the guidance of the intellectually weak in the paths of righteousness, and that they may be restrained from wicked acts (106).

There are two kands of action – good and evil; the effect of evil action is that men suffer acute pain (107).

And, O Devi! those who do good acts with minds intent on the fruits thereof go to the next world, and come back again to this, chained by their action (108).

Therefore men will not attain final liberation even at the end of a hundred kalpas so long as action, whether good or evil, is not destroyed (109).

As a man is bound, be it by a gold or iron chain, so he is bound by his action, be it good or evil (110).

So long as a man has not real knowledge, he does not attain final liberation, even though he be in the constant practice of religious acts and a hundred austerities (111).

The knowledge of the wise from whom the darkness of ignorance is removed, and whose souls are pure, arises from the performance of duty without expectation of fruit or reward, and by constant meditation on the Brahman (112).

He who knows that all which is in this universe from Brahma to a blade of grass is but the result of Maya, and that the Brahman is the one and supreme Truth, has this (113).

That man is released from the bonds of action who, renouncing name and form, has attained to complete knowledge of the essence of the eternal and immutable Brahman (114).

Liberation does not come fram japa, homa, or a hundred fasts; man becomes liberated by the knowledge that he himself is Brahman (115).

Final liberation is attained by the knowledge that the Atma (Soul) is the witness, is the Truth, is omnipresent, is one, free from all illuding distractions of self and not-self, the supreme, and, though abiding in the body, is not in the body (116).

All imagination of name-form and the like are but the play of a child. He who put away all this sets himself in firm attachment to the Brahman, is, without doubt, liberated (117).

If the image imagined by the (human) mind were to lead to liberation, then undoubtedly men would be Kings by virtue of such kingdoms as they gain in their dreams (118).

Those who (in their ignorance) believe that Ishvara is (only) in images made of clay, or stone, or metal, or wood, merely trouble themselves by their tapas. They can never attain liberation without knowledge (119).

Can men attain final liberation by restriction in food, be they ever so thin thereby, or by uncontrolled indulgence, be they ever so gross therefrom, unless they possess the knowledge of Brahman? (120).

If by observance of Vrata to live on air, leaves of trees, bits of grain, or water, final liberation may be attained, then snakes, cattle, birds, and aquatic animals should all be able to attain final liberation (121).

Brahma-sad-bhava is the highest state of mind; dhyana-bhava is middling; stuti and japa is the last; and external worship is the lowest of all (122).

Yoga is the union of the embodied soul and the Supreme Soul," Puja is the union of the worshipper and the worshipped; but he who realizes that all things are Brahman for him there is neither Yoga nor Puja (123).

For him who possesses the knowledge of Brahman, the supreme knowledge, of what use are japa, yajna," tapas, niyama, and vrata? (124).

He who sees the Brahman, Who is Truth, Knowledge, Bliss, and the One, is by his very nature one with the Brahman. Of what use to him are puja, dhyana, and dharana? (125).

For him who knows that all is Brahman there is neither sin nor virtue, neither heaven nor future birth. There is none to meditate upon, nor one who meditates (126).

The soul which is detached from all things is ever liberated; what can bind it? From what do fools desire to be liberated? (127).

He abides in this Universe, the creation of His powers of illusion, which even the Devas cannot pierce. He is seemingly in the Universe, but not in it (128).

The Spirit, the eternal witness, is in its own nature like the void which exists both outside and inside all things, and which has neither birth nor childhood, nor youth nor old age, but is the eternal intelligence which is ever the same, knowing no change or decay (129-130).

It is the body which is born, matures, and decays. Men enthralled by illusion, seeing this, understand it not (131).

As the Sun (though one and the same) when reflected in different platters of water appears to be many, so by illusion the one soul appears to be many in the different bodies in which it abides (132).

As when water is disturbed the Moon which is reflected in it appears to be disturbed, so when the intelligence is disturbed ignorant men think that it is the soul which is disturbed (133).

As the void inside a jar remains the same ever after the jar is broken, so the Soul remains the same after the body is destroyed (134).

*The knowledge of the Spirit, O Devi! is the one means
of attaining final liberation; and he who possesses it is
verily – yea, verily – liberated in this world, even yet
whilst living, there is no doubt of that (135).*

*Neither by acts, nor by begetting offspring, nor by wealth
is man liberated; it is by the knowledge of the Spirit, by
the Spirit that man is liberated (136).*

*It is the Spirit that is dear to all; there is nothing dearer
than the Spirit;O Shive! it is by the unity of Spirits that
men become dear to one another (137).*

*Knowledge, Object of knowledge, the knower appear
by illusion to be three different things; but if careful
discrimination is made, Spirit is found to be the sole
residuum (138).*

*Knowledge is Spirit in the form of intelligence, the object
of knowledge is Spirit whose substance is intelligence, the
Knower is the Spirit Itself. He who knows this knows the
Spirit (139).*

*I have now spoken of knowledge which is the true cause
of final liberation. This is the most precious possession of
the four classes of Avadhutas (140).*

Shri Devi said:

*Thou hast spoken of the two stages in the life of man –
namely, that of householder and mendicant; what is this
wonderful distinction of four classes of Avadhutas which
I now hear? (141).*

*I wish to hear and clearly understand the distinctive fea-
tures of the four classes of Avadhutas: do Thou, O Lord!
speak (about them) truly (142).*

Shri Sadashiva said:

*Those Brahmanas, Kshatriyas, and other castes who are
worshippers of the Brahma-mantra should be known to
be Yatis, even though they be living the life of a householder (143).*

*O Worshipped of the Kulas! those men who are sancti-
fied by the rites of Purnabhisheka should be known and
honoured as Shaivavadhutas (144).*

*Both the Brahma and Shaiva Avadhutas shall do all
acts in their respective states of life according to the way
directed by me (145).*

They should not partake of forbidden food or drink un-

less the same has been offered to the Brahman or offered in the Chakra (146).

O Beauteous One! I have already spoken of the customs and Dharmma of the Kaulas, who are Brahma Avadhutas, and of the Kaulas who have been initiated. For Brahma and Shaiva Avadhutas, bathing, eating evening meals, drinking, the giving of charities, and marital intercourse should be done according to the way prescribed by the Agamas (147-148).

The above Avadhutas are of two classes, according as they are perfect or imperfect. Beloved! the perfect one is called Parama-hangsa, and the other or imperfect one is called Parivrat (149).

The man who has gone through the Sangskara of an Avadhuta, but whose knowledge is yet imperfect, should, by living the life of a householder, purify his spirit (150).

Preserving his caste-mark and practising the rites of a Kaula, he should, remaining constantly devoted to the Brahman, cultivate the excellent knowledge (151).

With his mind ever free from attachment, yet discharging all his duty, he should constantly repeat "Ong Tat Sat," and constantly think upon and realize the saying,

"Sah aham" (152).

Doing his duties, his mind as completely detached as
the water on the lotus leaf, he should constantly strive
to free his soul by the knowledge of Divine truth and
discrimination (153).

The man, be he a householder or an ascetic, who commences any undertaking with the Mantra "Ong Tat Sat,"
is ever successful therein (154).

Japa, homa, pratishtha, and all sacramental rites, if
performed with the Mantra "Ong Tat Sat," are faultess
beyond all doubt (155).

What use is there of the various other Mantras? What
use of the other multitudinous practices? With this
Brahma Mantra alone may all rites be concluded (156).

Ambika! this Mantra is easily practised, is not prolix,
and gives complete success, and there is no other way
besides this great Mantra (157).

If it be kept written in any part of the house or on the
body, then such house becomes a holy place and the
body becomes sanctified (158).

O Deveshi! I am telling Thee the very truth when I say that the Mantra "Ong Tat Sat" is superior to the essence of essences of the Nigamas, the Agamas, and the Tantras (159).

This most excellent of Mantras, "Ong Tat Sat," has pierced through the palate, the skull, and crownlock of Brahma, Vishnu, and Shiva, and has thus manifested itself (160).

If the four kinds of food and other articles are sanctified by this Mantra, then it becomes useless to sanctify them by any other Mantras (161).

He is a King among Kaulas, who sees the Great Being everywhere, and constantly makes japa of the great Mantra "Tat Sat" (i.e., Ong Tat Sat), acts as he so inclines, and is pure of heart withal (162).

By japa of this Mantra a man becomes a Siddha; by thinking of its meaning he is liberated, and he who, when making japa, thinks of its meaning, becomes like unto the Brahman in visible form (163).

This Great, Three-footed Mantra is the cause of all causes; by its sadhana one becomes the Conqueror of Death himself (164).

O Maheshani! the worshipper attains siddhi in
whatsoever way he makes japa of it (165).

He who, renouncing all acts (rites), has been cleansed by
the Sangskara of a Shaiva Avadhuta, ceases to have any
right to worship Devas, to perform the Shraddha of the
Pitris, or to honour the Rishis (166).

Of the four classes of Avadhutas, the fourth is called the
Hangsa (Parama-hangsa). The other three both practise
yoga and have enjoyment. They are all liberated and are
like unto Shiva (167).

The Hangsa should not have intercourse with women,
and should not touch metals. Unfettered by restrictions,
he moves about enjoying the fruits of his meritorious
acts done in previous lives (168).

The fourth class, removing his caste-marks and relinquishing his household duties, should move about in this
world without aim or striving (169).

Always pleased in his own mind, he is free from sorrow
and illusion, homeless and forgiving, fearless, and doing
harm to none (170).

For him there is no offering of food and drink (to any

Deva); for him there is no necessity for dhyana or dharana, the Yati is liberated, is free from attachment, unaffected by all opposites, and follows the ways of a Hangsa (171).

O Devi! I have now spoken to Thee in detail of the distinctive marks of the four classes of Kula-Yogis, who are but images of Myself (172).

By seeing them, by touching them, conversing with them, or pleasing them, men earn the fruit of pilgrimage to all the holy places (173).

All the shrines and holy places which there are in this world, they all, O my Beloved! abide in the body of the Kula-Sannyasi (174).

Those men who have worshipped Kula Sadhus with

Kula-dravya are indeed blessed and holy, have attained their desired aim, and have earned the fruit of all sacrifices (175).

By mere touch of these Sadhus the impure becomes pure, the untouchable becomes touchable, and food unfit to be eaten becomes fit to be eaten. By their touch even the Kiratas, the sinful, the wicked, the Pulindas, the Yavanas, *and the wicked and ferocious, are made pure; who else but they should be honoured? (176-177).*

Even those who but once worship the Kaulika Yogi with Kula-tattva and Kula-dravya become worthy of honour in this world (178).

O Thou with the lotus face! there is no Dharmma superior to Kaula-Dharmma, by seeking refuge in which even a man of inferior caste becomes purified and attains the state of a Kaula (179).

As the footmarks of all animals disappear in the footmark of the elephant, so do all other Dharmmas disappear in the Kula-Dharmma (180).

My Beloved! how holy are the Kaulas! They are like the images of the holy places. They purify by their merepresence even the Chandalas and the vilest of the vile (181).

As other waters falling into Ganga become the water of Ganga, so all men following Kulachara reach the stage of a Kaula (182).

As water gone into the sea does not retain its separateness, so men sunk in the ocean of Kula lose theirs (183).

All beings in this world which have two feet, from the Vipra to the inferior castes, are competent for Kulachara (184).

Those that are averse to the acceptance of Kula-Dharmma, even when invited, are divorced from all Dharmma and go the downward path (185).

The Kulina who deceived those men who seek for Kulachara shall go to the hell named Raurava (186).

That low Kaula who refuses to initiate a Chandala or a Yavana into the Kula-Dharmma, considering them to be inferior, or a woman out of disrespect for her, goes the downward way (187).

The merit acquired by a hundred Abhisheka, by the performance of a hundred Purashcharana, ten million times that merit is acquired by the initiation of one man into the Kula-Dharmma (188).

All the different castes, all the followers of the different Dharmmas in this world, are, by becoming Kaulas, freed from their bonds, and go to the Supreme Abode (189).

The Kaulas who follow that Shaiva-Dharmma are like places of pilgrimage, and possess the soul of Shiva. They worship and honour one another with affection, respect, and love (190).

What is the use of saying more? I am speaking the very truth before Thee when I say that the only bridge for the crossing of this ocean of existence is the Kula- Dharmma and none other (191).

By the following of Kula-Dharmma all doubts are cut through, all the accumulation of sins is destroyed, and the multitude of acts is destroyed (192).

Those Kaulikas are excellent who, truthful and faithful to the Brahman, in their mercy invite men to purify them by Kulachara (193).

Devi! I have spoken to Thee the first portion of the Maha-nirvana Tantra for the purification of men. It contains the conclusions of all Dharmmas (194).

He who hears it daily or enables other men to hear it becomes freed from all sins, and attains Nirvana at the end (195).

By knowing this King among Tantras, which contains the essence of essence of all the Tantras, and is the most excellent among the Tantras, a man becomes versed in all the Shastras (196).

*The man who knows this Maha-Tantra is freed from the
bonds of actions. Of what use is it to him to go on pilgrimage, or to do japa, yajna, and sadhana? (197).*

*Kalika! he who knows this Tantra, is conversant with all
the Shastras, he is pre-eminent among the virtuous, is
wise, knows the Brahman, and is a Sage (198).*

*There is no use of the Vedas, the Puranas, the Smritis,.
the Sanghitas, and the various other Tantras, as by
knowing this Tantra one knows all (199).*

*All the most secret rites and practices and the most
excellent knowledge have been revealed by me in reply
to Thy questions (200).*

*Suvrata! as Thou art my most excellent Brahmi Shakti,
and art to me dearer than life itself, know Thou that the
Mahanirvana Tantra is likewise (201).*

*As the Himalaya is among the Mountains, as the Moon
is among the Stars, as the Sun is among all lustrous
bodies, so this Tantra is the King among Tantras (202).*

*All the Dharmmas pervade this Tantra. It is the only
means for the acquirement of the knowledge of Brahman. The man who repeats himself or causes others to*

repeat it will surely acquire such knowledge (203).

In the family of the man in whose house there is this most excellent of all Tantras there will never be a Pashu (204).

The man blinded by the darkness of ignorance, the fool caught in the meshes of his actions, and the illiterate man, by listening to this Great Tantra, are released fromthe bonds of karmma (205).

Parameshani! reading, listening to, and worshipping this Tantra, and singing its praise, gives liberation to men (206).

Of the other various Tantras each deals with one subject only. There is no other Tantra which contains all the Dharmmas (207).

The last part contains an account of the nether, earthly, and heavenly worlds. He who knows it (along with the first) undoubtedly knows all (208).

The man who knows the second part with this book is able to speak of the past, present, and future, and knows the three worlds (209).

There are all manner of Tantras and various Shastras, but they are not equal to a sixteenth part (in value) of this Mahanirvana Tantra (210).

What further shall I tell Thee of the greatness of the Mahanirvana Tantra? Through the knowledge of it one shall attain to Brahma-nirvana (211).

End of the Fourteenth Joyful Message of the First Part of the Mahanirvana, entitled, "The Consecration of Shiva-linga and Description of the Four Classes of Avadhutas."